Safe

FIREFIGHTING

First Things First

Steve Kidd

John Czajkowski

Garry Briese

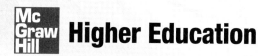

Higher Education

Boston   Burr Ridge, IL   Dubuque, IA   Madison, WI   New York   San Francisco   St. Louis
Bangkok   Bogotá   Caracas   Kuala Lumpur   Lisbon   London   Madrid   Mexico City
Milan   Montreal   New Delhi   Santiago   Seoul   Singapore   Sydney   Taipei   Toronto

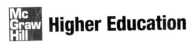

Higher Education

SAFE FIREFIGHTING 1: FIRST THINGS FIRST

Published by McGraw-Hill, a business unit of The McGraw-Hill Companies, Inc., 1221 Avenue of
the Americas, New York, NY 10020. Copyright © 2007 by The McGraw-Hill Companies, Inc. All rights reserved.
No part of this publication may be reproduced or distributed in any form or by any means, or stored in a
database or retrieval system, without the prior written consent of The McGraw-Hill Companies, Inc., including,
but not limited to, in any network or other electronic storage or transmission, or broadcast for distance learning.

Some ancillaries, including electronic and print components, may not be available to customers outside the United States.

 This book is printed on recycled, acid-free paper containing 10% postconsumer waste.

1 2 3 4 5 6 7 8 9 0 QPD/QPD 0 9 8 7 6

ISBN-13   978–0–07–297913–8
ISBN-10   0–07–297913–5

Publisher, Career Education: *David T. Culverwell*
Senior Sponsoring Editor: *Claire Merrick*
Editorial Coordinator: *Michelle L. Zeal*
Outside Developmental Services: *Julie Scardiglia*
Executive Marketing Manager: *James F. Connely*
Senior Marketing Manager: *Lisa Nicks*
Senior Project Manager: *Kay J. Brimeyer*
Senior Production Supervisor: *Laura Fuller*
Lead Media Project Manager: *Audrey A. Reiter*
Senior Media Producer: *Renee Russian*
Cover/Interior Designer: *Laurie B. Janssen*
(USE) Cover Image: *John Czajkowski, Delve Productions*
Senior Photo Research Coordinator: *John C. Leland*
Supplement Producer: *Tracy L. Konrardy*
Compositor: *Carlisle Publishing Services*
Typeface: *10/12 Melior*
Printer: *Quebecor World Dubuque, IA*

Medicine is an ever-changing science. As new research and clinical experience broaden our knowledge,
changes in treatment and drug therapy are required. The authors and the publisher of this work have
checked with sources believed to be reliable in their efforts to provide information that is complete and
generally in accord with the standards accepted at the time of publication. However, in view of the possibility of
human error or changes in medical sciences, neither the authors nor the publisher nor any other party who has
been involved in the preparation or publication of this work warrants that the information contained herein is in
every respect accurate or complete, and they are not responsible for any errors or omissions or for the results
obtained from use of such information. Readers are encouraged to confirm the information contained herein
with other resources. For example and in particular, readers are advised to check the product information sheet
included in the package of each drug they plan to administer to be certain that the information contained in this
book is accurate and that changes have not been made in the recommended dose or in the contradictions for
administration. This recommendation is of particular importance in connection with new or infrequently used drugs.

ww.mhhe.com

The Fire Service is constantly evolving, with firefighting techniques changing almost daily. Firefighters must face the challenge of this ever-
changing, dynamic work environment throughout their careers. The authors and the publisher of this work have checked with sources believed to
be reliable in their efforts to provide information that is complete and generally in accord with the standards accepted at the time of publication.
However, in view of the possibility of human error or changes in firefighting technology and practices, neither the authors nor the publisher nor
any other party who has been involved in the preparation or publication of this work warrants that the information contained herein is in every
respect accurate or complete, and they are not responsible for any errors or omissions or for the results obtained from use of such information.
Readers are encouraged to confirm the information contained herein with other resources.

We dedicate every word in this book to your safety.
We hope you do the same.

Steve Kidd

John Czajkowski

Garry Briese

About the Authors

Steve Kidd worked for 28 years with Orange County Fire Rescue Division, Florida, where he retired as a Company Officer. Along with John Czajkowski, he coauthored a 25-part Fire Service video training series and drill guide as well as the popular vehicle rescue video training series, *Carbusters!* Steve is a Technical Editor for *FireRescue Magazine* and has written numerous articles and a regular monthly column on fire and rescue-related topics over the past 20 years.

John Czajkowski worked for 31 years with Orange County Fire Rescue Division, Florida, where he retired as a Company Officer. He was a Charter Member of the Transportation Emergency Rescue Committee of the IAFC (International Association of Fire Chiefs) and lectured on vehicle rescue at many events, both in the United States and abroad. With Steve Kidd, he coauthored a 25-part Fire Service video training series as well as the popular vehicle rescue video training series, *Carbusters!* He has written many articles on Fire Service and rescue topics for several national fire publications.

Garry Briese is the Executive Director of the International Association of Fire Chiefs, having come to that position after serving in a similar post with the Florida College of Emergency Physicians. He has served with volunteer, combination, and career fire departments, is an original member of the *Carbusters!* extrication team, and has coauthored two textbooks for First Responders. He is a well-known speaker and instructor and is considered to be one of the thought leaders for today's fire and emergency services.

Brief Contents

Contents

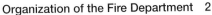
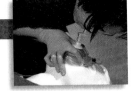

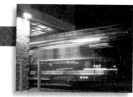
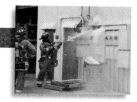
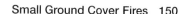
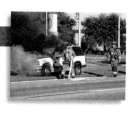

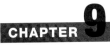

CHAPTER 9

Supply Hose Lines   185

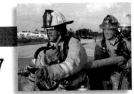

CHAPTER 10

Large Attack Lines   217

CHAPTER 11

Single-Family-Dwelling
Fires   241

Foreword

A book about *safe* firefighting ... wow. I thought to myself, they'll bombard the bookstores when that one comes out ... *not*. But then I realized that we are deep within some major changes in the Fire Service.

We are in the middle of some very positive changes in our business. And the primary change or renaissance we are experiencing is the fact that "we" are actually looking at—and taking action on—injury and death on the job. The Fire Service suffers almost one hundred and a dozen dead firefighters annually: about half from medical causes and the other half from driving too fast, not using seat belts, blowing stop signs and red lights, falling out (or off) of the apparatus, and experiencing building collapses, flashovers, burns, trauma, and other tragic events. We also suffer up to 100,000 serious injuries each year. *We have a problem. But who is really impacted by this "problem"?*

So often we accept our deaths as part of the job. Sometimes they are, but that is rare. You know and I know that it is a *rare* event when we are attempting to save a life and one or more of us die. Much more often than not, we die when we drive dumb, when we don't belt up, when we don't think about risk/benefit when going in, and when we are unhealthy. Heroes? Yes. All firefighters are heroes due to the very nature of the job. But heroic deaths? They are few and far between. We just don't talk about that, and as honorable a profession—career or volunteer—as this is, we do honor *all* firefighters who go before us, as we should. But we all know the real facts. And finally, we are starting to deal with it.

So what is the answer? *Training.* That's the *answer* and it is just that simple. And that is the *challenge*—not so simple.

There is a clear line between stupidity and bravery. There are many firefighters who have gone before us who have died horribly tragic but heroic deaths while attempting to save a life. Sometimes that is what must happen. But it is rare—*very rare.* The great majority of American firefighter line-of-duty deaths are clearly avoidable and can be avoided without any negative impact on the services you, as a firefighter, Officer, or Chief, provide. *Safe Firefighting: First Things First* will not negatively impact your love for

the job, your ability to provide service, or your "feeling" like a firefighter. What it will do is allow you to continue to *enjoy* being a *live* firefighter instead of having your spouse, kids, parents, and whoever else loves you watch you get fed through an IV for the rest of your life—or visit your grave. After all, once we are dead, we are dead. It's our family members—with a hard focus on our children, spouse, parents, and siblings—who suffer long after we are buried. And they spend the rest of their lives wondering if "that" death was "worth it" or not ... and so often they know the truth as we know it.

Firefighter training. That's the answer and one of the most exciting tools we now have. A critical part of that solution is this series, *Safe Firefighting.* It's the "non-sexy" name of this series *and* it is the culture we are starting to become—slowly. But we are getting there.

Why this book? Because this book *is* different. It helps us focus on what really matters—and what is just not *that* important. Make no mistake about it—this book was written 100% outside the box.

This is what matters: Identifying the fire "problem" on the scene, getting water on the fire, venting, staffing, protecting ourselves first, arriving in one piece, having applicable building construction info, understanding and applying "go in/don't go in," and having competent command officers. What doesn't matter: How a smoke detector works and what the inside of a hydrant looks like. This can be important info and may be worthwhile to know, but this info won't save your life as a firefighter. *Identifying the fire problem on the scene, getting water on a fire, knowing when to and when not to go in, and properly venting a structure* <u>*will.*</u>

There are heroes in our business. Some are recognized for risks that mattered and some are the ones who do work behind the scenes so that we can all come home safely. The writers of *Safe Firefighting*—Steve Kidd, John Czajkowski, and Garry Briese—fall into the second category. Steve, John, and Garry have decades of dirty, hands-on fire and rescue experience. And they have already impacted our business. But they decided to do more. They understood the need for a "new approach" in training firefighters—one way off the "traditional" scale—and they did something about it.

Safe Firefighting is not for all firefighters. Some will kick, scream, and whine about this approach and will refuse to consider changing. That's good. It will help the rest of us identify who gets it—and who doesn't.

Does this book suggest you can't go inside anymore? Not at all. Does it imply you will no longer be able to save life and property? Of course not. Does it stop us from performing as an effective and aggressive department or company? Absolutely not. This book takes all that and puts it in perspective to ensure that the right components exist so that we can do the job, based upon our ability to survive more often—much more often than we have in our past.

Billy Goldfetter
Deputy Fire Chief
Loveland-Symmes Fire Department
City of Loveland and Symmes Township, Ohio

Preface

Welcome to the Fire Service! This training program has been developed to help your instructors train you to be a competent, safe firefighter.

Firefighting is rewarding work and will give you great satisfaction in helping your community in times of emergency. Your community relies on and, indeed, expects the best possible work from you in any emergency. They really have no one else to turn to. When a fire or rescue emergency occurs, the Fire Service must answer the call, with the goal being that all of our members survive without injury or death and all of the victims are given the best possible chance for survival.

Firefighting is dangerous work and it is probably more dangerous than it has to be. There is a long tradition of regarding firefighters as heroes. There are instances in which firefighters are heroes, and we will not diminish those who have made sacrifices for their community. However, we must train and work so that any firefighter death or injury is one too many. We can never accept that it just happens or that firefighters sometimes die because they are heroes doing heroic things. Remember, you have a family that depends upon you and needs you just as much as your community does.

Firefighting is important work. It requires training and preparation. Experienced firefighters are hard to replace. You are needed alive, healthy, and working. Death and injuries to firefighters have devastating effects on both the community and the Fire Department. Your goal should be to do the very best job at all times. Returning alive and well and ready to answer the next call is important to us all.

At the end of the day, we want a thinking firefighter—one who is ready to adapt to changes, and willing to use new and safer techniques. Just as important, we want a firefighter who will also carry on a tradition of quality and dedication that will make his or her community and, indeed, our nation, a much safer place to live and work.

Program Description

Our curriculum is divided into three main levels of training, each progressively building upon the previous one as you proceed. The outcome we all want is a competent firefighter—a firefighter who will safely and efficiently perform the best possible job.

This program contains the most up-to-date and innovative information available today and is a unique learning system that provides skills training and review through the DVD that accompanies each book.

Safe Firefighting 1: First Things First

The first part of your training is provided in this manual and DVD. This material is the initial orientation and training for firefighter recruits who will not be going inside to fight a structural fire. It will empower you to assist with most exterior firefighting and emergency rescue operations. At this level, you will need close supervision and will have only the capabilities to assist the next two levels of firefighters trained in this program. By providing condensed training to the newest firefighter recruit, the fire department can get personnel safely involved in some Fire Department emergency operations sooner, while you complete more advanced training. This approach is a great help for fire departments that are in dire need of personnel, particularly volunteer departments.

Throughout the entire three-part series, you will be taught what you need to know in context. You will quickly find out that we are basing our information on scenarios, which will allow us to branch off to specific skills that will also be needed on other fire emergencies. By doing this, we hope to make the training interesting and pertinent to the job.

Your department may have more requirements after you start working with them. In fact, they probably will have more training for you, including learning how to do things "their way." Our goal is to get the most effective and important training to the firefighter at each level of training with the unnecessary "fluff" removed.

Safe Firefighting 2: Inside Operations

Inside Operations is the second book and DVD in the series. This intermediate level of training prepares the firefighter recruit to be qualified to fight an interior structural fire as part of a team. He or she will still be expected to be under direct supervision during firefighting operations.

With the information provided at this level, the firefighter recruit will also get in-depth training in responding to and handling more types of fire and vehicle crash emergencies. At the end of Safe Firefighting 2, our goal is to have a firefighter who works well with the firefighting crew, uses safe and effective techniques, is able to recognize dangerous situations, and responds in a manner that is safe for him- or herself and the public.

Safe Firefighting 3: Leading the Team

With the information provided at this level, firefighters will become capable of leading a firefighting crew during a fire scene operation. They will be able to identify the type of emergency at hand, select the best method to deal with the fire, and supervise a firefighting crew.

Firefighters at this level of training will be indirectly supervised by the Incident Commander, but, by and large, will be able to make their own decisions for handling their part of the emergency. These personnel will also learn how to handle more types of fire and emergency situations through added scenario-based training.

By learning from the printed matter, DVD, and CD, as well as through a lot of skills practice with your instructors, we want to give you the best and most interesting training possible today. Our goal is that our program will get the recruit through each level quickly and effectively with the desired result. Safety will never be compromised and will always be stressed in all training and demonstrations.

Steve Kidd
John Czajkowski
Garry Briese

Guided Tour

Features to Help You Study and Learn

What You Will Learn in This Chapter Each chapter opens with an overview of the topics covered in the chapter.

What You Will Be Able to Do This chapter-opening feature lists the skills the reader will have after reading the chapter and practicing the skills.

Reality! These brief readings present a combination of real-life situations and motivational introductions by the authors that set the stage for the training in the chapter, stressing the reasons firefighters need to learn the materials.

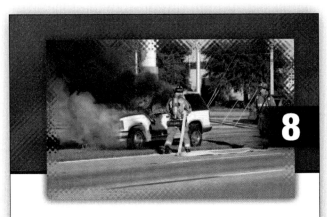

Passenger Vehicle Fires

What You Will Learn in This Chapter

In this chapter we will introduce you to vehicle fire operations, starting with personal protective equipment (PPE) and proper safety zones at vehicle fires. Then we will discuss vehicle design and burn characteristics. We will conclude the chapter with extinguishment techniques for vehicle fires.

We should also mention what you will not learn in this chapter. Fighting fires that involve a single automobile or light truck is much different from fighting fires in cargo-type vehicles or large, over-the-road equipment. Large vehicles often carry dangerous cargo and, at the very least, large amounts of flam-

What You Will Be Able to Do

After reading this chapter and participating in the practical skills sessions, you will be able to

1. Participate as a team member in setting up a typical safety zone and the traffic control needed at the scene of a vehicle fire.
2. Demonstrate how to chock the wheels and remove the keys of a vehicle involved in a fire.
3. Explain the safety risks of a vehicle fire and the importance of wearing full PPE and SCBA at a vehicle fire.
4. Describe the burn characteristics of the passen- of a fire

165

Reality!

Safety Lesson: A NIOSH Report

Wear Your Gear, Even on Small Fires!

On August 1, 2002, a firefighter in South Dakota was severely burned while fighting a fire that was consuming a wheat field. He had responded directly to the fire in his personal vehicle (POV) where he met up with another firefighter whose POV, a pickup truck, was equipped with a 75-gallon water tank and a gasoline-driven pump. According to the NIOSH report, although numerous firefighters responded to the scene, there was no Incident Command System established. The firefighters on the scene dispersed on their own as they arrived on the scene. The victim and the firefighter with the pickup truck talked on the scene and agreed that the victim would spray water from the bed of the truck while the other firefighter drove.

The two firefighters proceeded through a gate and into the field near the encroaching head of the fire. While fighting the fire, the victim was wearing tennis shoes, denim jeans, a T-shirt, and a baseball cap. A sudden gust of wind blew fire and smoke over the truck. The driver immediately pulled the truck forward and to the right. It is unknown if the victim fell from the truck as a result of being overcome by the fire and smoke or from the sudden forward movement of the truck. He ran about 200 yards, where he encountered a barbed wire fence and became entangled in the barbed wire. Other firefighters rushed to his aid, and the victim was evacuated by a medical helicopter to the burn center, where he died 5 days later from his injuries.

Follow-Up

NIOSH Report #F2002-37

After this incident was reviewed and evaluated, the NIOSH investigative report recommended that the following practices be implemented:

- Ensure that firefighters follow established procedures for combating ground cover fires.
- Develop and implement an Incident Command System.
- Provide firefighters with personal protective equipment (PPE) that is appropriate for wildland fires and is also NFPA 1977 compliant.
- Provide firefighters with appropriate wildland firefighter training.

Small Ground Cover Fires

Firefighters are called upon to perform many different jobs, including extinguishing **ground cover fires**. Ground cover fires occur in grassy vacant lots, rural wooded areas, parks, and even in the median areas on roadways (Figure 7-1). These fires are quite different from building fires. Ground cover fires are more like large Class A trash fires in that the fuel is spread out over a wider area. The tactics that firefighters use to extinguish these fires must take into consideration such elements as weather conditions, the humidity level, the type and arrangement of foliage, natural and manmade **firebreaks**, and the direction the fire travels as it burns.

In the United States, urban and suburban areas have been encroaching more and more on the wildland areas surrounding them. This spread is referred to as the **wildland/urban interface**. In this interface there is little or no separation between homes and even commercial buildings and the heavily wooded areas they are near. Property loss can result when large wildfires occur and outstrip local firefighting capabilities.

At this point in your training, we are going to limit our discussion to small ground cover fires. Even though we see and hear about the massive fires that occur in vast wildland areas, most ground cover fires are less

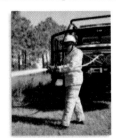

FIGURE 7-1 Ground cover fires are very common, even in urban areas. Most are small enough to be extinguished with a small hose line.

Safety Lesson: A NIOSH Report   Provided as appropriate to the text chapters, this feature details true, documented events reported to NIOSH about injuries and fatalities to firefighters on the job. This feature also includes recommendations to prevent similar tragic events.

View It!   This icon indicates the chapter skills presented on the DVD located in the back of the book.

Practice It!   This feature provides step-by-step instructions and photographs that detail many of the day-to-day individual skills firefighters will use.

Evolution   Here the reader will find step-by-step instructions and photographs that detail an essential firefighting process. The steps and photos work together to depict an evolution of tasks.

is similar to a task you may be doing on the emergency scene, you will probably need to take similar safety preparations before doing the task. For example, if you wear eye protection when using a saw on the emergency scene, you should do the same while using a saw in the fire station.

Use safe practices when handling tools and equipment. If you are not sure how to safely use a tool, don't use it. Ask for help and let someone show you the safe way to operate it. Consult user manuals and be sure to read, understand, and follow all safety precautions.

If routine station maintenance duties require you to work above the floor level—for example, from a ladder—then you should have someone with you as a safety person and you should use the proper equipment for the job (Figure 1-20). Most ladders carried on a fire truck are designed to be used on soft ground—not on slick hard floors—so don't go for the easy-to-grab ladder on the truck instead of taking the

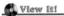

View It!

Go to the DVD, navigate to Chapter 3, and select *SCBA: Donning the Facemask.*

Practice It!

Donning the Facemask

Donning the facemask is the final step you take before you begin breathing from the system. Use the following steps when donning a facemask:

1. It makes no difference whether you don the mask by placing your chin in first and dragging the straps over your head or whether you use the ball-cap method (Figure 3-38). In the ball-cap method, you hold the straps on the back of your head and drag the mask down over your face (Figure 3-39). The main thing to remember is to have nothing between the rubberized face piece and your skin. The straps should be adjusted so that the mask fits snugly against your face. You should cover all remaining exposed skin once the mask is in place.

FIGURE 3-38

FIGURE 3-39

2. Start with your protecti... around your neck and ... Center the harness on ... any hair that may be be... mask. Starting with the ... them two at a time unti... (Figure 3-40).

3. Check the seal by cove... mask and inhaling gent... should not feel any lea... your face (Figure 3-41).

Evolution 11-1

Maneuvering a Small Attack Line During an Exterior Attack

This drill has been developed to practice the skills necessary to establish a water supply and to apply water from the exterior to a simulated single-family-dwelling fire using a small attack line. The firefighters will be working either to establish the water supply or to deploy, set up, and apply a fire stream to the simulated building fire (Figure 11-61). The drill should be repeated, switching firefighter positions so that each person can practice the training drill in both positions.

Training Area: Open area; level ground free of trip hazards

Equipment: Equipped pumper

Training burn building or other acquired building

Sustained water supply source, or static or water main system with hydrant

PPE: Full protective clothing and scba, on and ready for use

1. A fully equipped pumper with a crew consisting of a driver, a Company Officer, and two firefighters is positioned away from the water supply and simulated dwelling fire. All individuals are appropriately protected in PPE with their seatbelts on and ready to respond. A signal is given and the pumper responds to the simulated fire.

2. The pumper positions at the water supply source. A firefighter dismounts safely and removes any equipment necessary to establish a connection to the water supply, including supply hose lines. The firefighter signals for the pumper to proceed with a layout of supply hose while approaching and positioning at the simulated fire.

3. When the pumper positions at the fire, the second firefighter safely dismounts and receives orders from the Company Officer to deploy a small attack line and prepare to flow water onto the building from a safe area.

4. After establishing a connection to the water source, the first firefighter walks next to the supply hose line, straightening it out as he or she approaches the fire scene. This firefighter then arrives at the fire scene, locates the Company Officer, and receives orders to assist the second firefighter on the small attack line.

5. While the two firefighters are flowing water from the small attack line, they are directed to reposition it several times. They will also be directed to change the flow pattern of the stream.

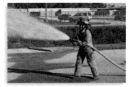

FIGURE 11-61 Using a small attack line, firefighters will establish a water supply or apply water to a simulated building fire from the outside.

6. When the drill has been completed, the crew will properly relieve pressure, disconnect, drain, and reload all the supply and attack hose. They should trade positions and repeat the drill.

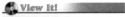

View It!

Go to the DVD, navigate to Chapter 11, and select *Exterior Attack, Large Attack Line.*

Exterior Fire Attack   271

Safety Tips! This feature provides information firefighters should use to keep themselves safe while performing their varied duties.

Tips! Here the reader will find information to perform his or her duties more effectively.

Boxed Information These boxes feature additional, specialized information for firefighters.

Key Words Key words are bolded in the text and also appear with their definitions in boxes following their first mention so that readers can learn the terminology specific to firefighting. These terms, along with their definitions, are also provided alphabetically in the glossary at the back of the book.

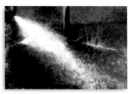
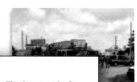

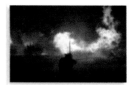
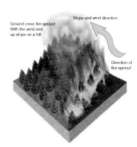

Do It!   This feature summarizes the key information covered in the chapter, focusing on what the firefighter recruit should do after reading the chapter.

Prove It   This assessment section includes knowledge and skills assessments.

Knowledge Assessment   This documentation tear-out sheet is a multiple-choice quiz the firefighter recruit can take and submit to his or her Instructor or Company Officer. Each quiz allows the reader to ensure that he or she has mastered the information before moving on to the next chapter.

Skills Assessment   This documentation tear-out sheet allows the firefighter recruit to demonstrate to his or her Instructor or Company Officer the skills acquired after reading the text and practicing the skills.

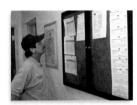

If an emergency call comes into the fire station, be prepared to take down the information and notify your dispatch, or transfer the call to the appropriate dispatch office for processing.

If the call requires an immediate response, get the proper information as dictated by your department's policy. At a minimum, you should request the following information: the emergency type and location, and the caller's name, address, and phone number.

FIGURE 1-25   Right-to-know information must be made available to all members of the fire department in their work area at the fire station. This information may be located on bulletin boards in the fire station. It should include information about hazardous materials and processes.

tric door openers may be located in fire apparatus activated by the driver. Bay doors should have electronic eye safety switches installed that stop doors from closing when they detect obstructions under the door.

Do It!

Your First Day

Everyone's first day in a new position or job is difficult. You will meet many new people and will be learning about your new job. Treat this first day as a challenge that is just the first step as a firefighter. Study how the supervision system works. Learn how to use the telephone and radio communications. Be eager to jump in and lend a hand on any job around the fire station as well as out on emergency scenes. Be cheerful and positive. A smile will take you a long way in making friends and fitting in.

Once you begin to be accepted as a part of the

Prove It

Knowledge Assessment
Signed Documentation Tear-Out Sheet

Entry-Level Firefighter—Chapter 4

Name: _____

Fill out the ten-question quiz below, the Knowledge Assessment Sheet, by circling the correct answer for each question. When finished, sign it and give to your instructor/Company Officer for his or her signature. Turn in this Knowledge Assessment Sheet to the proper person as part of the documentation that you have completed your training for this chapter.

1. The fire attack hose line system begins at the _____ and ends when the stream of water coming from the end of the nozzle effectively reaches the base of the fire.
   a. nozzle
   b. apparatus pump panel
   c. fire hydrant
   d. base of the fire

2. The size of the f _____ the vol
   a. increase
   b. have no affe
   c. reduce
   d. eliminate

3. The inner diame
   a. ¾ inch to 2 in
   b. 2 to 3 inches
   c. ¾ to 1⅛ inch
   d. 1 to 3 inches

4. Booster hose c
   disconnecting
   a. True
   b. False

5. Most couplings
   a. Clockwise
   b. Counterclock

6. Unlike booster l
   a. disconnected
   b. flowed
   c. rolled
   d. drained

Prove It

Skills Assessment
Signed Documentation Tear-Out Sheet

Entry-Level Firefighter—Chapter 4

Name: _____

Fill out the Skills Assessment Sheet below. Have your instructor/Company Officer check off and initial each skill you demonstrate. When finished, sign it and give to your instructor/Company Officer for his or her signature. Turn in this Skills Assessment Sheet to the proper person as part of the documentation that you have completed your training for this chapter.

Skill	Completed	Initials
1. Describe the components of a fire attack hose line system.	_____	_____
2. Demonstrate how to connect and disconnect hose lines.	_____	_____
3. Describe the application of different hose tools and accessories used with attack lines.	_____	_____
4. Demonstrate methods for rolling and carrying fire hose.	_____	_____
5. Explain good techniques for hose maintenance and care.	_____	_____
6. Explain and demonstrate how fire nozzles operate.	_____	_____
7. Demonstrate how to deploy and load booster lines.	_____	_____
8. Demonstrate how to properly hold and utilize a flowing booster hose.	_____	_____
9. Demonstrate how to deploy and load other jacketed attack lines.	_____	_____
10. Demonstrate how to hold and utilize a flowing small attack line.	_____	_____

Student Signature and Date _____   Instructor/Company Officer Signature and Date _____

105

Supplements

For the Student

Student DVD

- DVD of firefighting skills packaged in the back of the text
  - More than 75 essential skills demonstrated by video.
- Includes Digital Flashcards
  - 220 flashcards for self-study.

For the Instructor

Instructor CD

- PowerPoint Slides.
  - More than 300 Powerpoint Slides
- Lesson Plans
  - Full-color lesson plans in PDF format.
- Instructor's Computerized Test Bank

Acknowledgements

The authors and publisher wish to thank the following individuals and organizations for their assistance with this project:

Glen Ellman, *photographer*
Alex Menendez, *videographer and photographer*
George Mullins, *technical advisor*
Casselberry Fire Department, Florida
Central Florida Fire Academy
Ocoee Fire Department, Florida
Orange County Fire/Rescue Department, Florida
Seminole County Fire Division, Florida

Reviewers

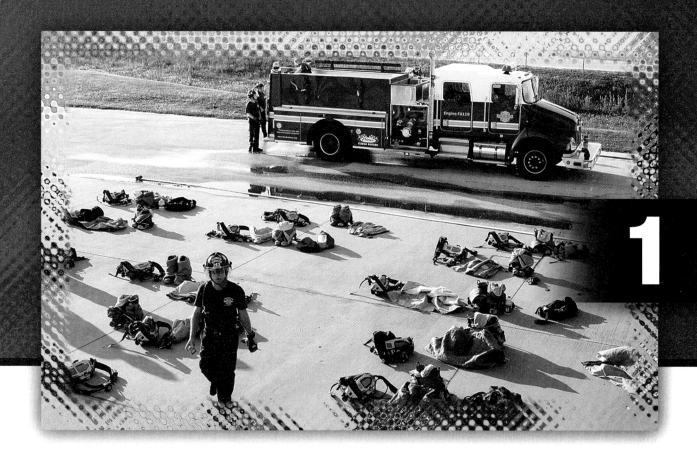

Welcome to the Fire Service

What You Will Learn in This Chapter

This chapter will introduce you to the Fire Service. You will learn how a typical fire department is organized and governed. You will also take a look at how we organize our operations at a fire or other type of emergency. The chapter ends with a look at your safety while at the fire station and suggestions for your first day as a firefighter.

What You Will Be Able to Do

After reading this chapter, you will be asked to tour the fire station so you will know where to find things that are important to your safety. After reading the chapter and taking the tour, you will be able to

1. Properly notify the Station Officer that you are in the station.
2. Locate all emergency exits.
3. Secure the station.

4. Locate and use important information about any hazardous materials that are found in the fire station.
5. Receive and transfer incoming phone calls to the fire station.

Beginning Your Career

It is important that you are successful while you are introduced to the inner workings, organization, and safety considerations of the Fire Department. As you will read in this chapter, the Fire Department maintains a rank structure that is utilized in both emergency and nonemergency operations. It is important for you to understand how this structure operates and where you will fit into it.

There are courtesy considerations and fire station manners that, if followed, will help you make a good first impression. Be a good listener when you first start out. There is so much you need to learn, even after you have completed all of your recruit training.

You also need to understand that safety is just as important around the fire station as it is at your own home or business. Perhaps there is an even more important reason for being safe at the fire station: It is the property of your community, built with everyone's money.

Remember, everyone wants you to succeed. Your instructor, your new supervisor, and your fellow firefighters will all contribute a serious investment of time and effort to ensure that you will be successful while you are in the fire service.

Unique North American Fire Service Terminology

Apparatus usually refers to Fire Service firefighting vehicles, like engine company units, truck company units, and rescue company units. You will see these terms used further in the text as *fire apparatus* (meaning any rolling piece of equipment), *fire engine* (a conventional pumper truck), *truck, ladder,* or *aerial apparatus* (meaning aerial or ladder truck), and *rescue apparatus* (meaning rescue truck). We use these terms frequently and you will undoubtedly hear them in your training sessions.

Organization of the Fire Department

Your fire department is no different from any other organized group of individuals with a common goal. Everyone has a job to do, and all must work within the Fire Department organization and management system. It is important for you to become familiar with the basic workings of your fire department's organization. All Fire departments share some similarities.

Some fire departments are staffed by full-time, paid firefighters (paid department), while others may be fully staffed by volunteers (volunteer department) who respond when there is a call for help. Some departments are a combination of paid and volunteer staff (combination department) in which a paid staff is available for the initial response to an alarm that is augmented with volunteers. A varia-

tion to these types of departments includes firefighters who are paid a small stipend to remain available in an area during designated hours so that they can respond quickly to an emergency. This type of department is referred to as a paid-on-call department.

Basic Work Groups: The "Company"

The basic work groups of most fire departments are composed of the first level of work teams, which are known as the *company*. The crew of each company consists of the team assigned to the apparatus or job task. The firefighters on a crew are usually managed by a first-line supervisor who may hold the rank of Senior Firefighter, Sergeant, Lieutenant, or Captain, depending on the organization and tradition of your department. Regardless of what rank your fire department designates for this lead role, the person in charge of the company is the Company Officer.

Companies are usually designated according to the type of their apparatus and the job they generally perform on the emergency scene. Traditionally, the crews are divided into engine companies, ladder or truck companies, and rescue or squad companies. There are also many specialized work groups such as **hazardous materials** (hazmat) units and technical rescue companies, and other specialized companies (Figures 1-1, 1-2, and 1-3). The list can go on and on. It is important for you to become familiar with the various company-level work groups in your fire department. You will need to understand how they are staffed and the specific functions each one has at the emergency scene.

KEY WORD

hazardous materials (hazmat)   Materials and processes that present a hazard to human health through poisoning, chemical and thermal burns, radioactivity, explosiveness, chemical reactivity, or carcinogenic exposure.

Engine Companies

Engine companies are the most common type of Fire Service company and have the general fire and rescue task responsibilities; however, they may also be utilized for rescue or truck operations if the need arises (Figure 1-4). These units usually carry a supply of water, a hose to connect to a sustained water supply, and a pump to push the water supply through hose lines to the nozzles for fire extinguishment

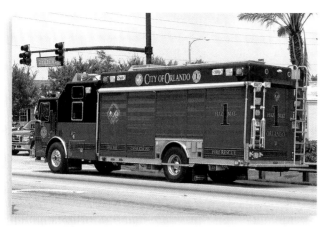
FIGURE 1-1   A hazardous materials unit.

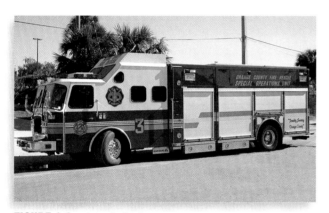
FIGURE 1-2   A technical rescue company.

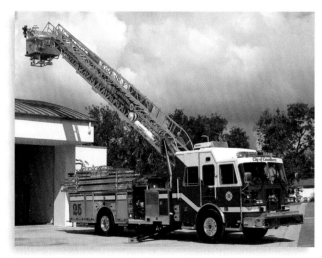
FIGURE 1-3   An aerial ladder unit (truck company).

(Figure 1-5). The firefighting crew is usually led by the Company Officer.

In many areas of the United States, the engine company is cross-trained to handle many of the jobs encountered on the emergency scene. The jobs that

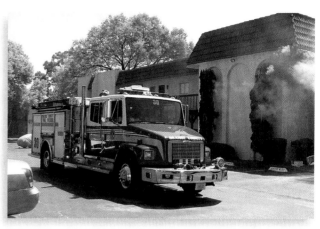
FIGURE 1-4   Engine companies have their own pump and carry water, manpower, equipment, and hose to the fire emergency.

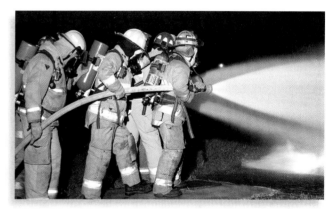
FIGURE 1-5   An engine company firefighting crew and Company Officer.

are handled on the emergency scene are based on the needs and capabilities of each community served by each fire department. Smaller departments are often required to have engine companies deliver many varied types of service to their community. The larger the fire department, the more likely it is that the companies will be more specialized into engines, rescues, and trucks.

Truck Companies

Compared to engine companies, truck companies have a more specialized function of additional fire and rescue task responsibilities. They also have elevated fire attack capabilities (Figure 1-6). They may or may not be equipped with their own **water supply.** They also have special training to deliver advanced **ventilation** and **forcible entry** techniques when needed on the emergency scene. Truck companies can provide fire **overhaul** and **salvage** capabilities and add personnel to assist in the overall firefighting effort.

water supply The water used for extinguishing fires that is carried to the fire by apparatus; pumped from static sources like ponds, rivers, and lakes; or obtained from pressurized water delivery systems through water mains and fire hydrant access points.

ventilation Techniques applied to building fires that allow smoke and hot gases to escape from a building involved in a fire. These techniques may also be utilized for atmospheres hazardous to health and life (such as a hazardous gas release inside a building).

forcible entry Methods of gaining access into a locked or obstructed building or vehicle by applying tools to physically dislodge and open a gate, doorway, or window.

overhaul The techniques and methods applied on an emergency fire scene that lessen the progress of the fire damage. The fire scene is checked for fire extension and hidden fires that are then extinguished. These techniques and methods include measures that help make buildings safe after a fire.

salvage Measures taken by firefighting personnel that help reduce property damage to rooms and content during and after a fire.

Rescue Companies

Rescue companies usually do not have a pump, water, or hose. Their primary function is to perform rescue at a fire as well as to assist in other firefighting activities. They may be called upon to rescue citizens as well as Fire Service personnel on the emergency scene. In some fire departments, these units are staffed by firefighters trained as **Emergency Medical Technicians (EMTs)** and **Paramedics,** which greatly enhances the emergency rescue and medical care capabilities of the department.

Technical rescue operations, like those situations that involve the rescue of victims trapped in unusual or special circumstances, are primarily handled by a rescue or truck company with specially trained personnel and with assistance from engine companies (Figure 1-7).

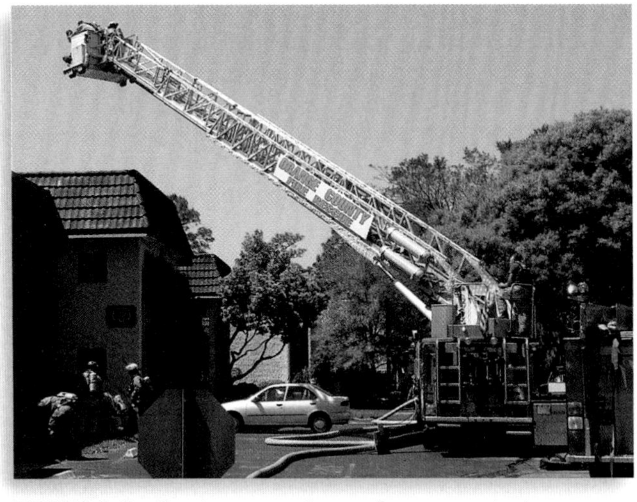

Emergency Medical Technician (EMT) A person trained in emergency prehospital care at a level above basic and advanced first aid.

Paramedic A prehospital emergency care provider who is trained at a level above Emergency Medical Technician.

technical rescue Any rescue discipline requiring specialized knowledge, skills, and tools. Technical rescue includes water, vehicle, rope, building collapse, trench, and confined space rescue.

Company Officers

The Team Leader or Company Officer in charge of the unit may be predesignated for each company, or the team for each unit may be assembled as firefighters arrive on the emergency scene. This latter scenario is more common in a volunteer fire department than in a fully paid or combination-type department. As a new

FIGURE 1-6 Truck companies perform many tasks, including forcible entry, ventilation, and overhaul and salvage capabilities. They also provide an elevated fire attack capability.

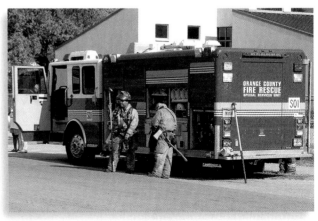

FIGURE 1-7 Some fire departments have Special Rescue units that provide technical rescue capability for the community.

firefighter, it is very important for you to learn who is in charge of these companies. It most likely will be your Company Officer on the emergency scene and therefore will be the people who will directly supervise your actions (Figure 1-8).

Chain of Command

The operations are organized by an established **chain of command.** This chain of command is the management plan for any emergency operation (Figure 1-9).

▬▬ KEY WORD ▬▬▬

chain of command The organization of supervisory levels within a fire department, generally utilized for both emergency and nonemergency operations.

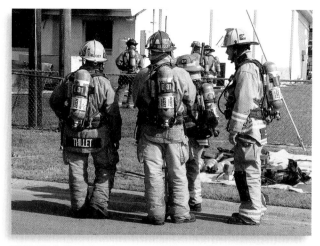

FIGURE 1-8 The Company Officer will most likely be your immediate supervisor. He or she will be the engine company team leader.

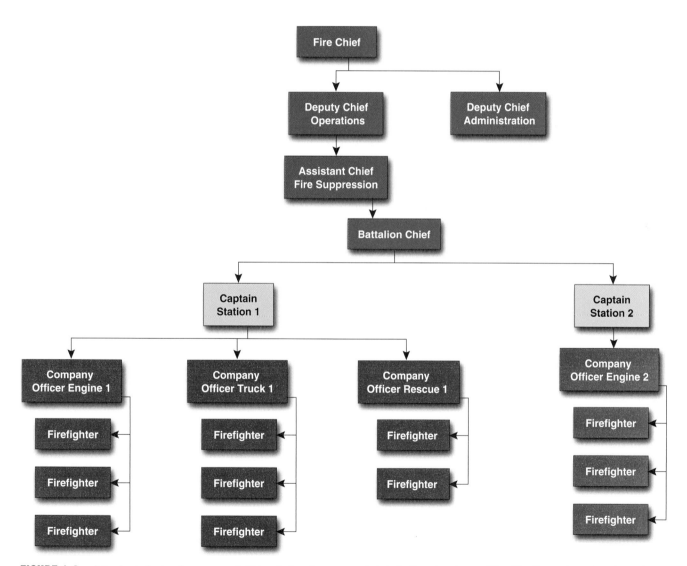

FIGURE 1-9 A typical chain of command. This chain of command details the structure of the Fire Department as it works at a typical emergency operation.

Mid-Management

The individual companies are supervised as a group by the next layer of supervision in the fire department. These ranks have many names, but they are mid-management personnel and may be designated as Captains, Battalion Chief, District Chief, or, in some instances, Assistant Chief. This all depends on the organizational makeup of your department.

In most cases, midlevel supervisors manage two or more Company Officers and serve as the commanders of emergency incidents involving two or more companies.

Upper Management

There is a lot more to a fire department than the basic companies. Many organizations are divided into divisions or bureaus that cover emergency and nonemergency operations. There can also be an Emergency Medical Division that handles the delivery of **Emergency Medical Services (EMS)** by the department, if provided. Either an Assistant Chief or a Deputy Chief, who answers directly to the Fire Chief, manages most divisions. An Assistant or Deputy Chief usually manages large incidents that involve several companies working on the scene.

▬ KEY WORD ▬▬▬▬▬▬▬

Emergency Medical Services (EMS)   A group of organizations that provide emergency medical prehospital care to the community.

Department Divisions

A larger fire department may be further divided into divisions that serve under the command of a division head. For now, let's concentrate on the typical divisions you may encounter.

Administration Division   Besides emergency operations, fire departments also have nonemergency work groups under their administration. Larger departments may have an Administration Division that coordinates nonemergency operations like supply and facility maintenance.

Fire Prevention Division   A good fire prevention program is an excellent approach to increasing firefighter safety. A Fire Prevention Division performs fire inspections and assists in building code enforcement. They may also handle arson investigations of suspicious fires and the delivery of public fire education programs. Fire prevention is a very important job of the fire service for its community. In recent years, more emphasis has been placed on the delivery of good fire prevention programs for the public.

Training Division   A Training Division provides recruit training and ongoing training programs for firefighters. These programs include weekly drill training for volunteer departments and daily training programs for paid firefighters. The Training Division also provides assistance for Company Officers so that they can provide training to their work groups.

Communications Division   Probably one of the most important divisions within any emergency agency is the Communications Division. The main role of the Communications Division is to operate the alarm office. In this office, call takers receive the initial call for help, process the information, and dispatch the appropriate units to handle the situation (Figure 1-10). Fire departments today communicate through many more ways than a simple telephone and two-way radio. Pagers, e-mail, and cell telephones are very common in most fire departments. All of these communications channels are coordinated by the Communications Division.

The Fire Chief

Almost all fire departments are led by a Chief Officer, Fire Commissioner, Fire Chief, or Fire Administrator. This individual is the top person in the chain of command as well as the manager of the fire department. There might be staff personnel who work with this individual to administer the department. This person may have many other jobs to perform, depending on the size and scope of the individual fire department he or she manages.

In volunteer fire departments, the Chief can be an elected position, for a specific length of time, such as one or two years. Some departments use a governing board to appoint their Chief.

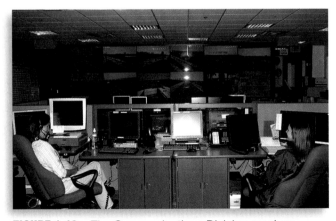

FIGURE 1-10   The Communications Division receives emergency calls, processes the information, and dispatches the appropriate fire units to the scene. This division is vital to Fire Department operations.

In some paid or volunteer fire departments, the Chief may be hired or appointed by the local government. Regardless of how the individual is placed in the position, this person is the chief executive of the organization. You should make it a point to identify the Chief of your department.

Governing Bodies

Fire departments are often under the control of local government (Figure 1-11). This governing body can be a city or county council with elected representatives serving on a board. Some fire departments may be part of another organization such as a private industry—for example, an **Industrial Fire Brigade.** Some other fire departments may be part of a government entity, such as a military fire service or federal forestry service. There may be a board of fire commissioners that approves budgets and defines policy. In volunteer fire departments, the governing board may be called a Board of Directors.

Today, more and more is being required of fire departments by the communities they serve. Most fire departments deliver some level of Emergency Medical Services to their community. In addition, responsibility for hazardous material incident mitigation is often given to the local fire department.

The Fire Service is usually the first emergency agency to arrive and begin initial steps to handle disasters, both natural and manmade. On the national level, fire departments are also an integral part of the United States' Homeland Defense response strategy.

■■■ KEY WORD ■■■

Industrial Fire Brigade   An organization similar to a fire department that protects a single business or business complex. This organization is generally privately funded and operated.

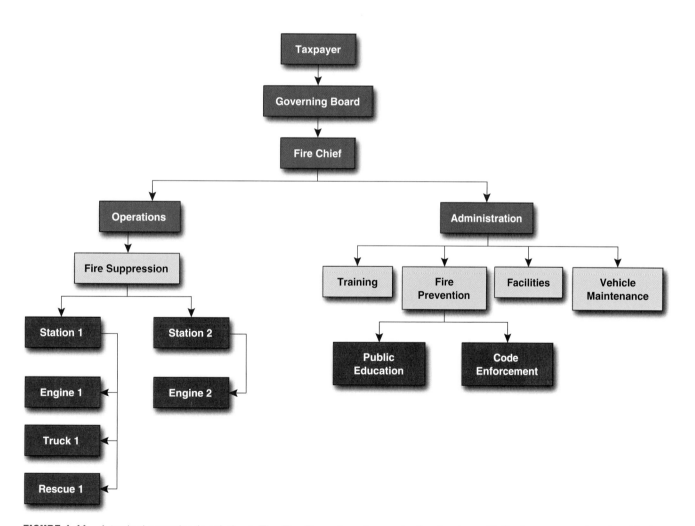

FIGURE 1-11   A typical organizational chart. The Fire Department organization begins with the taxpayer and ends with the newest firefighters, covering all branches of the organization.

Introduction to Incident Command

At first glance, the fireground or emergency scene may seem to be in total chaos (Figure 1-12). Watching firefighters working inside a burning structure while others outside work furiously to break windows, stretch hose lines, and control the scene may make you wonder how they know what to do and when to do it. As chaotic as it may seem, the emergency operations at a fire or rescue event are usually well coordinated through the use of an **Incident Command System (ICS).** When you become familiar with the basic framework of a typical Incident Command System, fireground operations will make a lot more sense to you.

When you arrive at the scene of an emergency, you operate under the command of your Company Officer. The Company Officer is responsible for your safety as much as you are; therefore, the Company Officer wants to keep in close contact with you at all times. The first rule of any emergency operation is that there is absolutely *no* room for **freelancing** of any type. Do not wander away from your team for any reason, even if you are not working at the moment. After you complete the Exterior Operations level portion of your training, you will be assigned tasks that can be completed in a safe area outside the burning building. If, for some reason, you are assigned to a Company Officer who is not familiar with you, be sure the officer knows your level of training so that you are not assigned duties that are beyond the scope of your training (Figure 1-13).

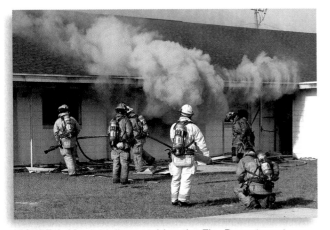

FIGURE 1-12 Initially, watching the Fire Department working at an emergency may seem chaotic. However, after you become more familiar with the Incident Command System, it will make more sense to you.

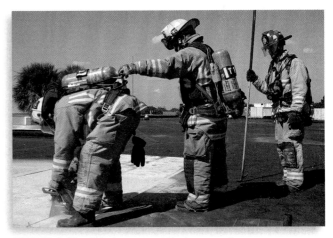

FIGURE 1-13 It is important that you make sure your Company Officer knows your level of training so that you are not assigned duties beyond your capabilities.

KEY WORDS

Incident Command System (ICS) An organization of supervision at an emergency that designates supervisory levels and responsibility.

freelancing Working independently of the Incident Command System, without the knowledge of the Incident Commander. *Freelancing* is seen as a negative term and is usually associated with an unsafe activity.

The Incident Commander

If the situation requires more than one company to handle the problem, an Incident Command System is established. Under the Incident Command System, a single officer, the **Incident Commander,** coordinates the different companies operating on the scene. This coordination enhances everyone's safety, reduces any redundant actions on the scene, and, most of all, coordinates the radio communications, keeping the radio chatter to an efficient minimum. To accomplish this, all of the on-scene radio communications are directed between operating companies and the Incident Commander (Figure 1-14). Only the Incident Commander talks directly to the communication center.

The first arriving person, most often the officer on the first arriving unit, should establish the Incident Command System. On the radio, the arrival report may sound something like this: *"Engine 1 on the scene, heavy fire showing from the first floor of a single-story, wood-frame house. Engine 1 establishing command."* Now everyone who is responding can develop a mental picture of what is burning and knows exactly who is in charge. As more companies arrive, the command and control of the event is passed to

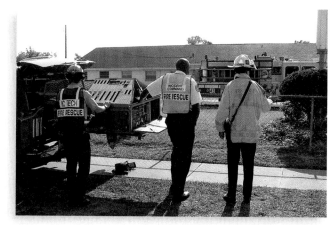

FIGURE 1-14 At a typical emergency scene with an Incident Command System established, all radio communications are made through the Incident Commander and not directly with the dispatchers.

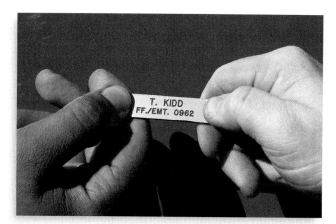

FIGURE 1-15 PAS tags allow the Incident Command System to track firefighters at an emergency scene. Immediately after you arrive at the scene, your Company Officer hands these tags to the Incident Commander.

higher-ranking officers so that the Company Officer can keep his or her crew intact.

■ KEY WORD ■

Incident Commander (IC) The person in charge of an emergency operation command structure and consequently in charge of the emergency incident at hand.

Personnel Accountability System

The Incident Commander uses a **personnel accountability system** to track each individual who is operating on the scene. Personnel accountability systems allow the Incident Commander to group individuals by crews and track them by job assignments. A firefighter gives a tag that indicates his or her name to the Company Officer (Figures 1-15 and 1-16). The Company Officer groups the tags for everyone on the crew and hands them to the Incident Commander or the Commander's designee so that everyone operating on an emergency scene is accounted for at all times.

■ KEY WORD ■

personnel accountability system An identification system used to track fire department units as well as personnel on the emergency scene.

Working Groups

If the emergency situation is particularly large and includes several companies operating simultaneously,

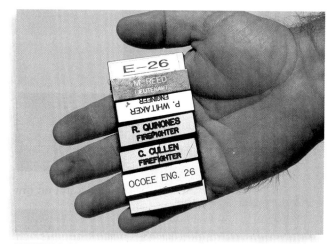

FIGURE 1-16 The PAS tag indicates your name and is grouped with other members of your firefighting team. A team is usually identified by the company designation for the fire unit.

the Incident Commander will probably divide the operating crews into separate groups that are each led by a group supervisor. Depending on local practices, these groups are called *sectors, branches, divisions,* or *work groups.* On the radio, a typical order may sound something like this: "*Command to Engine 1, report to the Fire Attack Branch for outside ventilation duties*" (Figure 1-17).

In order to establish uniform terminology, many agencies have decided to recognize the National Incident Management System (NIMS), which prefers the terms *division, branch,* and *group.* However, many departments still use the term *sector* to describe the smaller divisions of responsibility at an emergency. It is important that you become completely familiar with the terminology used by your department and other departments in your area.

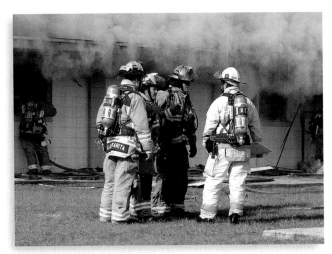

FIGURE 1-17 Several individual teams of firefighters may be assigned to a subdivided area of the emergency scene called a *branch,* and the branch is supervised by a Fire Officer.

Codes and Standards

There are many codes and standards that your fire department utilizes as guidelines in almost every aspect in which it operates. Is it vital that an Exterior Operations level firefighter like yourself be thoroughly knowledgeable about these many standards and rules? Not really, but you do need to know that they exist and that many times your fire department operates a certain way because of these standards and rules.

National Fire Protection Association (NFPA)

Probably the main source for Fire Service standards comes from the **National Fire Protection Association (NFPA).** This organization writes standards that cover everything from the boots you wear to the types of hose and nozzles you use. The training program you are taking now is covering areas of knowledge identified by NFPA Standards.

■ KEY WORD ■

National Fire Protection Association (NFPA) An organization that sets fire codes and standards recognized by most fire department organizations in the United States.

Occupational Safety and Health Administration (OSHA)

The rules of the federal **Occupational Safety and Health Administration (OSHA)** also greatly affect the fire service. They mainly deal with safety issues in emergency as well as nonemergency operations.

■ KEY WORD ■

Occupational Safety and Health Administration (OSHA) A federal governmental agency that establishes regulations that apply to many aspects of employee safety at the workplace.

National Institute for Occupational Safety and Health (NIOSH)

The **National Institute for Occupational Safety and Health (NIOSH)** is another safety regulator used in the Fire Service. This federal agency sets standards for tools and techniques and also investigates many line-of-duty Fire Service injuries and deaths. (See "Safety Lesson: A NIOSH Report" later in this chapter.)

We will point out national standards and codes where necessary. For now you need to know that they exist and that they govern many of the procedures and kinds of equipment used by the fire service.

■ KEY WORD ■

National Institute for Occupational Safety and Health (NIOSH) A federal agency concerned with improving employee safety in the workplace.

Fire Department Rules and Regulations

Every organization has a set of rules and regulations that guide how that organization operates. Your department may have rules and regulations, standard operating guidelines or procedures, or organizational bylaws that both govern how things are done and provide guidance.

For you as an Exterior Operations level firefighter, it is probably important that you identify these guidelines and start to learn them as they apply to you. They include things such as how you are to respond to an emergency call, the protective equipment to be used at each type of call, and the Incident Command System procedures.

Routine, day-to-day activities such as training, equipment checkout procedures, and station duty assignments are also included in the rules and regulations. Every fire department has its routine, or nonemergency, operations that are scheduled daily. They also have their emergency operations, which can happen at any time. You will spend much more time at the fire station in routine operations than you will on actual emergencies.

Fire Stations

Fire stations are unique buildings in the community. They contain the fire and rescue units and equipment used to respond to emergencies (Figure 1-18). The firefighters who respond on those units may be working in the stations, as in a full-time paid department, or they may respond to the station facilities to answer emergency calls, as in volunteer fire departments. In every community, fire stations are a source of pride and honor.

Fire stations, in fact, are owned by the citizens of the community, and the public feels at ease going into their fire station for help. In times of public emergencies and disasters, fire stations may be the only functioning public buildings in the community. People tend to go to their local fire station for help and information during these times.

These buildings usually have vehicle bays that house the various fire and rescue apparatus, a workshop area for tool and equipment maintenance, and a living area for firefighters and the public (Figure 1-19).

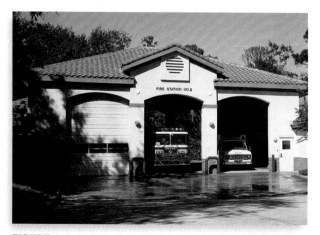

FIGURE 1-18 Fire stations are spaced throughout the community and are an integral part of any neighborhood.

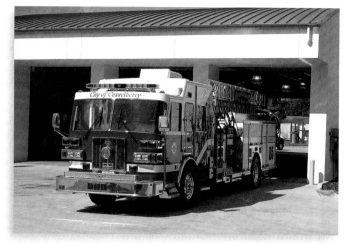

FIGURE 1-19 Fire stations house vehicles and can contain offices, living areas, storage areas, and public meeting areas.

The living area (day room or ready room) usually has some sort of kitchen and dining area, a training or lounge area (sometimes called a ready room), and offices. In fire stations that are staffed around the clock, dorm facilities for on-duty crews may be provided. Additional meeting and activity rooms, government offices, and fire emergency communications facilities may be attached, depending on the design and needs of the community.

Be sure to ask someone to show you around the fire station and get to know the building and facilities. Take note of exit locations, emergency notification procedures, and fire extinguisher locations. Find out who is normally in charge of the facility and introduce yourself to that person.

Station Safety

We are going to discuss fire station safety by covering three areas: (1) station safety for firefighters, (2) right-to-know requirements, and (3) station safety for visitors.

Station Safety for Firefighters

As you continue your training, you will learn a great deal about safety on the emergency scene. You'll become familiar with when to put on your safety gear and how to safely extinguish various types of fires. Your safety at the fire station is just as important as scene safety. Unfortunately, many individuals assume that safe practices can be sidestepped in the nonemergency circumstances of the station. However, many injuries and even deaths occur during nonemergency routines at the fire station.

To begin with, we must all keep the following rule in mind: *If the action you are taking at the fire station* is similar to a task you may be doing on the emergency scene, you will probably need to take similar safety preparations before doing the task. For example, if you wear eye protection when using a saw on the emergency scene, you should do the same while using a saw in the fire station.

Use safe practices when handling tools and equipment. If you are not sure how to safely use a tool, don't use it. Ask for help and let someone show you the safe way to operate it. Consult user manuals and be sure to read, understand, and follow all safety precautions.

If routine station maintenance duties require you to work above the floor level—for example, from a ladder—then you should have someone with you as a safety person and you should use the proper equipment for the job (Figure 1-20). Most ladders carried on a fire truck are designed to be used on soft ground—not on slick hard floors—so don't go for the easy-to-grab ladder on the truck instead of taking the time to use a proper stepladder. Don't be tempted to use the fire truck as a work platform by climbing up on the hose bed to do something as simple as changing a light bulb. It is too easy to walk off the side of the truck or fall as you are climbing up or down. Bottom line: *Use the proper tool for the job.*

Next, if there is a safety hazard that might be pointed out to the public at a fire inspection, the same rules apply at the fire station. A frayed wire on an extension cord is dangerous whether in a business, home, or fire station—the rules don't change.

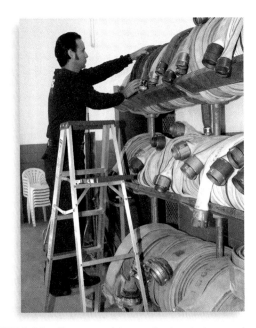

FIGURE 1-20 If you need to reach elevated areas in a fire station, use the proper ladder. Ladders on a fire truck may not be appropriate. Make sure to use the proper tools and equipment for the job at hand.

The National Institute for Occupational Safety and Health (NIOSH) conducts a program that is designed to determine the factors that cause or contribute to firefighter deaths and serious injuries suffered in the line of duty. This organization's intent is to help researchers and safety specialists develop strategies for preventing similar future incidents. Throughout this book, you will find examples of the lessons learned from some of these reports. It is our hope that you will take the time to read each lesson seriously, with the understanding that one or more firefighters have died in the reported incidents. We hope that you will learn something that can prevent you from suffering a similar fate. You can access the NIOSH reports on the Internet at http://www.cdc.gov/niosh/firehome.html or call 1-800-35NIOSH.

Safety Lesson

A NIOSH Report

An In-Station Accident

Accidents and injuries can happen to almost anyone, almost anywhere. The sad truth is that most accidents could have been prevented if everyone involved had been aware of the hazard associated with their actions as well as the proper safety steps one should take to prevent harm from those hazards. Fire and EMS departments are in the business of taking care of the victims of accidents; however, it is often the firefighter or EMS worker who is the injured person needing help.

On January 16, 2000, a 53-year-old male volunteer firefighter died after an extension ladder slipped out from under him while he was conducting routine maintenance work on the garage door at the firehouse. The victim and another firefighter had used a 14-foot fire service extension ladder to climb to the top of a rescue truck. They had used the rescue truck as a platform to work from as they assisted a civilian in changing the garage door opener. The victim had removed the existing door opener and was in the process of going to assist in readying the new door opener when the ladder slipped out from under him. The victim fell headfirst to the concrete floor.

When the victim fell to the floor, the second firefighter was left on top of the rescue truck with no way down but to jump. The civilian called 911 and attempted to render aid to the victim as the second firefighter jumped to the floor and ran next door to inform the victim's wife. Help arrived within minutes and the victim was transported to the local hospital via helicopter. He died the next day.

Follow-Up

NIOSH Report #F2000-07

The NIOSH investigative report concluded that three simple recommendations could have prevented this accident:

- Fire departments should ensure that ladders are used in accordance with existing safety standards.
- Fire departments should designate an individual as the fire station Safety Officer for all in-house maintenance to identify potential hazards and ensure that those hazards are eliminated.
- Fire departments should consider the use of mobile scaffolding, personal lifts, scissor lifts, or boom lifts instead of the top surface of a fire truck.

 Safety Tip!

Here are some safety tips for working in the fire station:

1. **Learn the layout of the station.**
   - Know how to exit the building and identify the exits.
   - Locate all the fire extinguishers and building fire systems.
2. **Practice good housekeeping.**
   - Keep all walkways and floors clear of clutter, spills, and trip hazards.
   - Keep the fire station and apparatus clean at all times.
   - Empty the trash often.
   - Keep all flammable materials in proper containers and cabinets.
3. **Keep the fire station secure.**
   - Keep unescorted visitors out of the vehicle bays.
   - Secure the station when no one is there.
   - Know how to report an emergency from the fire station.
4. **Maintain a safe attitude.**
   - Use care and proper protective gear when utilizing tools and equipment.
   - Always be careful working around apparatus in the vehicle bays.
   - There is no place for "horseplay" at the fire station.

Right-to-Know Requirements

As much as firefighters would like them to be, fire stations are no different from any other public access building in the community. Employers are required by law (OSHA) to inform their employees, including volunteers, about any hazardous materials operations or hazardous materials located at their workplace.

Fire stations post a public notice of right-to-know information for employees. They also should have files, kept on the property, that identify all hazardous chemicals, materials, and processes on site.

Regularly check the bulletin board for safety notices and information. Make it a point to become aware of any right-to-know information within the fire station. This information is posted in an area accessible to all employees. The person in charge of the station can tell you where this information is located.

Station Safety for Visitors

When the public comes into a fire station, they should be kept safe at all times. It is very important that they be greeted properly and asked if they can be assisted. A firefighter should stay with visitors until they have completed their business or have found the individual they are looking for.

Visitors should never be allowed to wander through the station by themselves. This likely leads only to trouble and may expose them to injury. By far the most dangerous place for the public is in the vehicle bays. Equipment may be out on the floors and vehicles may be entering or leaving the facility. An emergency call may come in and the vehicles will have to be used to respond quickly. Escort visitors to the vehicle bay area and lead them back into the office area of the fire station (Figure 1-21). Never leave visitors alone in the vehicle bay.

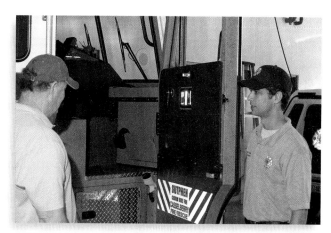

FIGURE 1-21 All visitors to a fire station should be escorted, especially in the vehicle bays.

Your Fire Station

Fire stations are multipurpose buildings that serve many functions in the community. When you visit a fire station for the first time, it is important that you introduce yourself to the person in charge and explain why you are there. As a new member, whether a volunteer or paid firefighter, you should then be shown the station.

Fire stations usually have a public access area that contains the entrance area or foyer, with offices used for things like communications and dispatch, staff functions like fire prevention and training, administrative offices for Chiefs, and offices for station crew supervisors.

Locate All Emergency Exits

While touring the station, look for all exits from the building (Figure 1-22). Just like any other building, fire stations can experience an emergency and a quick exit may be required. Assess the exit doorway. Does it have a lock or a latch? Will an alarm sound when you open it? Where does the exit door lead—to another interior space and then outside, or directly out of the station?

Find the Fire Extinguisher Locations

Fire extinguishers will probably be located near the office area, the kitchen and lounge areas, the vehicle bays, and the sleeping and meeting room areas.

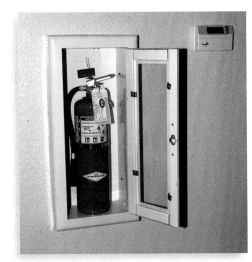

FIGURE 1-23 Learn the locations of the fire extinguishers in your station.

Check the types of extinguishers in each location (Figure 1-23).

Learn How to Secure the Station

During your station tour, be sure to ask about securing the fire station. You need to know how to properly lock as well as unlock the facility (Figure 1-24). Some stations issue keys to all personnel. Others may have lockbox devices with a combination lock or electronic cardkey access.

You should also ask about and learn the procedures for opening and closing vehicle bay doors. Elec-

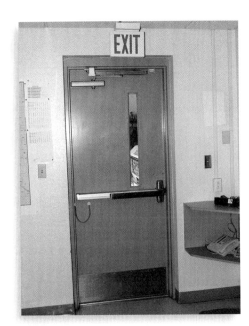

FIGURE 1-22 During your initial station tour, notice the locations of the exit doors.

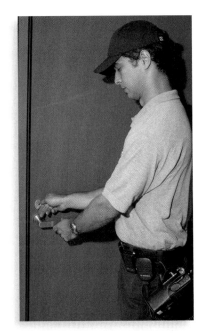

FIGURE 1-24 It is important to know how to secure the fire station.

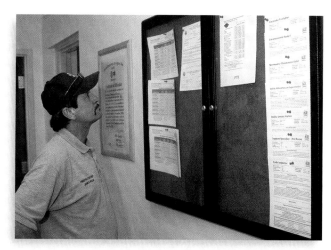

FIGURE 1-25 Right-to-know information must be made available to all members of the fire department in their work area at the fire station. This information may be located on bulletin boards in the fire station. It should include information about hazardous materials and processes.

tric door openers may be located in fire apparatus activated by the driver. Bay doors should have electronic eye safety switches installed that stop doors from closing when they detect obstructions under the door.

Locate Important Information About Any Hazardous Materials Found in the Fire Station

You should ask about any right-to-know information posted in the fire station. Find this location and note the processes and materials listed (Figure 1-25). Ask the person who is showing you around where these notices are located and how they are stored. Remember to read this information regularly so that you become familiar with it.

Learn How to Answer an Incoming Phone Call to the Fire Station

During your orientation visit to the fire station, it is important that you learn how to take a phone call. These calls are usually for fire department business, but occasionally they can be an emergency call for help. It is important to answer the phone in a professional, polite, and serious manner. Doing so conveys professionalism and reflects the respect you have for your community. A typical phone call reception should be, "*Hello, _____ Fire Department, (Your Name) speaking. How can I help you?*"

Always be ready to take a message or transfer the call to the appropriate person. Never hang up on a caller—always be prepared to give assistance.

If an emergency call comes into the fire station, be prepared to take down the information and notify your dispatch, or transfer the call to the appropriate dispatch office for processing.

If the call requires an immediate response, get the proper information as dictated by your department's policy. At a minimum, you should request the following information: the emergency type and location, and the caller's name, address, and phone number.

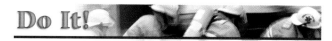

Your First Day

Everyone's first day in a new position or job is difficult. You will meet many new people and will be learning about your new job. Treat this first day as a challenge that is just the first step as a firefighter. Study how the supervision system works. Learn how to use the telephone and radio communications. Be eager to jump in and lend a hand on any job around the fire station as well as out on emergency scenes. Be cheerful and positive. A smile will take you a long way in making friends and fitting in.

Once you begin to be accepted as a part of the department, you will then begin to bond with your coworkers as you face the challenges of emergency work. This bonding will stay with you for the rest of your life—it is the invisible tie that binds all firefighters together. You have to depend upon each other to survive as well as to be successful in handling emergencies.

Always be the student. Set out to learn something every day you work at the fire department. Listen to others and be observant. Think before you speak or do anything. Most of all, never work outside your training and capability. Be safe at all times.

Our first chapter was intended to introduce you to the Fire Service. First we talked about how a typical fire department is organized and governed. Then we explained how fire departments manage themselves at emergency scenes. Finally, we described the makeup of a fire station and discussed fire station safety. You were also provided with skills training for notifying the Station Officer that you are in the fire station, how to locate all the emergency exits of a fire station, how to secure the fire station, and how to locate and use important information on any hazardous materials or processes in the fire station.

We hope that this first introduction into the Fire Service has inspired you to go on with your training and that you will be successful in becoming a safe firefighter for your community.

Prove It

Knowledge Assessment
Signed Documentation Tear-Out Sheet

Exterior Operations Level Firefighter—Chapter 1

Name: _____

Fill out the ten-question quiz below, the Knowledge Assessment Sheet, by circling the correct answer for each question. When finished, sign it and give to your instructor/Company Officer for his or her signature. Turn in this Knowledge Assessment Sheet to the proper person as part of the documentation that you have completed your training for this chapter.

1. NIOSH routinely investigates line-of-duty firefighter injuries and deaths.
   a. True
   b. False

2. The person who is in charge of an engine or truck company is commonly referred to as a
   1. Chief Officer.
   b. Division Chief.
   c. Company Officer.
   d. Firefighter.

3. Which of the following divisions conducts building inspections and enforces fire codes?
   a. Training
   b. Fire Prevention
   c. Supply
   d. Maintenance

4. Fire departments are often under the jurisdiction of
   a. local governments.
   b. state governments.
   c. the federal government.
   d. national agencies.

5. Complex fireground operations are usually controlled by
   a. a senior firefighter.
   b. an Incident Establishment System.
   c. an Incident Command System.
   d. a national standard.

6. Emergency personnel working at emergency scenes are usually tracked by some sort of
   a. personnel warning system.
   b. personnel accountability system.
   c. special transponders.
   d. radio frequencies.

7. In the Incident Command System, subdivisions of the command system are commonly referred to as
   a. sides.
   b. parts.
   c. sectors.
   d. divisions.

8. It is acceptable to allow visitors to the fire station to roam freely throughout the building.
   a. True
   b. False

9. A fire truck hose bed makes a great platform for working on lights at the ceiling of the fire station vehicle bay.
   a. True
   b. False

10. Any hazardous materials stored or used on the station property will be listed on the _____ kept in the fire station.
    a. right-to-know notice
    b. Internet listing
    c. rules and regulations
    d. Company Officer's desk

Student Signature and Date _____   Instructor/Company Officer Signature and Date _____

18

Prove It

Skills Assessment
Signed Documentation Tear-Out Sheet

Exterior Operations Level Firefighter—Chapter 1

Name: _____

Fill out the Skills Assessment Sheet below. Have your instructor/Company Officer check off and initial each skill you demonstrate. When finished, sign it and give to your instructor/Company Officer for his or her signature. Turn in this Skills Assessment Sheet to the proper person as part of the documentation that you have completed your training for this chapter.

Skill	Completed	Initials
1. Give the name of the person in charge of the station.	_____	_____
2. Describe the general layout of the fire station.	_____	_____
3. Describe the types and numbers of units in the vehicle bay areas.	_____	_____
4. State how many exits there are from the building.	_____	_____
5. Describe the locations of the exits.	_____	_____
6. Demonstrate how to answer a phone call and make an outgoing business call.	_____	_____
7. Demonstrate how firefighters can enter the locked fire station.	_____	_____
8. Demonstrate how to properly secure the fire station.	_____	_____
9. Demonstrate how to safely open and close the bay doors.	_____	_____
10. Show the location of the station bulletin board and the right-to-know information.	_____	_____

Student Signature and Date _____   Instructor/Company Officer Signature and Date _____

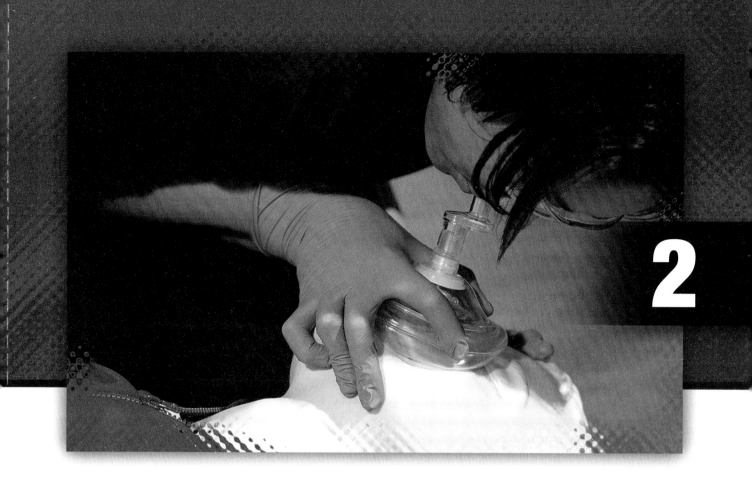

2

Basic First Aid and CPR

What You Will Learn in This Chapter

This chapter will introduce you to some fundamental first aid practices, which include a safe approach to the scene, the legal implications of your actions, and several steps you can take prior to the arrival of the Emergency Medical Services.

What You Will Be Able to Do

After reading this chapter and practicing the skills in a classroom setting, you will be able to

1. Describe some of the steps you can take in allowing a safe approach to a scene in which someone has been injured.

2. Describe the principles of the standard of care, consent, and abandonment.

3. Demonstrate the steps for ensuring infection control and body substance isolation.

4. Describe the ABCs of first aid.

5. Demonstrate the head tilt–chin lift and jaw-thrust maneuvers for opening a person's airway.

6. Demonstrate abdominal thrusts.

7. Demonstrate assessing a patient's carotid pulse.

8. Demonstrate rescue breathing.

9. Demonstrate proper chest compressions for a pulseless person.

10. Demonstrate the proper use of an automatic external defibrillator (AED).

11. Demonstrate the methods for applying direct pressure and a pressure dressing to control external bleeding.

12. Describe the signs and symptoms of shock and demonstrate the steps for managing a patient who is in shock.

13. Demonstrate the application of a cold compress.

14. Describe the severity of burns.

15. Demonstrate the treatment of a burn injury.

Reality!

Basic Emergency Care

Firefighters must respond to and handle all kinds of emergency situations. There are times when someone is injured and that person needs emergency first aid care on the scene. For this reason, it is important for all firefighters to have a basic knowledge of first aid, cardiopulmonary resuscitation (CPR), and infection and body substance isolation (BSI) techniques.

Safety Lesson

A NIOSH Report

An On-Scene Collapse

On November 2, 2001, a 62-year-old male volunteer firefighter collapsed at the scene of a vehicle fire as he was bringing a tool to the Chief. Despite immediate CPR at the scene and subsequent advanced life support both in the ambulance and at the hospital emergency department, the firefighter died.

Follow-Up

The NIOSH Investigative Report (Report #F2002-24) concluded with several recommendations, including that the fire department "Consider including an automatic external defibrillator as part of the basic life support equipment for fire department vehicles."

You will learn about automatic external defibrillators and CPR in this chapter.

First Aid Training

There are several levels of emergency medical certification that you can obtain, including the classifications **Emergency Medical Responder (EMR)**, Emergency Medical Technician (EMT), Advanced Emergency Medical Technician (AEMT), and Paramedic. In addition, fundamental lifesaving certifications are available in **cardiopulmonary resuscitation (CPR)** and automatic external defibrillator (AED) training. To what level you can expect to be trained during the next few years usually depends upon the level of emergency medical care your department provides. Because this text and the accompanying DVD provide training for the External Operations

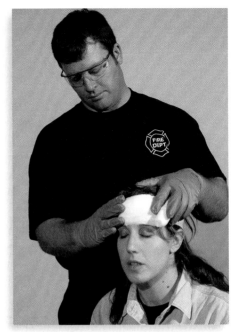

FIGURE 2-1 First aid is the care given to a patient prior to the arrival of higher trained and equipped prehospital emergency medical providers.

level of firefighting, we will concentrate on first aid, CPR, and the use of AEDs.

First aid is the care that a person, while acting alone or as part of a team, can reasonably give prior to the arrival of higher trained and equipped prehospital emergency medical providers (Figure 2-1). Assisting a person who is not breathing, controlling bleeding, providing initial treatment for burns, and assisting a person who is in shock are the fundamentals of first aid.

Knowing first aid is important in everyday life. Most people do not think about providing initial treatment until an injury occurs. With a little training, more lives can be saved. It is important that the actions we take fall within the standard of care that is associated with our level of training.

KEY WORDS

Emergency Medical Responder (EMR) A designation for an emergency professional trained in very basic first aid and rescue skills.

cardiopulmonary resuscitation (CPR) The process of providing breathing and blood circulation to someone who has stopped breathing and whose heart is not beating effectively.

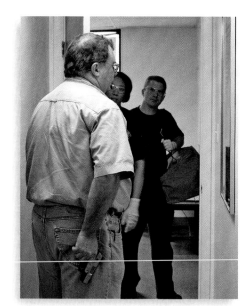

FIGURE 2-2 In order to protect yourself, be sure look for any hazardous conditions that may be present at the scene. You do not want to become a patient yourself.

Initial Approach

In providing first aid, your first responsibility is to yourself. Never rush in blindly to render aid without first assessing the scene (Figure 2-2). To be effective in your first aid efforts, you must first be aware of what caused the problem so that you can maintain a safe attitude in everything you do—otherwise, you can fall victim to the same fate. A good example is when a person is electrocuted. Although the victim may be severely burned and possibly not breathing, it is vital to your own safety that you take the first step of ensuring that the victim and his or her immediate area are not energized with electrical power before you begin to render aid. This may involve waiting for the power company to arrive to control the power. The same rules apply when any other danger is present.

Automobile crashes are particularly dangerous after the fact, due to traffic hazards. Therefore, your first step in rendering first aid at the scene of a traffic accident must be to make yourself visible by donning a reflective vest and controlling the traffic before you begin patient care. It is essential to the victim that you survive so you can render first aid—so, yes, ensuring your personal safety is the first step to rendering care.

It is always preferable that you make the scene safe when practical rather than move an injured pa-tient to a safer location. Moving a traumatized victim can cause further harm. However, there are times when moving the patient to a safe location is the only practical action to take—for example, when the patient is in danger of smoke inhalation or burns from an uncontrolled fire, or the patient is in water and is in danger of drowning. If you must move a trauma patient to a safer location, try your best to move the patient's spine as little as possible, keeping his head and neck in line with his body and in a neutral position as you go.

Gain Consent

When people are injured, those around them often panic. Being trained in first aid and providing a calm, reassuring presence goes a long way toward calming all those involved. Unfortunately, there will be times when not everyone who needs your help will want it. This is often the case when someone is injured during a violent act or while under the influence of alcohol or illicit drugs. Law enforcement personnel should stabilize any potentially violent scene before you approach the area. Even when there is no act of violence or personal hazard present, some people simply do not want to be helped. Your next step is to establish a "connection" with the patient and gain her **consent** for the treatment you are about to render. Just speaking in a calm, respectful tone is usually all it takes. Introduce yourself to the patient and ask her name. Explain what you are about to do and ask the person if it is all right with her to do it.

In most cases, you should take the time to seek the patient's permission before you touch the patient. If the person is a minor and his or her parent or guardian is not present to give their consent, then it is implied that you have permission to treat the child. If the patient is unconscious, heavily intoxicated, or otherwise unable to make an informed decision, then he is unable to give his informed consent for treatment. In this case, it is implied that you have permission to help the patient. However, if the person is conscious and unruly, you should try to keep the patient calm to prevent him from doing more harm. In this case, you should wait for law enforcement and/or more highly trained medical providers to arrive to assist you, except in the following situations: (1) when the injury is life-threatening, or (2) if more harm will come by delaying treatment for the time it would take for other emergency care providers to arrive.

Do No Harm

Having consent to treat a person does not allow you to do more than a careful person with your level of training should do at a given emergency. You should have a good reason for every action you take, and you can take those actions as long as they do no harm. For example, you are about to receive training about how to use direct pressure with a pressure dressing to control bleeding from an arm laceration. You should not take this process a step further by improvising a tourniquet, which could potentially starve the limb of oxygen and blood, causing the patient to ultimately lose the arm. Stay within the limits of your training.

Call for Additional Help

The second action you should take on nearly all emergencies is the following: *Call for additional help!* At this point in your training, any wound that requires more than a Bandaid® to control the bleeding should be assessed by someone with more medical training than you. After you are sure of your personal safety, activate EMS by calling for help. When you reach a dispatcher, be prepared to stay on the line for further instructions. Even though you will have some initial first aid training by the end of this chapter, many dispatch centers have certified Emergency Medical Dispatchers on duty who can give you more in-depth instructions for the situation.

Once you have begun treatment, it is your responsibility to stay with the patient until you are relieved by another medical provider with an equal or higher level of training. To do otherwise could be interpreted as **abandonment**, for which you can be held liable unless leaving the patient is the only way you can activate EMS.

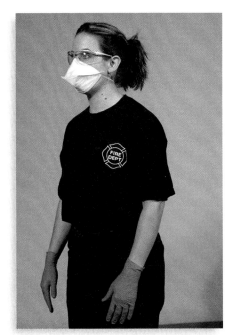

FIGURE 2-3 Practicing basic body substance isolation is not only required of emergency responders, it is also plain common sense.

Infection Control and Body Substance Isolation

Before we discuss bleeding control and CPR, we should spend a little more time on your personal safety and health (Figure 2-3). Since the 1980s, the fire and rescue community has been aware of the spread of AIDS (acquired immune deficiency syndrome) and HIV (human immunodeficiency virus) in the general population. There is probably a greater threat of infection by tuberculosis, hepatitis, and many other diseases. For example, **hepatitis C** can live within a dried clot of blood for as long as seven days. In addition, **tuberculosis** can be transmitted with a simple cough. These biological threats have resulted in regulations requiring proper awareness, isolation control, and protective measures. For this reason, all emergency responders are required to have training in **body substance isolation (BSI)** practices.

The most effective, and therefore the most important, step you can take to protect yourself from communicable disease is proper **handwashing**; this step also helps to prevent spreading germs. Washing your hands before and after contact with any patient, even if you are wearing gloves, and frequent handwashing throughout the day are vital habits to have. Properly washing your hands involves removing all jewelry, vigorously rubbing your hands together under warm water with soap, and taking care to wash the palms and backs of your hands, between your fingers, and your wrists. After washing, rinse your hands with your fingers pointing downward so that the germs flow off and away with the soap. Take care to avoid touching any part of the sink area with your clean hands, using a paper towel to turn off the faucet if necessary.

View It!

Go to the DVD, navigate to Chapter 2, and select *Handwashing.*

Practice It!

Proper Handwashing

Take a few minutes to practice the steps for properly washing your hands:

1. Remove all your jewelry (Figure 2-4).

FIGURE 2-4

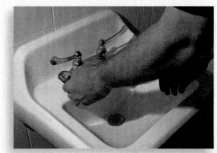

2. Wash your palms, the backs of your hands, between your fingers, and your wrists with warm water and soap for at least a minute. Rub them vigorously (Figure 2-5).

FIGURE 2-5

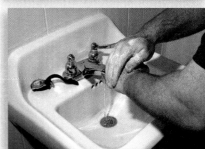

3. Dry your hands and use a paper towel to shut off the faucet, taking care not to touch any part of the sink with your bare hands (Figure 2-6).

FIGURE 2-6

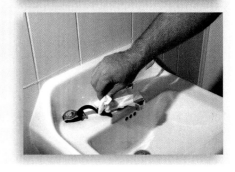

Infection Control Programs

When you respond as a firefighter, even if you are not trained as an emergency medical provider, you will eventually encounter the body fluids and airborne pathogens that contribute to the spread of infectious disease. You should be aware of the threats these diseases pose to you, how to protect yourself from them by using proper isolation protection, and how to effectively clean clothing that may have been in contact with body substances.

Your department should have an ongoing infection control program to address these issues. Requirements for an infection control program are defined in NFPA 1500, the Standard on Occupational Safety and Health, and are required by the Code of Federal Regulations (29 CFR 1910.1030). These requirements cover the following topics:

- Utilization of personal protective equipment
- Procedures and guidelines for infection control on the job
- Proper methods for disposing of contaminated items and medical waste materials
- How to clean and decontaminate exposures to yourself as well as to your equipment and clothing
- What to do if you have been exposed to infectious agents
- Medical considerations
- Immunization requirements

An awareness program addresses the many diseases, apart from the ones already mentioned, that can be spread by and contracted from contaminated biological exposure. It provides instruction in how to use universal precautions and the decontamination facilities in the fire station, as well as the proper notification practices to document your exposure.

Body Substance Isolation

Several types of contaminated materials provide avenues of disease exposure, including:

- Blood
- Airborne secretions (cough and sneeze)
- Body substances
- Human feces
- Body fluids
- Food
- Direct contact
- Used needles

Personal protective equipment (PPE) for infectious disease isolation includes items found in a

TABLE 2-1 Contents of a Typical Body Substance Isolation (BSI) Kit

- Splash-resistant eyewear
- Face protection devices
- Fluid-resistant garments
- Patient isolation garments, bags
- Sleeve protectors, shoe covers
- Emergency medical gloves
- Sharps container
- Contaminated wastes container

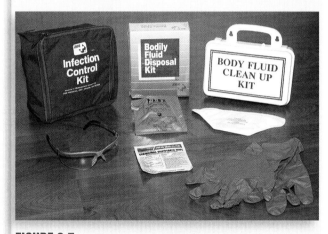

FIGURE 2-7

typical body substance isolation kit (Table 2-1 and Figure 2-7).

KEY WORD

personal protective equipment (PPE), medical Specially designed clothing and protective equipment that provides overall body protection. It includes head, eye, hand, foot, and respiratory protection. PPE is approved for the hazard that a firefighter or rescuer can expect to encounter in a particular working environment.

Universal Precautions

When you are dealing with or are exposed to body substances, it may be difficult to determine which material can be a potential risk to you. For this reason, we take **universal precautions** when potentially exposed to body substances. These precautions include wearing eye protection (splash-resistant eyewear), hand protection, (approved, nonlatex, disposable

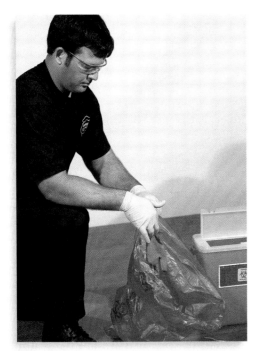

FIGURE 2-8 Always place disposable medical garments and gloves as well as any medical and biological waste in an approved biological waste container.

medical gloves), and other body protection (such as a splash-resistant gown) as needed.

After dealing with an emergency involving a potential infectious exposure, it is very important to properly dispose of protective gloves and garments. These items, along with any disposable medical waste (such as used dressings and bandages), should be placed in approved biological waste containers and bags for proper disposal. The containers are marked with a biological waste emblem. The waste bags are red with a **biological waste emblem** (Figure 2-8).

Nondisposable items should be properly cleaned and disinfected at a cleaning and disinfecting wash area approved by the fire station. This area has approved cleaning gloves, detergent disinfecting soap, and an antiviral solution. All items must be thoroughly washed and dried before placing them back into service.

When clothes and fire gear are exposed to blood-borne pathogens, they should be washed as soon as possible. This should be done by the fire department.

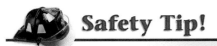 **Safety Tip!**

It is not recommended that firefighters take their exposed clothing and gear home to wash it in their home washing machines because home washing machines do not reach the high temperature necessary to do the job.

If you believe you have been directly exposed to an infectious disease, your department has a procedure to report and document the exposure. This procedure includes the proper way to document the exposure, who to direct your report to, and additional actions to be taken.

There are also several immunizations that can be taken to help reduce risks of infectious disease. Check the immunization requirements of your department. You may have already been immunized as part of your qualification for recruitment by the department.

■ KEY WORD ■

universal precautions Infection control practices, such as using eye and face protection, disposable gloves, and disposable outer garments, that can protect individuals from diseases that may be transmitted through blood and other body fluids.

The ABCs of First Aid

Life-threatening injuries or conditions almost always involve a person's airway, breathing, and/or blood circulation. We refer to this as the ABCs of emergency care: **A**irway, **B**reathing, and **C**irculation. Assessing a patient's ABCs allows you to know if there is an immediate danger to life. If the patient is talking, then you can properly assume that the patient has an open airway and is breathing and his blood is circulating. If you see obvious bleeding, then the patient's circulation will eventually become compromised, so that would be your first priority of care.

Airway Management Techniques

If you approach a patient who is sitting upright, is unable to speak, and is obviously not breathing, then you could surmise that the patient is probably not able to breathe because his airway is obstructed—possibly by a foreign body, which is often the case with a patient who is choking. In this case, your obvious priority is to open the patient's airway by using **abdominal thrusts.**

■ KEY WORD ■

abdominal thrusts An emergency maneuver used to clear an obstructed airway.

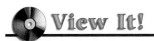
View It!

Go to the DVD, navigate to Chapter 2, and select *Abdominal Thrusts.*

Practice It!

Abdominal Thrusts

Use the following steps when performing abdominal thrusts:

1. Take proper BSI precautions and activate EMS.
2. Determine if the patient is choking and, if possible, obtain consent to treat him or her (Figure 2-9).

FIGURE 2-9

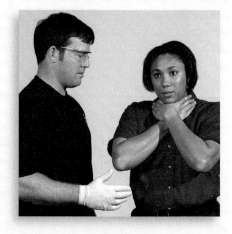

3. Stand behind the patient, wrapping your arms around the patient's waist while making a fist with one hand (Figure 2-10).

FIGURE 2-10

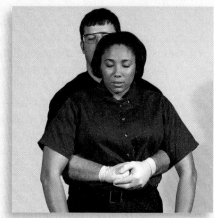

4. Grasp your fist with your other hand and place it into the patient's abdomen above the navel while avoiding the bottom of the patient's breastbone (Figure 2-11).

FIGURE 2-11

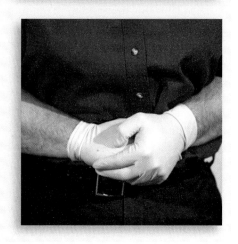

5. Thrust your fist inward and upward quickly and as many times as needed to expel the foreign body from the patient's airway (Figure 2-12).

FIGURE 2-12

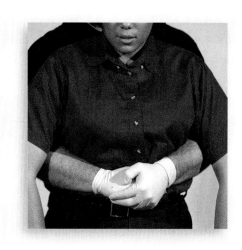

Upper Airway Management

Probably the object that most commonly occludes an unconscious person's airway is the tongue. When a person becomes unconscious, the muscles relax and the tongue can fall backward into the throat, occluding the airway (Figure 2-13).

If the patient is unconscious, check for the presence of spontaneous breathing by watching the patient's chest for movement and by listening closely for sounds of air passing through his nose and mouth. If the patient is not breathing, reposition his airway using either a head tilt–chin lift or a jaw-thrust maneuver. The head tilt–chin lift maneuver is very simple to accomplish; however, it involves manipulating the patient's head and neck a bit (Figure 2-14). Therefore, this maneuver is not recommended if the patient has been injured. It should also not be used if the patient has fallen in such a way as to potentially cause a neck injury or if there is trauma to the oral area. In these cases, a jaw-thrust maneuver should be used.

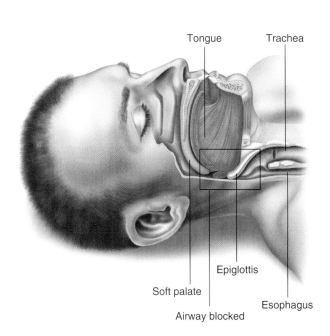

FIGURE 2-13 Airway blocked by tongue.

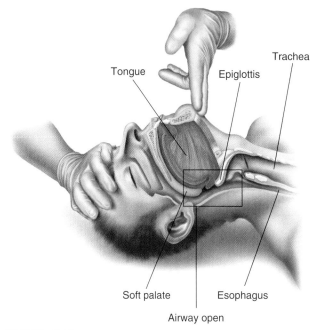

FIGURE 2-14 Head tilt-chin lift maneuver opens the patient's airway.

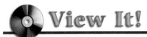 **View It!**

Go to the DVD, navigate to Chapter 2, and select *Head Tilt–Chin Lift Maneuver.*

 Practice It!

Head Tilt–Chin Lift Maneuver

Use the following steps when performing the head tilt–chin lift maneuver:

1. Take proper BSI precautions and activate EMS (Figure 2-15).

FIGURE 2-15

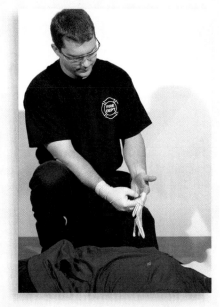

2. Place the patient on his back and kneel beside his head (Figure 2-16).

FIGURE 2-16

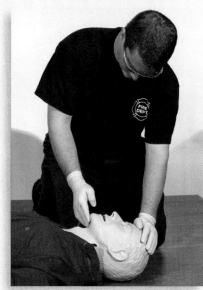

3. Place one hand on the patient's forehead and the other below the patient's chin. Now gently lift the chin and tilt the patient's head back (Figure 2-17).

FIGURE 2-17

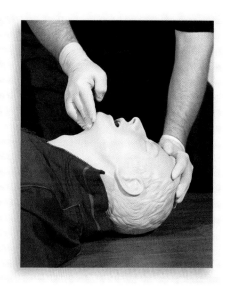

 View It!

Go to the DVD, navigate to Chapter 2, and select *Jaw-Thrust Maneuver.*

 Practice It!

Jaw-Thrust Maneuver

Use the following steps when performing the jaw-thrust maneuver:

1. Take proper BSI precautions and activate EMS (Figure 2-18).

FIGURE 2-18

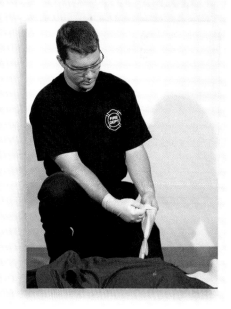

—Continued

2. Place the patient on his back and kneel above the patient's head (Figure 2-19).

FIGURE 2-19

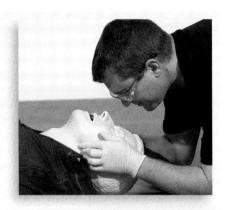

3. Place a hand on either side of the patient's head, with your thumb resting on the patient's cheekbones and your fingers underneath the patient's lower jaw. Your fourth and little finger of each hand should be behind the angled part of the patient's lower jaw, with the rest of your hand above the angle of the jaw (Figure 2-20).

FIGURE 2-20

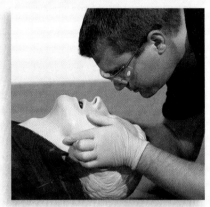

4. Thrust the patient's lower jaw forward with your fingers while using your thumbs for leverage (Figure 2-21).

FIGURE 2-21

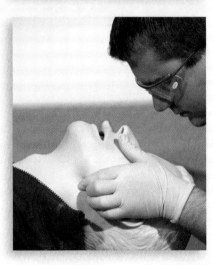

Once you have ensured that the patient's airway is open, you should check to see if he has started breathing on his own. Then assess the patient's pulse. If the patient is breathing and has a pulse, and he is not a victim of a traumatic injury, place him on his left side so that secretions can drain naturally from his mouth, thus helping to avoid further choking. This position is called the **recovery position.**

KEY WORD

recovery position Positioning a patient on his left side so that secretions can drain naturally from his mouth, thus helping to avoid further choking.

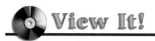
Go to the DVD, navigate to Chapter 2, and select *Pulse Check.*

Practice It!

Pulse Check

Use the following steps when performing a pulse check:

1. Place two fingers on the patient's "Adam's apple" and slide them downward to find your landmark. Do not use your thumb (Figure 2-22).

FIGURE 2-22

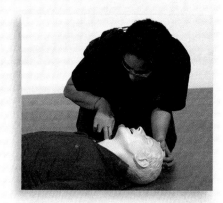

2. Apply gentle pressure until you feel the patient's pulse (Figure 2-23). Do not press too hard as this can occlude the pulse.

FIGURE 2-23

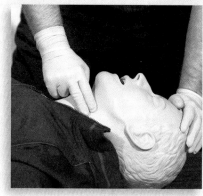

CPR

Cardiopulmonary resuscitation (CPR) is the foundation of emergency lifesaving skills. Virtually everyone should have some sort of CPR training. Opening the patient's airway (**A**irway), providing rescue breathing (**B**reathing), and applying chest compressions to force the patient's blood to circulate (**C**irculate) are vital for a cardiac arrest victim's chance of survival. CPR is a skill that requires certification, and the guidelines for CPR are updated frequently; therefore, detailed CPR guidelines are not provided in this text.

Airway

The fundamentals of providing adult CPR include the following: opening the airway, activating EMS, assessing for breathing, providing rescue breaths, checking a pulse, and providing chest compressions. We have already discussed the first steps: checking the patient's airway, assessing for breathing, and taking a pulse. Next we will practice the sequence by adding rescue breathing and chest compressions to the cycle. If your fire department does not provide CPR certification classes, you can contact the

American Heart Association or the American Red Cross for information on where you can obtain this certification.

■ KEY WORDS ■

American Heart Association An organization that provides certification and training for heart-related prehospital care such as CPR.

American Red Cross An organization that develops and provides certification of various levels of first aid training and CPR.

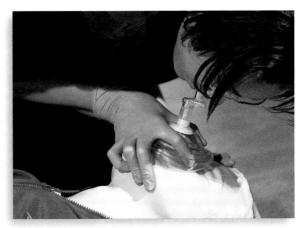

FIGURE 2-24 Pocket masks allow you to use the air in your own lungs to perform rescue breathing for the patient while providing protection for you.

Breathing

A pocket mask should be part of your first aid kit. Pocket masks come in two basic styles—the full face mask, which is rigid, and the smaller, folding mask that can fit in a small pouch on your keychain. Either type provides a barrier against body fluids, and mouth-to-mask ventilation is a better avenue for providing breaths than mouth-to-mouth breathing. While it isn't absolutely essential that you have a pocket mask for rescue breathing, the risks make it an essential element of a well-stocked BSI kit. If you do supply breaths mouth-to-mouth, you will need to follow appropriate exposure notifications, as previously discussed in this chapter.

When you first encounter an unconscious patient, you should perform three quick steps during the initial moments: (1) assess for scene safety, (2) don your BSI equipment (gloves and protective eyewear), and (3) activate EMS by instructing someone to call 911. The next steps you take involve establishing unresponsiveness in the patient, assessing the patient's need for CPR, and providing the necessary care. Before we put it into a full sequence, let's talk a little about rescue breathing and chest compressions.

Rescue breathing occurs when you literally provide air to the patient by blowing into the patient's mouth to fill the lungs. Equipped EMRs, EMTs, AEMTs, and Paramedics have very specific tools to do just this. However, if you are alone when you encounter the patient, you will only have a pocket mask,

so you will have to rely on the air in your lungs to provide the rescue breaths. Seal the patient's nose and mouth with the pocket mask (Figure 2-24). If you are using the folding type, pinch off the patient's nose as you open the airway with either the head tilt–chin lift or jaw-thrust method. Seal the mask's breathing tube with your mouth and deliver slow, purposeful breaths, watching for the patient's chest to rise. If it doesn't rise, reposition the patient's airway and try again.

Circulation

Chest compressions circulate the blood when you push down on the patient's breastbone (called the *sternum*), thus compressing the heart and lungs. The key to proper chest compressions is proper hand placement on the patient's chest. Place the heel of one hand squarely on the center of the patient's breastbone, about an inch or so above the bottom of the sternum. The object is to avoid pressing down on the lower tip of the breastbone as this can injure the patient and will also diminish the effectiveness of your compressions. Each compression should be 1½ to 2 inches deep on an average-size adult. Compressions should occur at a rate of approximately 100 per minute, stopping every 30 compressions to deliver 2 rescue breaths.

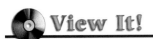 **View It!**

Go to the DVD, navigate to Chapter 2, and select *CPR Fundamentals*.

Practice It!

CPR Fundamentals

The following steps should be used when performing the fundamentals of CPR:

1. Assess the scene, take proper BSI precautions, and activate EMS (Figure 2-25).

FIGURE 2-25

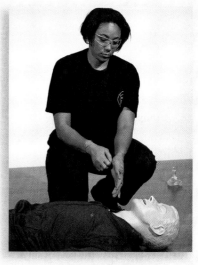

2. Open the airway (Figure 2-26).

FIGURE 2-26

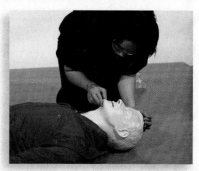

3. Assess breathing—look, listen, and feel (Figure 2-27).

FIGURE 2-27

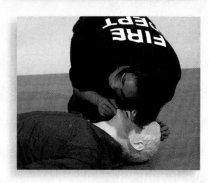

4. If the patient is breathing, place him in the recovery position (Figure 2-28).

FIGURE 2-28

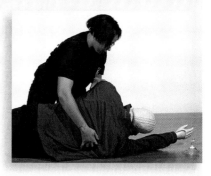

—Continued

5. If the patient is not breathing, give 2 rescue breaths at 1 second per breath (Figure 2-29).

FIGURE 2-29

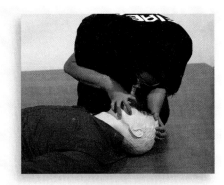

6. Assess for a pulse, taking no more than 10 seconds (Figure 2-30).

FIGURE 2-30

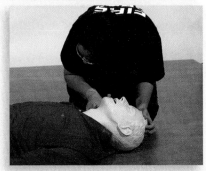

7. If there is no pulse, give 30 chest compressions (Figure 2-31).

FIGURE 2-31

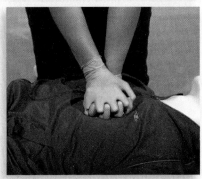

8. Open the patient's airway and give 2 rescue breaths (Figure 2-32). Repeat this cycle of breaths and compressions.

FIGURE 2-32

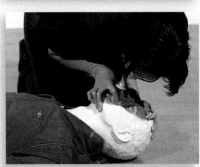

9. Assess for a pulse and breathing (Figure 2-33). Repeat the cycles until you are relieved by another rescuer, or an AED or EMS arrives.

FIGURE 2-33

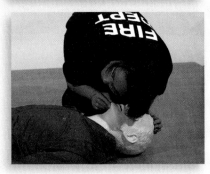

10. If the patient recovers, place him in the recovery position (Figure 2-34).

FIGURE 2-34

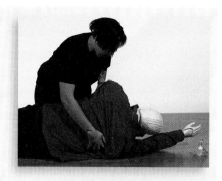

11. If the patient's circulation is present but the patient is not breathing, continue rescue breathing, delivering 1 breath every 5 to 6 seconds, and reassess the circulation every 2 minutes (Figure 2-35).

FIGURE 2-35

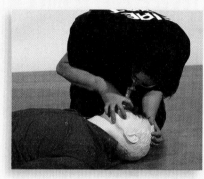

Automatic External Defibrillators (AEDs)

In addition to CPR, early defibrillation is recommended as a vital part of the initial treatment for a person in cardiac arrest. **Automatic external defibrillators (AEDs)** are becoming commonplace in government buildings, in shopping malls, and on passenger aircraft, and they are carried by many Emergency Medical Responders. AEDs are easy to learn and simple to use. They should be a part of your CPR certification training (Figure 2-36).

Automatic external defibrillators are just that—automatic. They are designed to give verbal instructions about their use, assess the patient's electrical heart activity, and automatically deliver a cardiac shock (defibrillation) only when necessary. An AED will not deliver a shock to someone who shouldn't be shocked. Early defibrillation is now viewed as being just as important as early CPR to the patient's chance of survival.

The key to using an AED is to properly place the sticky pads on the patient's chest and then ensure that no one is touching the patient when you have the machine assess the patient and deliver the shock. When you apply the pads, align them as indicated in the drawings on the pad's wrapper. Take the time to press them firmly against the patient's skin, making sure that the gel inside the pad makes good contact with the skin. AEDs that you will encounter in the field will have printed placement directions somewhere on the inside cover and will also provide additional verbal instructions with use.

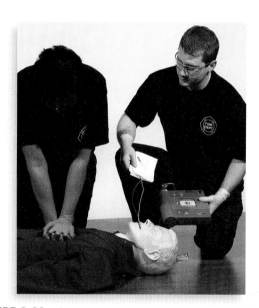

FIGURE 2-36 Automatic external defibrillators (AEDs) are becoming more common in public buildings. Your CPR training should include AED application.

KEY WORD

automatic external defibrillators (AEDs) Devices that are located in many types of public access areas and provide defibrillation (cardiac shock) in case of sudden heart attack with a loss of breathing and pulse.

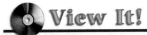

Go to the DVD, navigate to Chapter 2, and select *Automatic External Defibrillation.*

Practice It!

Automatic External Defibrillation

The steps below should be used to perform automatic external defibrillations. *Note:* This sequence begins with BSI in place.

1. Continue CPR while you turn on the AED and attach the AED pads (Figure 2-37).

FIGURE 2-37

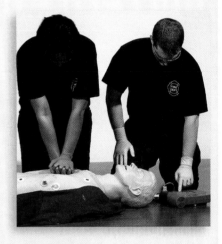

2. Direct the rescuer to stop CPR and ensure that everyone is clear of the patient (Figure 2-38).

FIGURE 2-38

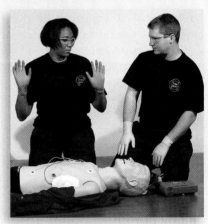

3. Initiate analysis of the patient by pushing the *analyze* button (Figure 2-39). If the AED does not detect a shockable rhythm, resume CPR for 5 cycles and check again. Continue until ALS providers take over or the victim starts to move.

FIGURE 2-39

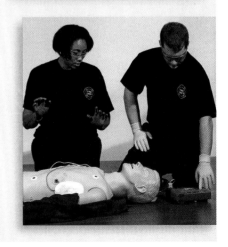

4. Deliver a shock (push the *shock* button) as indicated by the machine (Figure 2-40).

FIGURE 2-40

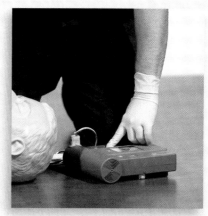

5. Assess for a pulse and direct the resumption of CPR if necessary (Figure 2-41).

FIGURE 2-41

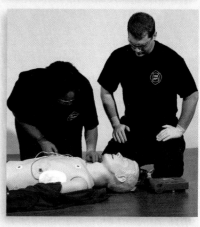

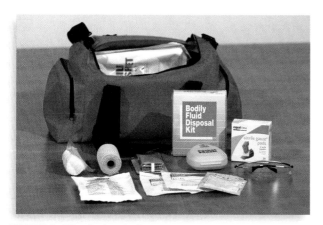

FIGURE 2-42   A simple first aid kit.

First Aid Supplies

An essential part of first aid is having the necessary supplies. A simple first aid kit should contain the following items (Figure 2-42):

- BSI kit
- Reflective traffic safety vest
- Pocket mask
- Sterile dressings
- Conforming gauze
- Adhesive tape
- Flashlight
- Scissors
- Disposable blankets

Controlling Bleeding

A person can tolerate a minimal amount of blood loss without suffering any significant consequences. However, even a small wound can cause a person to lose a dangerous amount of blood, so small wounds should not be taken lightly. Also, remember to take BSI precautions before you encounter any blood.

Most open bleeding can be controlled with direct pressure. A pressure dressing consists of a sterile dressing and a bandage to hold it in place. Take note of the size and depth of the wound before applying bandages so that you can relay this information to the appropriate medical personnel. To control the bleeding, cover the wound with one or several sterile dressings and apply direct pressure with your gloved hand. These steps should slow or stop the bleeding. Leave the pressure dressing in place once the bleeding has been controlled and wrap it with a gauze bandage. It is important that you don't pull the bandage away from the wound because doing so can pull away any clots that may have formed on the wound, starting the bleeding process again.

Once the pressure dressing is applied, if possible, elevate the wound to help slow the bleeding further. If you need more dressings because blood is soaking through them, apply the new dressings on top of the bandage and add another gauze bandage to hold it in place. Even though the bleeding may have been stopped by the pressure dressing, the patient should seek further medical attention.

 View It!

Go to the DVD, navigate to Chapter 2, and select *Applying a Pressure Dressing.*

 Practice It!

Applying a Pressure Dressing

Use the following steps when applying a pressure dressing:

1. Take BSI precautions and activate EMS (Figure 2-43).

FIGURE 2-43

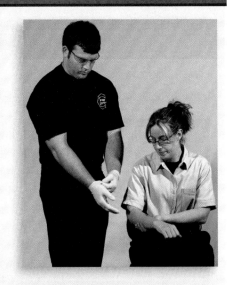

2. Inspect the wound for any loose debris and remove any debris from the surface of the skin (Figure 2-44).

FIGURE 2-44

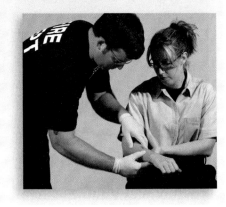

3. Cover the wound with a dry, sterile dressing and apply direct pressure with your hand (Figure 2-45).

FIGURE 2-45

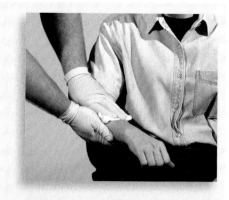

4. Once the bleeding has slowed, wrap the dressing with a stretch gauze bandage (Figure 2-46).

FIGURE 2-46

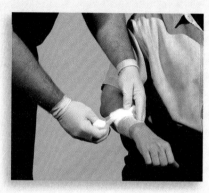

 View It!

Go to the DVD, navigate to Chapter 2, and select *Bandaging an Impaled Object*.

 Practice It!

Bandaging an Impaled Object

Use the following steps when bandaging an impaled object:

1. You may encounter a patient who has an object impaled through his skin (Figure 2-47). This object may be as simple as a nail or as complex as a piece of steel passing through the length of his body. In any case, *DO NOT REMOVE THE IMPALED OBJECT.*

FIGURE 2-47

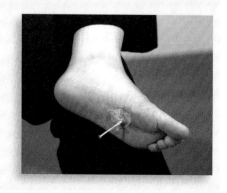

—*Continued*

2. Take BSI precautions and activate EMS (Figure 2-48).

FIGURE 2-48

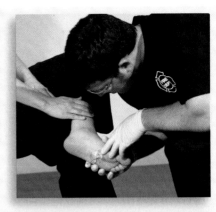

3. Take manual control of the impaled object (Figure 2-49). Inspect the wound for any loose debris and remove any debris from the surface of the skin. *DO NOT REMOVE THE IMPALED OBJECT.*

FIGURE 2-49

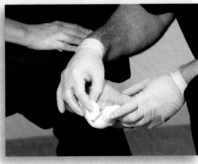

4. Place sterile dressings around the object and wrap a stretch gauze bandage around the object in a crisscross manner (Figure 2-50). You should secure the foreign object in place while applying pressure to the wound.

FIGURE 2-50

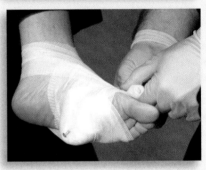

Bruises

Not all bleeding is external. Blunt trauma usually leaves a bruise, as do broken bones and sprains. The treatment for a simple bruise is the application of a cold compress. Chemical cold packs are the most common tool for treating bruises; however, something as simple as a bag of frozen vegetables from the kitchen will work well. Avoid placing the cold compress directly on the skin. A washcloth or sterile gauze dressing provides enough insulation to allow the cold to penetrate while preventing skin irritation from direct skin contact with extreme cold.

Shock Management

Shock occurs when the patient's circulation is compromised. It can be due to a heart condition, blood loss, internal bleeding, a head injury, or other medical causes. Shock requires advanced medical intervention. However, you can take some steps to help the patient between the time that you activate EMS and the arrival of advanced medical care.

You need to recognize the signs of shock. Some of the signs of shock include

- Pale, cool, clammy skin
- A rapid, weak pulse
- A hollow or sunken appearance to the eyes
- Shallow breathing
- Nausea, vomiting
- Dizziness and/or a diminished level of consciousness
- Unexplained or excessive thirst

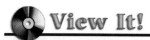

Go to the DVD, navigate to Chapter 2, and select *Shock Position.*

⇨ Practice It!

The Shock Position

Use the following steps to place patients in the shock position:

1. The best position for most shock victims is on their back. If the cause of a patient's injury could include a possible injury to the neck, it is important that you keep the patient's head and neck in position.

2. Ensure the ABCs and elevate the patient's feet about a foot off the ground if possible (Figure 2-51). Obviously, if the patient has a hip or lower leg injury, you should not elevate the patient's feet.

FIGURE 2-51

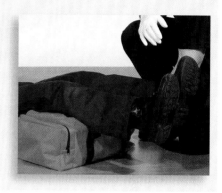

 View It!

Go to the DVD, navigate to Chapter 2, and select *Recovery Position.*

⇨ Practice It!

The Recovery Position

If the patient is vomiting or is about to vomit, the best position is on her side so that no vomit falls back into the airway, causing her to choke. Use the following steps to place patients in the recovery position:

1. Place the patient on her left side if possible to help prevent vomiting. This is called the recovery position (Figure 2-52).

FIGURE 2-52

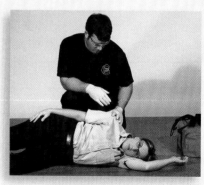

2. Maintain the patient's body temperature as much as possible until help arrives (Figure 2-53). Do not give the patient anything to eat or drink.

FIGURE 2-53

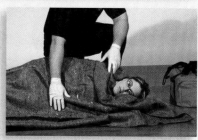

Burns

When you are on an emergency scene in which someone has a burn injury, you will hear various terminology. This terminology relates to the cause or type of burn, the extent or size of the burn area, and the severity of the burn damage to the skin.

Types of Burns

People can be burned in many different ways (Figure 2-54). They can be exposed to open flame, hot objects, or radiant heat from the sun or fire. These cause thermal burns. Examples of thermal burns include severe sunburn, burns to extremities from a flash fire, and burns to the hands from touching a hot object like a stovetop burner.

People can also receive burn damage to their respiratory tract from inhaling hot smoke or even chemical fumes. This is a serious condition, and patients with respiratory burns need to be transported rapidly to an emergency medical trauma care facility.

Individuals exposed to acid- or alkaline-based substances can sustain a chemical burn. An example of this type burn is a worker in a chemical processing plant who accidentally gets an acid product on his skin.

People can also receive burn injuries from electrical shock. Examples include an electrical utility company worker who touches a high-voltage electrical line and an individual who is struck by lightning. Smaller-voltage exposures can also cause minor burns to hands and fingers. One problem you may encounter when assessing someone who is burned from electrical shock is the difficulty in determining the extent of the burn. These burns might cause only a small damaged area on the skin but extensive damage to internal tissues and organs.

The Extent and Severity of Burns

The size of the burn is one of the determining factors for the extent of the burn injury. The larger the area of the body and the more skin damaged, the more severe the injury. The severity of burn injuries is also measured by the depth of the damage. Generally speaking, the deeper the burn damage, the higher the degree of injury.

Superficial burns are sunburn-like injuries. The damage is only to top layers of skin and will usually heal after a week (Figure 2-55).

Partial-thickness burns are accompanied by blistering of the burn area. These burns are deeper injuries of the skin and may take a few weeks to heal (Figure 2-56).

Full-thickness burns extend deeply into the skin and create damage to tissues below the skin. These burns require extended care. In many cases, full-thickness burns that cover a large percentage of the body can eventually result in the patient's death (Figure 2-57).

First Aid for Burns

Burn injuries present their own peculiar set of circumstances and treatments. The best first aid treatment is

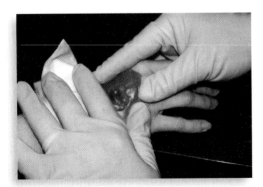

FIGURE 2-54 People can be burned in many different ways, including from thermal, chemical, and electrical sources.

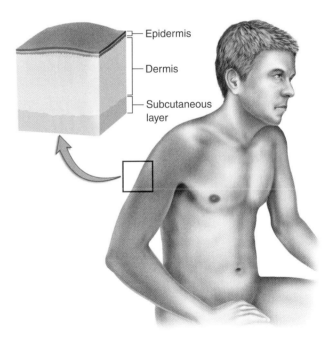

FIGURE 2-55 A superficial burn.

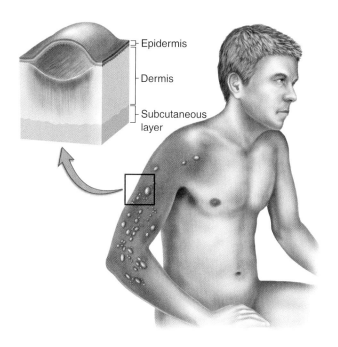

FIGURE 2-56   A partial-thickness burn.

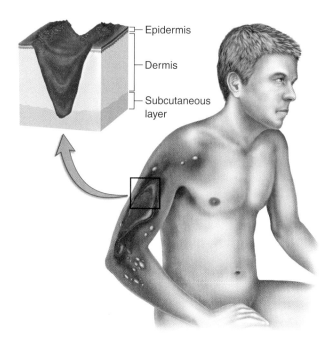

FIGURE 2-57   A full-thickness burn.

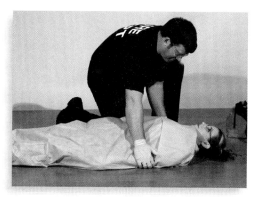

FIGURE 2-58   Burn blankets provide the best patient cover for burn patients.

simply cooling the area with water and covering the burn site with a dry, clean dressing with little or no bandaging. You should also keep the patient warm with a light, clean blanket (burn blankets provide the best patient cover) (Figure 2-58).

Care should be taken not to break any blisters. Also, never apply ointments or fluids except water to a burn injury.

Burn patients should be treated for shock and transported to an emergency trauma care facility.

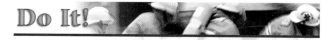

Advancing Your First Aid Skills

In this chapter, "Basic First Aid and CPR," you have learned many skills and techniques for rendering effective first aid. In your career as a firefighter, you can participate in much more in-depth training for all of the topics presented here. Providing some level of prehospital care is becoming more common for fire services in the United States, especially as they increase their responsiveness to their communities. We strongly suggest that you continue your education and training in EMS through advanced study.

Knowledge Assessment
Signed Documentation Tear-Out Sheet

Exterior Operations Level Firefighter—Chapter 2

Name: _____

Fill out the ten-question quiz below, the Knowledge Assessment Sheet, by circling the correct answer for each question. When finished, sign it and give to your instructor/Company Officer for his or her signature. Turn in this Knowledge Assessment Sheet to the proper person as part of the documentation that you have completed your training for this chapter.

1. Your first responsibility when approaching an injured person on an emergency scene is
   a. patient safety.
   b. your safety.
   c. controlling any bleeding.
   d. obtaining consent.

2. Which of the following terms applies to an injured minor whose parent or guardian is not present?
   a. *Nonconsenting*
   b. *Ineligible*
   c. *Implied consent*
   d. *Too risky*

3. Wearing splash-resistant eyewear, approved disposable medical gloves, and additional body protection when needed is an example of
   a. universal precautions.
   b. advanced first aid preparation.
   c. hazardous materials protection.
   d. excessive protection.

4. The *C* in the *ABCs of first aid* stands for
   a. cover.
   b. cancer.
   c. circulation.
   d. caution.

5. When performing abdominal thrusts, the breastbone is compressed by the fist.
   a. True
   b. False

6. If a person has fallen off a ladder and is not breathing, which maneuver should be used to open the airway?
   a. Head tilt
   b. Nose thrust
   c. Chin lift
   d. Jaw thrust

7. To control bleeding, place sterile dressings over the wound and
   a. call for help.
   b. apply direct pressure with your hand.
   c. loosely tape them in place.
   d. go for help.

8. Excessive bleeding can cause a person to go into shock.
   a. True
   b. False

9. When positioning a person in shock, if she is about to vomit, the patient should be placed _____.
   a. on her left side
   b. on her back
   c. on her stomach
   d. sitting upright in a chair

10. A burn patient with blistering over the burn site would have which of the following types of burn?
   a. Superficial
   b. Full thickness
   c. Partial thickness
   d. Shallow

Student Signature and Date _____   Instructor/Company Officer Signature and Date _____

Prove It

Skills Assessment
Signed Documentation Tear-Out Sheet
Exterior Operations Level Firefighter—Chapter 2

Name: _____

Fill out the Skills Assessment Sheet below. Have your instructor/Company Officer check off and initial each skill you demonstrate. When finished, sign it and give to your instructor/Company Officer for his or her signature. Turn in this Skills Assessment Sheet to the proper person as part of the documentation that you have completed your training for this chapter.

Skill	Completed	Initials
1. Demonstrate proper adherence to universal precautions, donning body substance isolation protection, and handwashing.	_____	_____
2. Describe the procedure for reporting body substance exposure.	_____	_____
3. Demonstrate abdominal thrusts to a standing patient.	_____	_____
4. Demonstrate the head–lift maneuver.	_____	_____
5. Demonstrate the jaw-thrust maneuver.	_____	_____
6. Demonstrate CPR.	_____	_____
7. Demonstrate AED operation.	_____	_____
8. Demonstrate how to control bleeding with a pressure dressing.	_____	_____
9. Demonstrate how to hold a dressing in place when applying a bandage to the arms and legs.	_____	_____
10. Demonstrate how to dress and bandage a head laceration.	_____	_____
11. Demonstrate how to dress and bandage a neck laceration.	_____	_____
12. Demonstrate how to apply a dressing and bandage to a wound involving an impaled object.	_____	_____
13. Demonstrate how to move a person with a leg wound into the shock position.	_____	_____
14. Demonstrate how to treat a burn injury to an extremity.	_____	_____

Student Signature and Date _____   Instructor/Company Officer Signature and Date _____

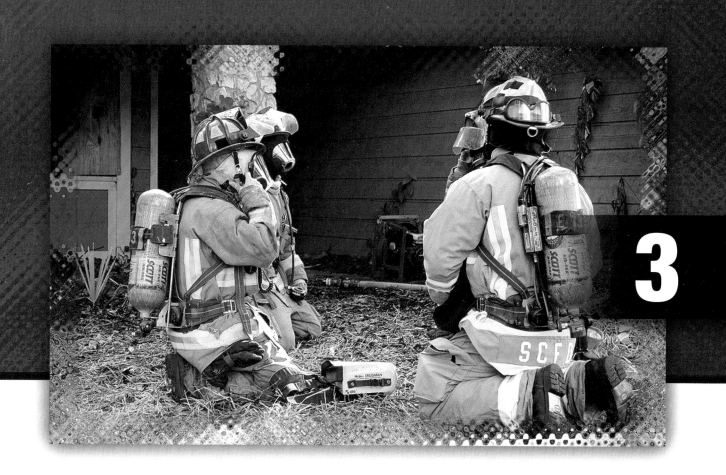

Protective Equipment

What You Will Learn in This Chapter

In this chapter you will learn how to use and care for the most important gear you will use—your personal protective equipment. This equipment includes protective clothing, a self-contained breathing apparatus, and a personal alert device that electronically signals to others that you are in trouble. You will also learn more about an important safety component of incident management that was introduced in Chapter 1: the personnel accountability system.

What You Will Be Able to Do

After reading this chapter and practicing the skills in a classroom setting, you will be able to

1. Describe the components of personal protective clothing used for structural firefighting.
2. Describe the components of an entire personal protective equipment ensemble used for structural firefighting.
3. Properly don and wear all of your personal protective clothing.
4. Describe the procedures for the care and cleaning of your personal protective clothing.
5. Describe the components of a self-contained breathing apparatus (SCBA).
6. Demonstrate the proper way to check and assemble an SCBA.
7. Properly don an SCBA from the seat-rack position.
8. Properly don an SCBA from the ground using the coat method.
9. Properly don an SCBA from the ground using the over-the-head method.
10. Properly check and employ a personal alert safety system (PASS) in both automatic mode and manual mode.
11. Report to your immediate supervisor or the Personnel Accountability Officer when responding to an emergency.

Reality!

Safety Lesson: A NIOSH Report

Personal Protective Clothing Is Essential!

On August 8, 1999, three volunteer firefighters were burned, one critically, while trying to control a fire involving a recreational vehicle (RV) that was parked next to a single-family dwelling. Two volunteer fire departments responded with two engines and a total of five personnel. Engine 1 arrived first, with a driver/operator and no other firefighters on board. The driver/operator deployed a booster line to protect the exposed side of the house and then turned his stream to the burning RV in an attempt to control the fire. Engine 2 arrived with three personnel, and a fourth volunteer arrived in his personal vehicle.

As the firefighters of Engine 2 were pulling hose from their truck, the RV's 50-gallon gasoline tank ruptured and its burning fuel spilled down the inclined driveway toward the firefighters of Engine 2. The intense fire lasted only about 15 seconds; however, it engulfed the firefighters as it ran down the sloped driveway toward them. Although at least two of the firefighters had placed their protective clothing in the truck prior to their response, none of the firefighters on the scene were wearing their personal protective clothing or breathing apparatus during the incident. Of the three who were burned, the critically injured firefighter died 8 days later from the full-thickness burns he received over 96% of his body—he had been totally engulfed in fire. The driver/operator of Engine 2 saw the flames coming toward the engine and was forced to flee. He received partial-thickness burns on his back. The other firefighter from Engine 2 received partial-thickness burns to his arms and legs as he attempted to outrun the flames.

Follow-Up

NIOSH Report #F99-34

Among other recommendations, the NIOSH investigative report concluded the following:

- Fire departments should develop and implement standard operating procedures (SOPs) that
  - Consider the available firefighting equipment, staffing, and resources within a community;
  - Outline how an incident management system will be best implemented within the specific community, given the anticipated staffing and equipment response levels;
  - Outline the proper positioning of fire apparatus on the fire scene; and
  - Outline the proper selection and use of hose line(s) for mounting an attack to control a fire.
- Fire departments should develop and implement a policy requiring the use of personal protective equipment and protective clothing.
- States and municipalities should provide adequate financial support and administrative leadership for fire departments, thus ensuring that adequate training and equipment are provided for firefighters.

Personal Protective Clothing

One of the first signs to a new firefighter recruit that he or she is really getting into the fire service is getting your firefighting gear. Images of firefighters working at a big fire, with all the excitement that goes along with it, are conjured up as each item is fitted and assigned. It is vitally important that you understand how **personal protective clothing (PPC)** protects you, how to use it properly, and the care you will be required to give it. Although at this point in your training you won't be going inside a burning building, the previous case study should impress upon you the importance of wearing your full protective gear at any hazardous incident.

▬ KEY WORD ▬

personal protective clothing (PPC)   Protective clothing worn by firefighters during emergency fire control operations. This ensemble includes protection for the eyes, head, hands, feet, and body.

Types of Protective Clothing

Many types of firefighting protective clothing are available today. Many of these are designed for specific uses. You will probably be issued a standard set of protective clothing for structural firefighting and perhaps another set for wildland firefighting (Figures 3-1 and 3-2). Other specialized sets of gear are required for emergency operations, such as hazardous materials operation (Figure 3-3). In this chapter, we are going to talk about structural firefighting only. You will be trained in the other types of protective clothing as you become qualified by your department to perform other types of emergency operations.

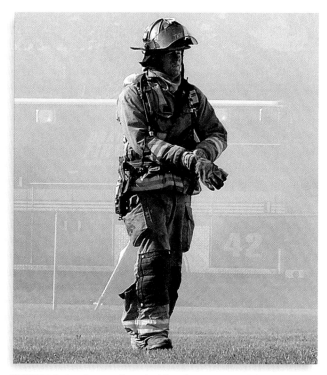

FIGURE 3-1 Protective clothing for structural firefighting.

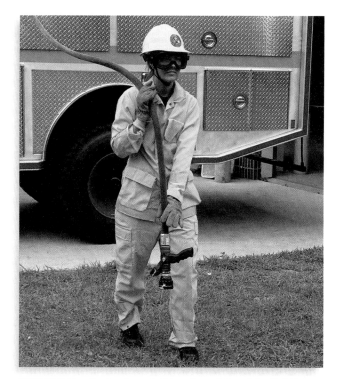

FIGURE 3-2 Protective clothing for wildland firefighting.

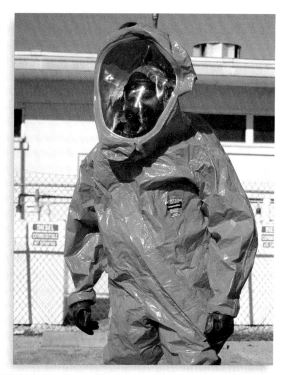

FIGURE 3-3 Protective clothing for a hazardous materials incident.

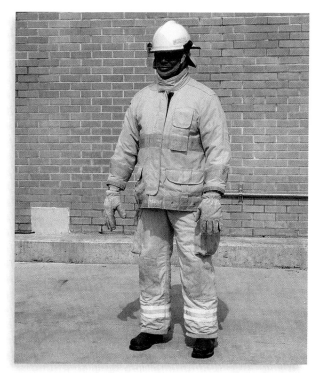

FIGURE 3-4 A firefighter in typical full personal protective clothing (PPC).

Components of Protective Clothing

Your protective clothing is a combination of several items, each of which must be in place with all the others before maximum protection is established (Figure 3-4). For example, if you do not have your gloves on at a fire, you are not fully protected and you are exposing yourself to injury.

The full set of protective clothing includes the following:

- Firefighter coat and pants
- Boots to protect your feet
- Gloves to protect your hands
- A hood to protect your head from heat
- A firefighter helmet for head protection
- A pull-down protective visor and goggles for eye protection

All of this clothing must pass rigorous tests and certifications. The clothing is very expensive, so it is important that you take care of it.

Protective gear must be comfortable to wear and as easy as possible to work in. Try to use care when being fitted for your gear. Properly fitting gear will significantly increase your protection in high-heat situations.

Coat and Pants

A firefighter's coat and pants are made up of three layers of protection. The first layer, the outer shell, is somewhat flame-retardant. It is not, by any means, flameproof. However, in a flash-fire type incident, it may give you a few seconds to get out of the heat and survive. An important component of the outer shell is the reflective trim, which makes you more visible to others when working in dark conditions.

The second and third layers of protection are in the inner liner, which is a combination of a thermal barrier and a moisture barrier (Figure 3-5). These barriers help protect you from excessive heat and water from the outside. They are also designed to allow your body to release some of the heat that builds up from exertion at the fire. For this reason, it is important that

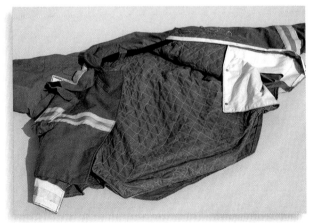

FIGURE 3-5 The inner liner is a combination of a thermal barrier and a moisture barrier that help protect the wearer from excessive heat.

you keep all the components of your coat and pants together; don't remove the liners.

Boots

Your boots are made of either rubber composite materials or leather. Their soles are resistant to puncture. Nails, the sharp edges of steel, and glass can wreak havoc on unprotected shoes and boots. These boots also have steel toes for added foot protection. The boots are heat resistant as well, and they do not let water in.

Gloves

Your gloves are designed to go with the coat. If your coat has built-in wristlets with a thumbhole, then your gloves do not need wristlets built into them (Figure 3-6). If your coat has no wristlets, then you need gloves that have that protection sewn into the glove (Figure 3-7). This type of glove is specially designed to protect against both heat and puncture while pro-

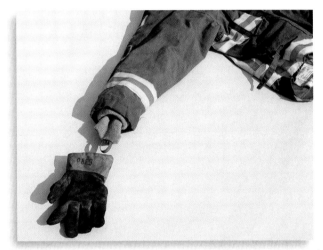

FIGURE 3-6 Gloves and coat with wristlets for structural firefighting.

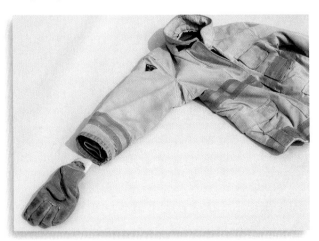

FIGURE 3-7 Gloves and coat without wristlets for structural firefighting.

viding as much dexterity as possible to the hands and fingers.

Hood and Helmet

Your fire hood provides protection to your exposed head and neck (Figure 3-8). It is somewhat flame-resistant.

A firefighter's helmet is uniquely designed. It is impact-resistant to protect the firefighter from falling objects, shield from water, and provide protection from heat. The suspension inside is provided to give you some impact resistance. More importantly, it provides ventilation for heat release from the top of your head. Reflective trim for visibility is a very important part of a firefighter's helmet.

The helmet also features a small, partial hood that is connected to the inner lining of the helmet. It is important that you always pull down this hood when you wear the helmet at a fire emergency to protect your ears and neck.

Your helmet also has a pull-down eye shield. This shield provides superficial eye protection for

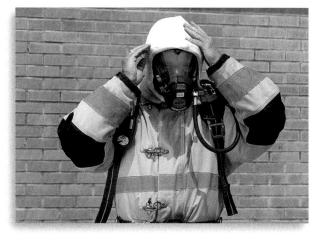

FIGURE 3-8 The firefighter's hood provides protection to the head and neck.

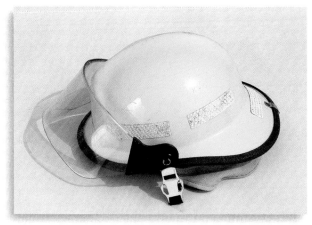

FIGURE 3-9 A typical structural firefighting helmet.

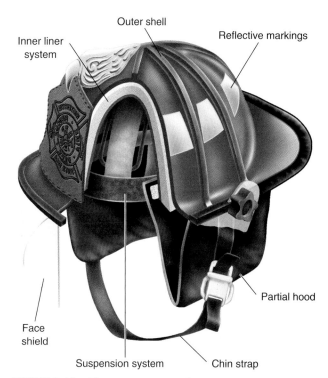

FIGURE 3-10 The components of a structural firefighting helmet.

instances in which you are in a hurry, or you are not wearing goggles or the face piece of your **self-contained breathing apparatus (SCBA).** Your eyes can still be exposed to objects flying up from underneath the pull-down eye shield. **The addition of safety-approved goggles or your SCBA face piece greatly enhances the eye protection you receive from the pull-down eye shield on your helmet (Figure 3-9).**

A helmet has an inner liner, a suspension system, a partial hood, a chin strap, and eye shields. It is important that all of these components are in good working order and are used at all structural fires (Figure 3-10).

▰▰▰ KEY WORD ▰▰▰

self-contained breathing apparatus (SCBA) Personal protective equipment worn by firefighters to provide respiratory protection in an atmosphere that is hazardous to life.

Other Protective Gear

Other protective gear, such as an SCBA and a personal alarm system, are additional devices that allow a firefighter to be completely protected. This additional gear is referred to as complete personal protective equipment and will be discussed in more detail later in this chapter.

Safety Tip!

WARNING: Fires are hot. Temperatures range from 500 to 1500 degrees Fahrenheit. When you start to feel the heat through your protective gear, you should immediately retreat to a cooler area! You are about to get burned! Even in your gear!

Donning Protective Clothing

Personal protective clothing is your lifeline at any emergency. Your fire department and Company Officer have standard guidelines for you to follow that advise you when to don the protective clothing and how much protective clothing will be necessary. At times, full protection is needed; at other times, you can dress down. Your Company Officer, the Incident Commander, or a designee will determine when to remove your gear. *When in doubt, keep your gear on.*

 ## View It!

Go to the DVD, navigate to Chapter 3, and select *Methods of Donning Personal Protective Clothing.*

Practice It!

Methods of Donning Protective Clothing

Most protective clothing for structural firefighting is easy to don and doff (that is, put on and take off). You will quickly become so accustomed to donning and doffing that they will become second nature to you. It is important to develop the correct habits for donning protective clothing so that they become automatic.

1. With the pants folded down around the boots, step into the boots and pull the pants up and into position with the suspenders. Close the front flap and adjust the waist as needed (Figure 3-11).

FIGURE 3-11

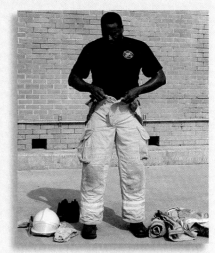

2. Put on the hood, pulling it down around your neck (Figure 3-12).

FIGURE 3-12

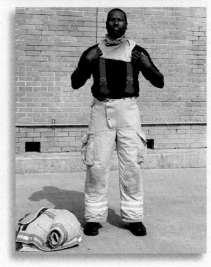

3. Now don the fire coat, fastening the front (Figure 3-13).

FIGURE 3-13

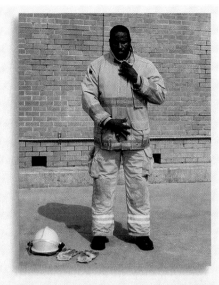

4. Next, pull up the hood so that it covers any exposed skin and place the fire helmet on your head, making sure that the partial hood on the helmet is in position. Attach the chinstrap (Figure 3-14).

FIGURE 3-14

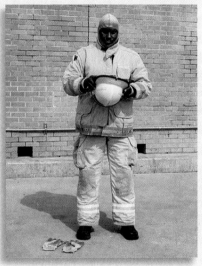

5. Pull down the face shield or put on protective goggles (Figure 3-15).

FIGURE 3-15

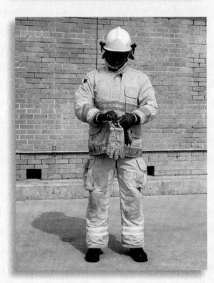

—Continued

6. Pull on the gloves (Figure 3-16).

FIGURE 3-16

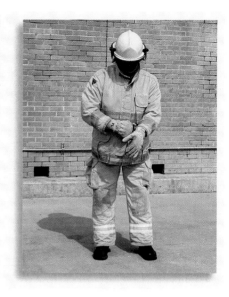

The Care and Maintenance of Protective Clothing

Because your protective clothing is so important to your safety and survival, you must know how to care for and maintain your gear. Your department has specific policies regarding this care and maintenance, but there are a few general rules.

Storing Personal Protective Clothing

Store your gear in a dry place that is easy to access yet protects the gear from the weather. Do not store your gear in the apparatus bay where it can collect diesel particulates.

Cleaning Personal Protective Clothing

Fire Service protective clothing should be cleaned a minimum of every 6 months. It is recommended that this cleaning be done professionally or at least in **professional-grade washers** operated by the fire department. Dirt and products of combustion will start to degrade the fire-resistance capabilities of the materials. It is important to wash this gear after every structural fire. Fire gear contaminated with petroleum products should be removed from service immediately and sent for professional cleaning.

This clothing should never be cleaned using chlorine bleach, which degrades the fire-protective qualities of the clothing materials. To prevent cross-contamination after washing the clothes, be sure to operate the washer several times, empty of clothes, to rinse it clean after washing the fire gear.

If the structural-fire clothing has been contaminated with **body substances,** follow recognized cleaning procedures to decontaminate the clothing. If the clothing is contaminated with biological or chemical contaminants, your department may have to dispose of the gear if it cannot be properly decontaminated.

Inspecting Personal Protective Clothing

Inspect all of your protective clothing, including boots, gloves, and helmet, for cleanliness and damage. Your coat and pants should be intact, with no rips, tears, or raveled threads. Reflective trim is very susceptible to tears, burns, and unraveled seams. Do not simply tear off the damaged portion of trim—the trim is an essential part of your safety. Go through the proper channels within your department to have your gear repaired using an approved repair method.

Boots should be watertight and not leaking water. If they leak, they should be repaired or replaced.

Helmets should have an operating chinstrap, be cleaned of debris, and be checked for scrapes and wear. Exposed fiberglass fibers, or exposed wire supports or unraveled threads on a leather helmet, are indicators that the helmet needs to be replaced. Extreme heat damage is indicated by severe color change or even deformation of the face shield or the helmet itself. In all cases, the helmet should be considered for replacement when any of these changes occur.

All of your safety gear is designed to give you maximum use and protection. Proper care and maintenance will ensure that you receive the most protection from your gear. Always follow the manufacturer's recommendations as well as your fire department's guidelines for caring for your protective fire gear.

Self-Contained Breathing Apparatus (SCBA)

Your personal protective clothing is designed to protect your skin. However, to complete your ensemble of **personal protective equipment (PPE)**, you must also protect your respiratory system. A self-contained breathing apparatus (SCBA) completes your protective gear. While every component of your PPE is essential, the SCBA is probably the most critical component of the ensemble when you are exposed to toxic smoke, hazardous gasses, and steam.

■ KEY WORD ■

personal protective equipment (PPE), *firefighting* The protective equipment firefighters wear when fighting fires, especially in a hazardous atmosphere. This gear includes a complete set of personal protective clothing with the addition of a self-contained breathing apparatus (SCBA) for respiratory protection.

SCBA Systems

An SCBA is the heaviest component of your PPE. The most common type of SCBA used for firefighting is the positive-pressure, open-circuit system. The **open-circuit system** provides clean, dry air from a compressed air cylinder at a pressure that is slightly above that of the surrounding air. The positive pressure of the air inside your mask helps reduce the incidence of toxins entering the facemask area—the pressure is constantly pushing out a small amount of air through any gaps between the mask and your skin, and this prevents toxins from pushing into the mask through those gaps. As you breathe, your exhaled air is exhausted through an exhalation valve on the face piece, which is necessary to prevent you from breathing the carbon dioxide that is present in your exhaled breaths. Because the exhaled air is expelled to the atmosphere and is not contained within

the mask, this type of breathing system is called an *open-circuit* system. The system is "open" because the air in the cylinder is consumed or "used up" as you breathe.

■ KEY WORD ■

open-circuit system A type of SCBA system that provides clean, dry air from a compressed air cylinder, through a regulator, at a pressure slightly above that of the outside atmosphere. Exhaled air is exhausted through a valve on the face piece.

Who Can Wear an SCBA

Before you don and use an SCBA, you need to take some important steps. First, you must be physically capable of bearing the weight of the gear. **You must pass a physical examination by a physician.** Next, you should undergo a "fit test" in which different sizes of air masks are fitted on your face and checked for leaks by a certified SCBA technician or industrial hygienist. It is recommended that your face be clean shaven because excess facial hair can cause leaks. Finally, you must undergo extensive training on the use of your SCBA before you enter any hazardous atmosphere.

SCBA System Components

The components of an SCBA system are featured in Figure 3-17.

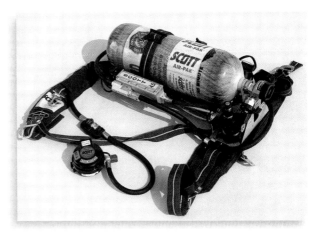

FIGURE 3-17 The components of a self-contained breathing apparatus (SCBA) system.

Cylinders

The air cylinders firefighters use come in different sizes and pressures, depending on the manufacturer and the type of systems purchased by your department. In general, the cylinders are referred to as *30-minute, 45-minute,* and *60-minute* cylinders. Do not let this unofficial rating deceive you into thinking that you can get a full 30 minutes of use out of a "30-minute" cylinder. In reality, a 30-minute cylinder may provide 20 minutes of air, but 15 minutes is the average. The rate at which you use the air in a cylinder depends on several factors, including your physical condition and size, the amount of physical activity you are performing, and the temperature in which you are working.

It is important to note that while a 60-minute cylinder won't provide a full 60 minutes of air, it *will* provide twice as much "working time" as a 30-minute cylinder. The air cylinder has a pressure gauge that indicates the amount of air pressure inside. A remote pressure gauge allows the wearer to check the cylinder pressure while wearing the SCBA. Newer units have a "heads-up display" inside the mask that gives you constant information on the amount of air remaining in the cylinder.

Although the added air supply will allow you to remain in a contaminated atmosphere longer, the extra air capacity that a 45- or 60-minute air cylinder provides should be considered "safety" air. It is not intended to allow you to work longer than you should before stopping to rest in a safe location. Because of the heat buildup and physical toll that firefighting presents, most agencies do not allow firefighters to work much more than 35 minutes in full protective clothing before they rest.

Alarms

An audible, low-air alarm will let you know when you are nearing the end of your available air. Many manufacturers now offer a vibrating and a visual alarm. Just as you might expect, the amount of breathing time you will get out of the system once the low-air alarm sounds depends on the same factors that come into play when determining the work time you will get from a cylinder. Without exception, the most important thing to remember is that when your low-pressure alarm sounds, it is time to leave the hazardous scene. . . . immediately!

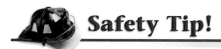

Safety Tip!

Proper air management is a must for firefighter safety. Maintain a constant awareness of the remaining air levels in the SCBA, keeping in mind the amount of time it will take you to reach a safe atmosphere. Waiting until a low-pressure alarm activates may be too late.

Regulators

The air contained in the compressed air cylinder is stored at a high pressure. The high-pressure air flows through a high-pressure hose to the regulator, where it is reduced to a usable pressure. On some SCBAs, the regulator connects directly to your facemask. On others, the regulator is on your waist belt and a low-pressure tube delivers the air at the regulated pressure to your facemask. Most regulators have an emergency bypass valve, which is red. As its name indicates, the emergency bypass valve allows high-pressure air to bypass the regulator in case of a failure. By slightly cracking open the emergency bypass valve, you will receive the remaining air in the cylinder at a fairly fast rate. If you ever encounter a reason to use this valve, do so to escape the hazardous area and immediately report the SCBA failure to an officer. You should take steps to ensure that the SCBA is not used again before a qualified technician repairs it.

Straps

The cylinder, high-pressure hose, low-air alarm, and regulator are connected to the backpack, which is fitted with harness straps. The harness has shoulder straps and a waist strap. Whenever you wear an SCBA, it is essential that all of the straps are properly fastened and adjusted.

Checking and Assembling an SCBA

Most fire departments carry their breathing apparatus already assembled and in racks, ready to use, on the fire truck. However, you should be familiar with the simple steps for connecting the air cylinder to the backpack and checking the SCBA to ensure its readiness for use. This check should be performed daily as well as before and after each use.

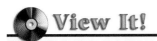
View It!

Go to the DVD, navigate to Chapter 3, and select *SCBA Visual Inspection.*

Practice It!

Visual Inspection of an SCBA

Use the following directions to visually inspect the various components of an SCBA:

1. *Face piece.* Check for cracks or tears in the rubber seal. Look for any debris that may be in the exhalation valve. Look for any loose clamps. Put the mask on and check the exhalation valve by exhaling gently while blocking the breathing tube with your hand (Figure 3-18).

FIGURE 3-18

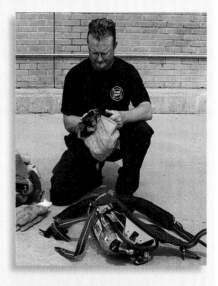

2. *Regulator.* Check for cleanliness and any signs of external damage. Operate the main-line valve and emergency bypass valve to check for smooth operation (Figure 3-19).

FIGURE 3-19

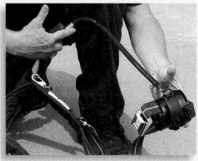

3. *High-pressure hose.* Look for external damage and check the O-ring on the coupling for damage or deformity (Figure 3-20).

FIGURE 3-20

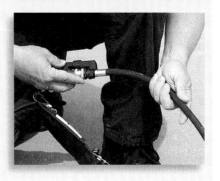

—Continued

4. *Harness straps.* Look for excessive wear to the straps and check all stitching for any obvious damage. Make sure that all hardware on the straps is clean and operable (Figure 3-21).

FIGURE 3-21

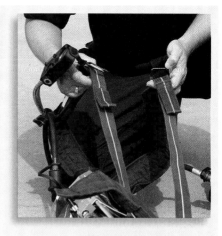

5. *Audible alarm.* Look for any obvious external damage (Figure 3-22).

FIGURE 3-22

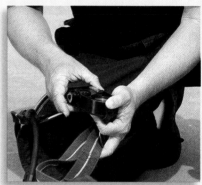

6 *Cylinder.* Look for any signs of damage, any gouges, or any abraded areas. Any deformity should be brought to the attention of the Company Officer. Check the pressure gauge and make sure that the cylinder is filled to the appropriate level. To check for accuracy, compare the cylinder gauge to the regulator gauge (Figure 3-23).

FIGURE 3-23

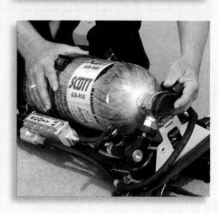

Donning and Doffing an SCBA

There are several acceptable methods for donning and doffing an SCBA, and none is better than any other in most cases. Your main concern should be to put the apparatus on safely and rapidly. The end result should be a properly adjusted and fastened harness assembly.

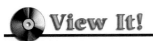 **View It!**

Go to the DVD, navigate to Chapter 3, and select *SCBA: Seat-Rack Donning.*

Practice It!

Seat-Rack Donning of an SCBA

This method of putting on an SCBA requires that you start with it in the seat rack.

1. **Do not take off your seat belt.** Place your arms through the shoulder straps, leaving the straps loose for the moment (Figure 3-24).

FIGURE 3-24

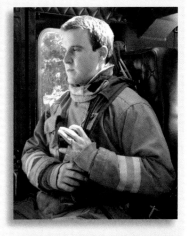

2. Fasten the waist belt, taking care to keep it separate from your seat belt, which should remain fastened any time the truck is in motion (Figure 3-25).

FIGURE 3-25

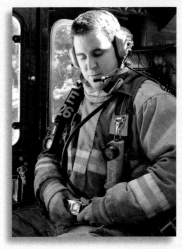

3. After the truck has come to a full stop and just before exiting the truck, unfasten your seat belt and adjust the shoulder straps to a good fit (Figure 3-26).

FIGURE 3-26

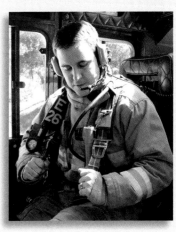

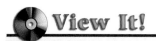
Go to the DVD, navigate to Chapter 3, and select *SCBA: Coat Method Donning.*

Practice It!

Coat Method Donning of an SCBA

This method of putting on an SCBA requires that you start with it on the ground.

1. Kneel behind the SCBA. Check the SCBA cylinder pressure to make sure the cylinder is full. Make sure that the main line valve and the emergency bypass valves on the regulator are closed. Open the main cylinder valve fully (Figure 3-27). Listen for the low-pressure alarm to sound briefly as the system is charged.

FIGURE 3-27

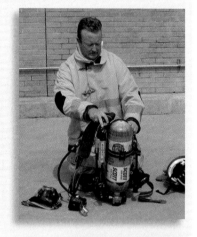

2. Check both the cylinder pressure gauge and the remote air pressure gauge. Make sure they are within 100 psi of each other. If they are not, do not use the SCBA (Figure 3-28).

FIGURE 3-28

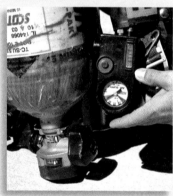

3. Grasp the shoulder strap that is on the same side as the air regulator and lift the pack off the ground, slinging it over your shoulder (Figure 3-29).

FIGURE 3-29

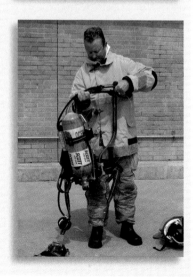

4. Place your other arm through the offside strap. Allow both of your hands to travel down the straps to the adjustment buckles, pulling the backpack snuggly to a comfortable position (Figure 3-30).

FIGURE 3-30

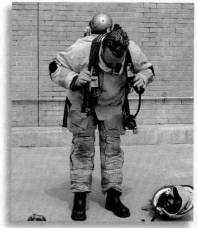

5. Clip the waist strap and adjust it to a snug, comfortable fit (Figure 3-31). At this point, most of the weight of the SCBA should be carried on the waist strap.

FIGURE 3-31

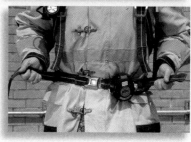

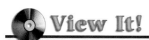 View It!

Go to the DVD, navigate to Chapter 3, and select *SCBA: Over-the-Head Method.*

Practice It!

Over-the-Head Donning of an SCBA

This method of putting on an SCBA requires that you start with it on the ground.

1. Kneel behind the SCBA. Check the cylinder pressure of the SCBA to make sure it is full. Make sure that the main line valve and the emergency bypass valves are closed on the regulator. Open the main cylinder valve fully (Figure 3-32). Listen for the low-pressure alarm to sound briefly as the system is charged.

FIGURE 3-32

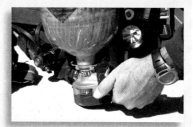

2. Check both the cylinder pressure gauge and the remote air pressure gauge. Make sure they are within 100 psi of each other. If they are not, do not use the SCBA (Figure 3-33).

FIGURE 3-33

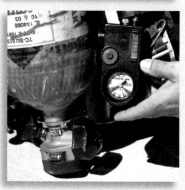

—Continued

3. Reach between the shoulder straps and the backpack, grasping the backpack on each side (Figure 3-34).

FIGURE 3-34

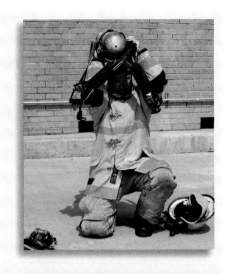

4. Lift the assembly over your head, allowing the SCBA to slide down your back with the shoulder straps falling into place (Figure 3-35). Allow both hands to travel down the straps to the adjustment buckles, pulling the backpack snuggly to a comfortable position (Figure 3-36).

FIGURE 3-35

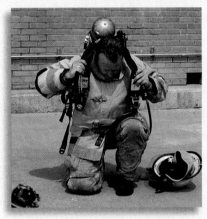

FIGURE 3-36

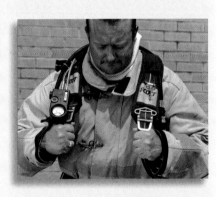

5. Clip the waist strap and adjust it to a snug, comfortable fit (Figure 3-37). At this point, most of the weight of the SCBA should be carried on the waist strap.

FIGURE 3-37

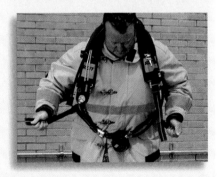

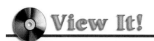
Go to the DVD, navigate to Chapter 3, and select *SCBA: Donning the Facemask.*

➡ **Practice It!**

Donning the Facemask

Putting the facemask on is the final step you take before you begin breathing from the system. Use the following steps:

1. It makes no difference whether you put the mask on by placing your chin in first and dragging the straps over your head or whether you use the ball-cap method (Figure 3-38). In the ball-cap method, you hold the straps on the back of your head and drag the mask down over your face (Figure 3-39). The main thing to remember is to have nothing between the rubberized face piece and your skin. The straps should be adjusted so that the mask fits snugly against your face. You should cover all remaining exposed skin once the mask is in place.

FIGURE 3-38

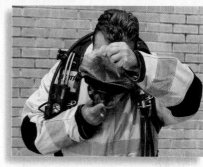

FIGURE 3-39

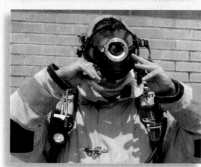

2. Start with your protective hood pulled down around your neck and your coat collar pulled up. Center the harness on your head and clear away any hair that may be between your head and the mask. Starting with the bottom straps, tighten them two at a time until you create a snug fit (Figure 3-40).

FIGURE 3-40

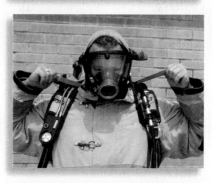

3. Check the seal by covering the opening in the mask and inhaling gently for 10 seconds. You should not feel any leaks as the mask squeezes to your face (Figure 3-41).

FIGURE 3-41

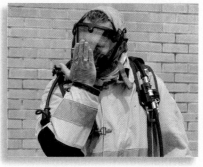

—Continued

4. Now check the exhalation valve by exhaling gently (Figure 3-42). Don't exhale too hard or you can damage your eardrums.

FIGURE 3-42

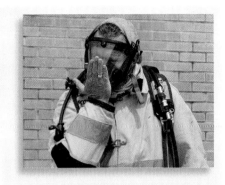

5. Now connect to your air supply and inhale to start the airflow (Figure 3-43).

FIGURE 3-43

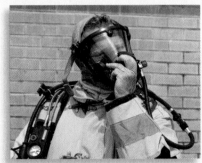

6. Pull your protective hood up and over the straps to cover any exposed skin (Figure 3-44). Make sure that the hood doesn't cover any part of the lens or the exhalation valve.

FIGURE 3-44

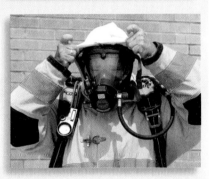

7. Now put your helmet on with the earflaps down and fasten the chinstrap snugly under your chin, taking care that it doesn't pass over the top of the low-pressure hose (if your SCBA is equipped with one) (Figure 3-45).

FIGURE 3-45

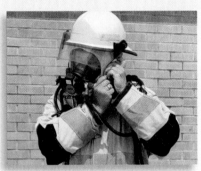

8. Now fasten your collar for a final bit of protection (Figure 3-46).

FIGURE 3-46

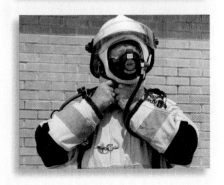

Practice It!

Breathing Compressed Air

You may feel a bit claustrophobic when you put an SCBA on the first time. Your entire PPE provides you with a protective environment that is new to you. It is not unusual for an inexperienced person to go through an entire 30-minute SCBA cylinder of air in less than 15 minutes.

1. Be aware of your breathing rate while working. You will get more than enough air from a properly functioning SCBA with each breath. However, excitement will cause you to breathe rapidly, thus cutting down your "working time" from the air supply.

2. Practice as often as you can with the SCBA so that you will remain comfortable in your "new environment" (Figure 3-47).

FIGURE 3-47

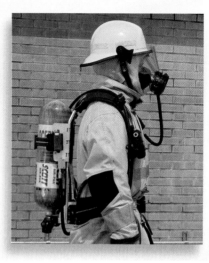

Returning an SCBA to "Ready-to-Use" Status

Remember: Most emergency equipment is only as good as the last person who used it. In other words, you should return the equipment to a "ready-to-use" status before you put it away. This is especially important with SCBAs. Returning an SCBA to ready-to-use status starts with the way you remove the mask when you are through using the apparatus. Simply grabbing the mask and dragging it over your head will eventually stretch the straps, diminishing their service life. Instead, loosen all the straps before gently removing the mask (Figure 3-48).

Once you have taken off the mask, loosen all the straps fully and clean the mask, following the man-

ufacturer's recommendations for sanitizing it. Make sure to thoroughly dry the mask before placing it back in service. Take care not to get water into a low-pressure air hose. If some water gets into the hose inadvertently, allow the hose to dry thoroughly before you use it again.

Loosen all the straps on the backpack and clean them with mild soap and water, and then allow them to dry. Inspect the straps and place a fresh air cylinder in the backpack. Perform an operational check of the entire SCBA and place it back into service (Figure 3-49).

Do not attempt to fill a compressed air cylinder unless you have received specific training from your

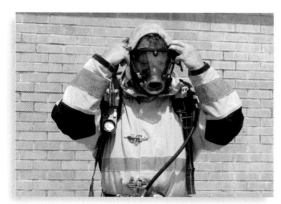

FIGURE 3-48 Make sure to loosen all straps and gently remove the mask to avoid stretching the straps.

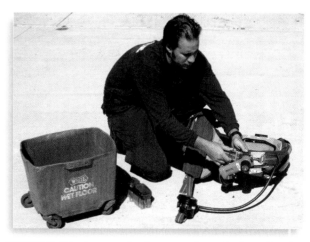

FIGURE 3-49 Loosen the harness straps before cleaning the mask with mild soap and water.

Self-Contained Breathing Apparatus (SCBA) **69**

agency in following the fill-station manufacturer's instructions. Compressed air cylinders must be inspected on a regular basis by a technician who is certified to do so. Although it is a very rare event, the failure of a compressed air cylinder usually has catastrophic results and can be deadly, so make sure to follow the manufacturer's guidelines *exactly*.

Personal Alert Safety System (PASS)

It is very easy to become disoriented when working in a smoke-filled environment. A **personal alert safety system (PASS)** is a small electronic device that is designed to detect your movement or your lack of movement. It sounds a very loud alarm if it determines that you have remained stationary for a predetermined length of time. The purpose of this device is to signal to other firefighters that you need help and to give them an audible signal that helps them in locating you. All PASS devices feature two modes of operation: (1) a manual activation mode in which you can activate the alarm when you need help, and (2) an automatic activation mode, which will sound a pre-alert in the form of a short, lower-volume signal to let you know that the PASS device has sensed you aren't moving. The pre-alert signal is designed to help prevent false alarms. The PASS will go into a full alarm mode within seconds of sounding the pre-alert.

There are many different brands and types of PASS devices available. However, the two main differences are in the way you turn on the device. An ordinary PASS must be switched on before you enter a hazardous atmosphere (Figure 3-50). An *integrated* PASS is built into your SCBA and is automatically turned on when you open the air cylinder to use the breathing apparatus (Figure 3-51). Because it is very important to use every safety device available to you when you enter a hazardous atmosphere, it is important to ensure that the PASS is on and working whenever you use an SCBA, regardless of the way it is turned on.

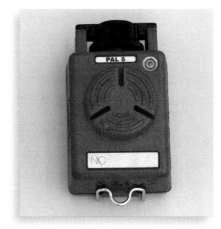

FIGURE 3-50 An ordinary PASS must be switched on before you enter a hazardous atmosphere.

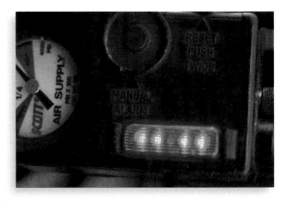

FIGURE 3-51 An integrated PASS is automatically turned on when the air cylinder on the SCBA is opened for use.

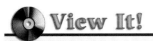 **View It!**

Go to the DVD, navigate to Chapter 3, and select *Personal Alert Safety System.*

Practice It!

Inspecting a Personal Alert Safety System

Note: The following steps are the general operating procedure for a PASS. Follow all of the manufacturer's directions for operating your particular device.

1. Inspect the outside of the unit for any deformities and for cleanliness (Figure 3-52).

FIGURE 3-52

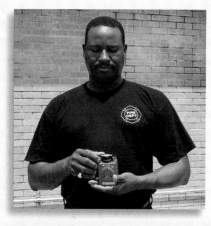

2. Turn on the device and listen for a signal that indicates that it is armed (Figure 3-53).

FIGURE 3-53

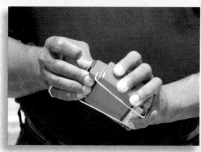

3. Shake the device when you hear the pre-alert to make sure that it returns to a ready state (Figure 3-54).
4. Leave the device motionless. It should sound a pre-alert within 30 seconds.
5. Allow the device to remain motionless until it again sounds a pre-alert signal and then allow it to go into a full alarm mode.

FIGURE 3-54

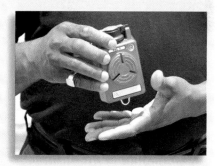

6. Reset the alarm to a ready state (Figure 3-55). Now check the alarm's manual alert switch for operation.
7. Turn the device off.

FIGURE 3-55

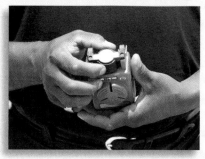

It is extremely important that you turn off the PASS when you are not in a hazardous atmosphere. It is also important for you to control the PASS when training with your SCBA. False alarms can desensitize other firefighters into assuming that someone simply forgot to turn off his or her PASS.

Reporting to Command

Another item that is essential to every firefighter's safety is a personnel accountability system. In this system, the Incident Commander or a designee accounts for every person as they enter and exit a hazardous area or environment. To keep track of everyone, the Accountability Officer will use some form of a tracking system in which each firefighter reports to his or her Company Officer, who then reports to the Accountability Officer.

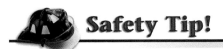

Safety Tip!

One of the most important components of the personnel accountability system—and probably the most important to *your* safety—is that you never work alone in a hazardous area. Anyone wearing an SCBA must work as part of a team of at least two people. While it is important that you learn how to "self-rescue," there is often nothing more important to your safety than a partner. SCBA masks limit your visibility, and the protective seal provided by your PPE isolates many of your senses. Therefore, working within a group means that everyone looks out for each other's safety. NEVER WORK ALONE WHEN WEARING AN SCBA!

Practice It!

Personnel Accountability System

The following steps are components of the personnel accountability system:

1. To make this procedure easy to use on the emergency scene, most fire departments assign each firefighter some type of accountability tag (Figure 3-56).

FIGURE 3-56

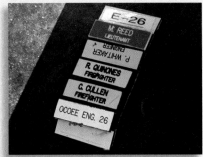

2. Each individual firefighter's tag is grouped with the rest of the tags from that company to form a "passport" for that company.

3. The passport is then given to the Accountability Officer, who keeps track of the entire company as a group or as individuals, according to their assignments at the emergency scene (Figure 3-57).

FIGURE 3-57

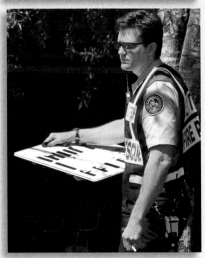

Safety Tip!

While personnel accountability is a very important function of command, the accountability system is only as good as the individual firefighter on the scene. It is your responsibility to give your accountability tag to your Company Officer before you board the fire apparatus in responding to an emergency. If you are a volunteer who arrives on the scene in your personal vehicle, then you should report to the command post, give your accountability tag to the Accountability Officer, and wait for a job assignment. *DO NOT FREE-LANCE!* Even the most seasoned fire veteran must work within the Command system.

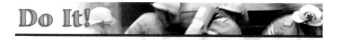

Do It!

Be Safe!

In this chapter you learned how to use and care for the most important gear you will use, your personal protective equipment. This gear includes protective clothing, an SCBA, and a personal alert device (the PASS), that electronically signals others when you are in trouble. You also learned an important safety component of incident management, the personnel accountability system. This information is important. Hopefully you have gained important skills in using this protective gear and understand its importance to your overall safety on the fire emergency scene.

Prove It

Knowledge Assessment

Signed Documentation Tear-Out Sheet

Exterior Operations Level Firefighter—Chapter 3

Name: _____

Fill out the ten-question quiz below, the Knowledge Assessment Sheet, by circling the correct answer for each question. When finished, sign it and give to your instructor/Company Officer for his or her signature. Turn in this Knowledge Assessment Sheet to the proper person as part of the documentation that you have completed your training for this chapter.

1. A firefighter's protective clothing is made up of several pieces, all of which must be in place for maximum protection.
   a. True
   b. False

2. How many layers of protection are provided in a set of structural firefighting coat and pants?
   a. Two
   b. Four
   c. Three
   d. Five

3. Maximum eye protection is provided by the pull-down face shield on a fire helmet.
   a. True
   b. False

4. At a minimum, how often should your fire service protective clothing be cleaned?
   a. Every 6 months
   b. Every 6 weeks
   c. Every 4 months
   d. Every 5 months

5. A complete ensemble of personal protective equipment is not complete without
   a. a uniform shirt.
   b. a self-contained breathing apparatus.
   c. flameproof socks.
   d. a personal accountability tag.

6. Which of the following is *not* a contributing factor to your rate of air use when breathing from the air bottle of your SCBA?
   a. Your physical condition
   b. The amount of physical activity you are performing
   c. The temperature in which you are working
   d. The PASS timer

7. The _____ knob opens the emergency bypass valve on your self-contained breathing apparatus.
   a. green
   b. red
   c. blue
   d. yellow

8. Which of the following is the final step of putting on your SCBA before breathing from the system?
   a. Putting on your gloves
   b. Putting on your helmet
   c. Putting on your facemask
   d. Putting on your hood

9. A personal alert safety system (PASS) has an audible alarm that detects your movement and
   a. the SCBA air tank level.
   b. your radio signal.
   c. your lack of movement.
   d. the atmospheric pressure.

10. Which of the following phrases best describes what the personnel accountability system provides to firefighters and crews working on an emergency scene?
    a. A tracking system
    b. An alarm system
    c. A strategy system
    d. An alert device

Prove It

Skills Assessment
Signed Documentation Tear-Out Sheet

Exterior Operations Level Firefighter—Chapter 3

Name: _____

Fill out the Skills Assessment Sheet below. Have your instructor/Company Officer check off and initial each skill you demonstrate. When finished, sign it and give to your instructor/Company Officer for his or her signature. Turn in this Skills Assessment Sheet to the proper person as part of the documentation that you have completed your training for this chapter.

Skill	Completed	Initials
1. Describe the components of personal protective clothing used for structural firefighting.	_____	_____
2. Describe the components of an entire ensemble of personal protective equipment used for structural firefighting.	_____	_____
3. Properly put on and wear all of your personal protective clothing.	_____	_____
4. Describe the procedures for the care and cleaning of your personal protective clothing.	_____	_____
5. Describe the components of a self-contained breathing apparatus (SCBA).	_____	_____
6. Demonstrate the proper way to check and assemble an SCBA.	_____	_____
7. Properly put on an SCBA from the seat-rack position.	_____	_____
8. Properly put on an SCBA from the ground.	_____	_____
9. Properly put on an SCBA from the ground using the over-the-head method.	_____	_____
10. Properly check and employ a personal alert safety system (PASS) in both automatic mode and manual mode.	_____	_____
11. Describe what you need to do when you use the personal accountability tag • When you ride the apparatus • When you drive your personal vehicle to the scene	_____	_____

Student Signature/Date _____   Instructor/Company Officer Signature/Date _____

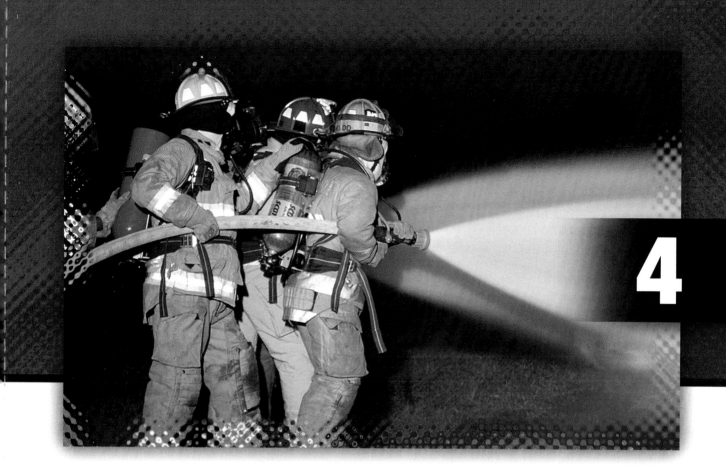

Preconnected Attack Lines

What You Will Learn in This Chapter

This chapter will introduce you to various small hoses, nozzles, and equipment. It will also show you how fire hose is loaded and pulled off the fire apparatus. You will learn how to hold and flow a small fire attack hose under full operating pressure.

What You Will Be Able to Do

After reading this chapter and practicing the skills in a classroom setting, you will be able to

1. Describe the components of a fire hose system.
2. Demonstrate how to connect and disconnect hose couplings.
3. Describe the application of different hose tools and accessories that are used with fire hose.
4. Demonstrate the methods for rolling and carrying fire hose.
5. Explain good hose maintenance and care techniques.

6. Explain and demonstrate how fire nozzles operate.
7. Demonstrate how to deploy and load booster hose.
8. Demonstrate how to properly hold and utilize a flowing booster line.
9. Demonstrate how to deploy and load a preconnected attack line.
10. Demonstrate how to hold and utilize a flowing small attack line.

Reality!

Fire Hose

This chapter provides our first discussion about hose. The subject of fire hose is broken down into two categories: *attack* and *supply*. The **attack line** is used to carry the water from the pump to the fire. The **supply line** is used to move water from its source—for example, a fire hydrant, tanker truck (also known as a tender), or pond—to the pump. In this chapter, we will discuss the fire hose that is used to attack and extinguish most fires, the preconnected attack line.

The preconnected attack line is your primary fire-extinguishing tool as well as your main lifeline. It protects you by allowing you to put a water barrier between you and the fire. Additional protection is provided in that you can follow the fire attack line out of an unsafe area to the pumper or to a safe area. In this way, it automatically marks your trail for a safe retreat—in most cases.

For these reasons, you must understand the importance of becoming familiar with, and well trained in, the applications and use of fire attack lines. They are the primary tool you will use to extinguish most fires and they are your lifeline for safe firefighting.

KEY WORDS

attack line The hose that is used to carry the water from the pump to the fire.

supply line The hose that is used to move water from its source—for example, a fire hydrant, tanker truck (also known as a tender), or pond—to the pump.

Fire Service Terminology

It is important that you understand the terminology you will hear when you are working with fire hose:

- *Hose* refers to a section of hose. This term may also indicate multiple sections of hose.
- *Fire hose* refers to a section of hose used for firefighting purposes in the fire service. It can also refer to multiple sections of fire hose.
- *Hose line* refers to one or more sections of hose being utilized for any of the following reasons:
  - To deliver a water supply to the fire **apparatus** pump
  - To deliver water from the pump to the nozzle, which converts the water into a fire stream that flows toward the seat of the fire
  - To protect any exposures to a fire
- *Attack line* refers to a hose line used to deliver a fire-extinguishing stream to the seat of the fire. It includes the nozzle at the end of the hose line.
- *Small attack line* refers to a fire attack hose line that is ¾ inch to 2 inches in diameter.
- *Large attack line* refers to a fire attack hose line that is 2 ½ inches or more in diameter.

- *Supply line* indicates a hose line used to deliver a supply of water from a water supply source to the fire apparatus pump.

KEY WORD

apparatus Rolling equipment (such as an engine, a truck, or a rescue unit) that is used in the Fire Service.

Attack Lines

When we speak about attack lines, we are really talking about a hose system. It is a system because it is made up of several pieces of equipment, sections of hose, and a nozzle used by firefighters to apply water to the desired location. This system ultimately functions to extinguish the fire. With a proficient knowledge of the system, its components, and how they work together, as a firefighter, you will work safely and effectively.

An attack line begins at the pump on the fire *apparatus* and ends at the stream of water that comes from the end of the nozzle (Figure 4-1). It results in a **fire stream** that effectively reaches the base of the fire. The pump on the apparatus is designed to deliver enough water through the system to provide an effective stream of water to the fire. The pump panel is where the flow of water through the attack lines is regulated both for volume (how much water) and pressure (how fast it moves) (Figure 4-2). The volume is expressed in gallons per minute (gpm) and the pressure is expressed in pounds per square inch (psi). These two forces help determine the amount of water and the reach of the fire stream coming from the nozzle.

KEY WORD

fire stream The flow of water from the open end of a fire nozzle that reaches the desired location (that is, the fire).

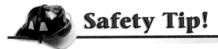 **Safety Tip!**

When handling fire hose, always wear at least head, eye, hand, and foot protection. Full bunker gear is preferable.

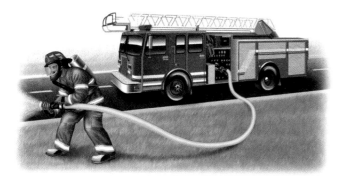

FIGURE 4-1 A fire attack line system starts at the pump and ends at the nozzle tip.

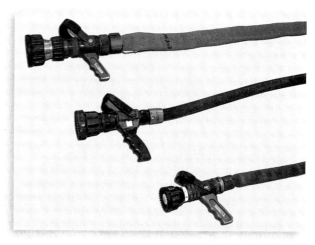

FIGURE 4-3 A 1-inch booster hose line and a 1¾-inch attack line. Small attack lines are ¾ to 2 inches in diameter and are usually carried in a preconnected configuration on the fire truck.

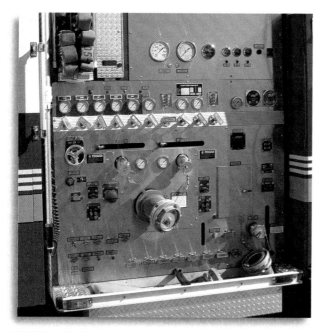

FIGURE 4-2 The pump panel on the fire apparatus is where the water supply coming into the pump and the water flow going into the fire attack lines is controlled.

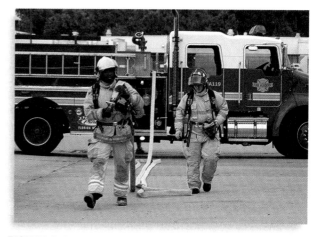

FIGURE 4-4 The most commonly used preconnected fire attack lines are small attack lines. These lines are 1½, 1¾, to 2 inches in diameter.

As you can see, there is a great deal to learn about hose and water and how we use them to put out fires. There will be much more detailed training provided in later parts of this text as well as in the other parts of this training curriculum that you can use as your training advances.

Small Attack Lines

Small attack lines have a diameter of ¾ inch to 2 inches, which is measured on the inside diameter of the hose. They are usually categorized as booster lines, which are on a reel and are seldom removed from the truck, and preconnected attack lines. Technically, both fall under the category of preconnected lines because they are carried on the truck already connected to the pump with the nozzle attached and arranged in a way so that they can be quickly deployed for use (Figure 4-3).

Preconnected Attack Lines

The most common type of fire attack hose lines you will use for fighting fires are 1½ inches, 1¾ inches, and 2 inches in diameter (Figure 4-4). These attack hose lines primarily come in lengths of 50 feet and are usually made of multilayered, jacketed hose material. They can also be made of lightweight, synthetic, rubberized materials (Figure 4-5).

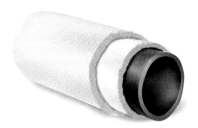

FIGURE 4-5 Construction of a typical 1¾-inch fire attack hose line.

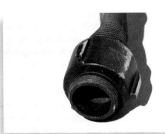

FIGURE 4-6 Typical threaded male hose coupling.

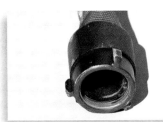

FIGURE 4-7 Typical threaded female hose coupling.

The couplings are male (exposed threads) and female (threads inside a swivel end)—one of each, at opposite ends of the hose (Figures 4-6 and 4-7). The male coupling is one piece—a sleeve with threads on the outside of the end. The female coupling has two parts—a sleeve and a swivel on the sleeve that contains the hose gasket. The threads are on the inside of the swivel end. The design of the threads is standard throughout most of the Fire Service in the United States and is referred to as **national standard threads (NST).**

Rocker lugs or rocker pins on the couplings provide a grip point for a spanner wrench. Spanner wrenches (or "spanners") are used to grip the rocker lugs of overtightened couplings to break them free. Standard couplings are designed to screw together in a clockwise direction. Conversely, they are loosened by being turned counterclockwise. Resist the temptation to overtighten couplings with spanners, as doing so compresses the gasket and can cause leaks rather than prevent them. Couplings should be hand-tight.

One lug on each of the couplings is usually marked with a Higbee indicator, which is a small notch cut into one of the lugs (Figure 4-8). The Higbee indicator helps you align the threads for proper tightening. Align the Higbee indicators across from each other and the couplings should tighten smoothly without cross-threading.

There are other types of hose couplings available. These couplings provide quick-connect features that allow rapid connecting of hose lines (Figure 4-9). Check with your department about connecting and disconnecting techniques if your department uses this type of fire hose.

Attack lines can be found in a few basic configurations on the fire apparatus. They can be loaded in specific hose bed areas and preconnected together and to the fire apparatus pump via a discharge port. They may also be preconnected into a bundle for use as a high-rise pack. This bundle makes it easier to carry fire attack hose up to higher floor levels of a multistory building when fighting a fire. Spare sections of hose may also be carried rolled and stored in a disconnected configuration and used to extend existing preconnected attack lines.

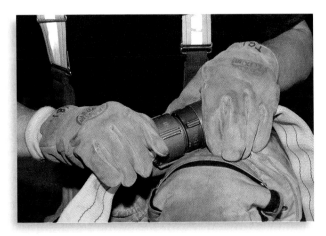

FIGURE 4-8 On threaded hose couplings, align the Higbee cuts on each coupling before you screw them together.

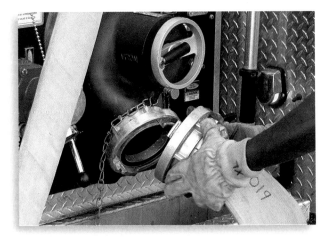

FIGURE 4-9 Quick-connect couplings, shown here on large-diameter supply hose.

■ KEY WORD ■

national standard threads (NST) A nationally recognized Fire Service specification that established the number and size of threads used in fire hose couplings. This specification is recognized throughout most of the United States.

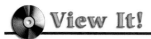 View It!

Go to the DVD, navigate to Chapter 4, and select *Small Attack Line Stretch.*

 Practice It!

Stretching Small Attack Lines

Small attack lines are usually preconnected in lengths of 100 to 200 feet and are loaded in hose bed areas of the fire apparatus. Because small attack lines are loaded in many different configurations, you need to learn about and practice with the methods your fire department uses to pull the load and deploy the lines.

The following techniques can be used to pull and stretch any preconnected, small attack line:

1. Pull the correct hose load, grasping the loops that extend beyond the hose bed in which the hose is loaded (Figure 4-10). Then either back away from the apparatus until the hose clears the hose bed and then turn and walk toward the fire, or walk away from the apparatus with the line feeding off your shoulder. The method used depends upon the type of hose load.

FIGURE 4-10

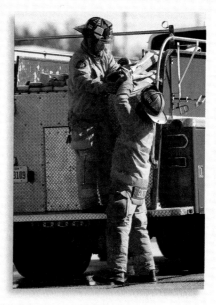

2. Hold the loops firmly as you walk away from the apparatus, letting go of the loops as you feel a tug from the apparatus (Figure 4-11). Keep as much slack as you can; you need this slack to maneuver the hose at the fire. When you reach your preliminary position outside the hazardous area, drop the excess hose and arrange it in long loops. It is best to get as much into position as possible before the attack line is charged with water. The attack line is more difficult to move after it is charged.

FIGURE 4-11

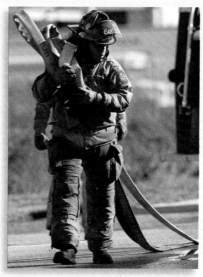

—Continued

3. Signal the driver when you are ready for water to fill the hose. Slowly open the nozzle to let out excess air and to adjust the nozzle to the desired pattern and flow (Figure 4-12). Then close the nozzle before advancing the line.

FIGURE 4-12

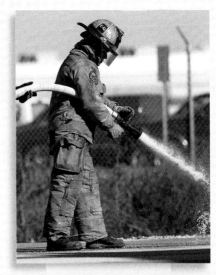

4. A second firefighter or the pump operator should walk the deployed attack line, straightening any kinks in the line (Figure 4-13).

FIGURE 4-13

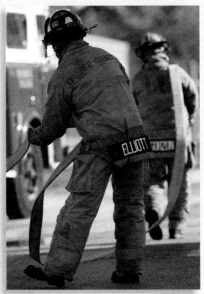

5. Maneuver the charged attack line into position and open the nozzle slowly, directing the water to the desired point on the fire (Figure 4-14).

FIGURE 4-14

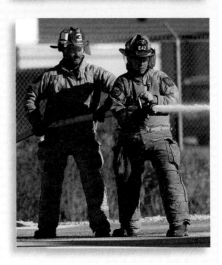

6. Larger attack lines flow much more water than smaller lines. Therefore, they are handled differently and require more strength and skill to maneuver into position. Many times they require two firefighters for best operation and positioning. Much more **nozzle reaction** is present with these lines, which is a reaction to the volume and pressure of the water flowing from the nozzle. Anticipate this force and brace your body against the hose line at your hip and knee. Lean into the hose line with your body (Figure 4-15).

FIGURE 4-15

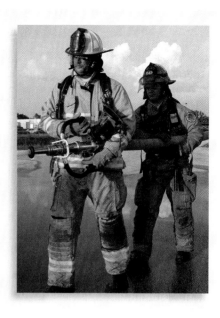

 View It!

Go to the DVD, navigate to Chapter 4, and select *Loading Small Attack Lines.*

 Practice It!

Loading Small Attack Lines

Small preconnected attack lines can be loaded in a "ready-for-use" manner using several different styles of loads. Because different methods of loading attack lines are used by different fire departments, we will cover only the main steps for working as a team member while loading an attack line. The various types of hose loads are described in the next level of this curriculum. For now we will concentrate on general methods you can follow to assist with the process.

Use the following guidelines when loading small attack lines:

1. Confirm that the water has been shut off at the apparatus pump. Open the nozzle to allow any water pressure to be released. Then take the nozzle off the hose line (Figure 4-16)

FIGURE 4-16

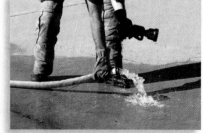

2. Disconnect the sections of hose and drain each section of hose. If the hose is to be loaded on the scene, stretch the lines out and reconnect them after they have been drained. Assist in loading the hose into its storage location and reattach the nozzle (Figure 4-17). *Note:* If the hose is to be replaced at the fire station, drain and roll it for secure storage on the apparatus. When you return to the fire station you may be required to clean it before loading the hose.

FIGURE 4-17

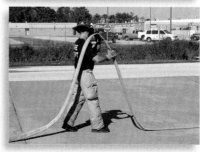

Booster Attack Lines

Most booster attack hose is made of multiple layers of hard, synthetic rubber materials. These lines generally come in 100-foot lengths and are stored on the apparatus prewound on hose reels. These hose reels can be located in several places on fire apparatus, including inside compartments, or near the hose bed or behind the cab of the fire apparatus (Figure 4-18). Lightweight booster lines have a rubber liner and a cloth jacket for reinforcement. They also have a helix-coiled wire that gives the hose its permanent round shape.

Booster attack lines are attached together with male and female couplings (Figure 4-19). The female coupling is made of a sleeve and a swivel with a gasket located inside the swivel. Make sure these gaskets are in place when connecting the sections of any fire hose. The male coupling is constructed of one piece and has exposed threads. These threads need to be protected from damage. Never drag exposed male couplings across the ground, as doing so will damage the threads.

Booster hose line couplings usually have small grip points that are recessed. They require a special type of spanner wrench called a Barway spanner for disconnecting and connecting (Figure 4-20).

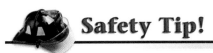 **Safety Tip!**

Booster lines do not provide sufficient water flow for interior fire attack, dumpsters, or to extinguish a well-involved car fire. Booster lines should be used only for small to medium exterior fires, such as trash fires or field fires that involve grass or very low brush. Think of a booster line as a utility line, not an attack line.

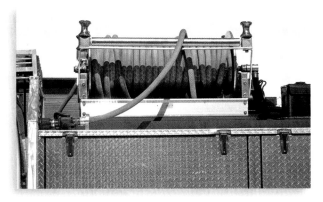

FIGURE 4-18 Booster line hose reels can be located in several different places on fire trucks.

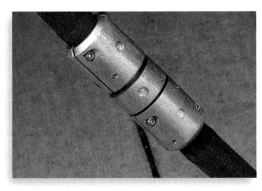

FIGURE 4-19 Booster line couplings, with the male and female connected.

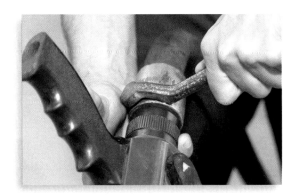

FIGURE 4-20 Barway spanner wrenches are specially designed for booster line hose couplings.

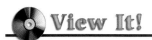
View It!

Go to the DVD, navigate to Chapter 4, and select Booster Attack Line Stretch.

Practice It!

Stretching Booster Attack Lines

Use the following steps to stretch a booster hose:

1. Grasp the nozzle and step down from the apparatus, and then turn toward the fire. Stop a short distance from the apparatus and grab some slack line to take with you. If someone else is advancing with the nozzle, grab the hose about 25 feet behind him or her and help pull the line (Figure 4-21).

FIGURE 4-21

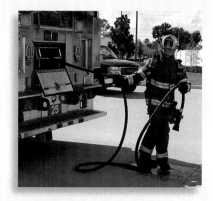

2. When you are near the fire but in a safe area, stop and point the nozzle at the ground and slowly open it (Figure 4-22). Doing so bleeds trapped air from the hose and ensures that you have water and the desired stream pattern at the nozzle before approaching the fire.

FIGURE 4-22

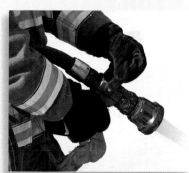

3. Shut off the nozzle and hold the line under your arm and the nozzle at a comfortable level, keeping a hand on the operating valve as you approach the fire (Figure 4-23).

FIGURE 4-23

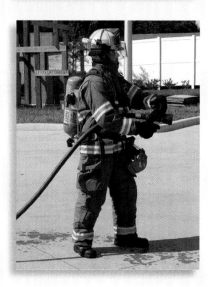

—Continued

4. Now flow water onto the base of the fire to extinguish it (Figure 4-24). Make sure to hold the flow of water until the fire is completely extinguished.

FIGURE 4-24

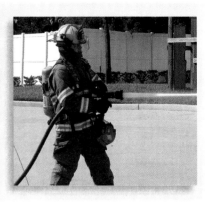

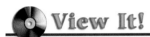

View It!

Go to the DVD, navigate to Chapter 4, and select *Loading Booster Attack Lines.*

Practice It!

Loading Booster Attack Lines

In loading a booster attack line, always wear gloves when handling the line to protect your hands from any glass or other sharp edges that may have become embedded in the hose. You will also need to have a rag handy to remove any dirt from the hose as you load it.

Use the following steps to load a booster attack line:

1. Bring the nozzle end back to the apparatus at the hose reel. Load the booster line by operating the hose reel rewind button and rolling the hose back onto the reel. Try to keep the roll as neat as possible—and never allow the nozzle to scrape along the ground, as doing so can damage the nozzle (Figure 4-25).

FIGURE 4-25

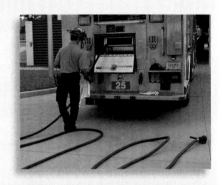

2. Allow the line to pass through a rag held by your gloved hand to wipe away dirt and grime (Figure 4-26). Inspect the hose for any obvious cuts or other damage as it passes through your hand.

FIGURE 4-26

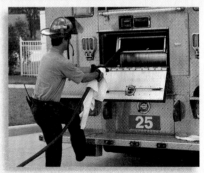

3. Make sure the nozzle is secure and that its valve is in the *off* position.

One-Inch Jacketed Attack Lines Your fire apparatus may be equipped with a jacketed attack line that is 1 inch in diameter. Many departments have started using this small-diameter hose instead of booster lines for trash fires and small grass fires. Consequently, 1-inch jacketed hose is commonly referred to as a *trash line*. These lines can be located in a special hose bed area or in a compartment on the fire apparatus. They may or may not be already preconnected to the apparatus pump. Their design features a single, synthetic jacket, with a male coupling at one end and a female coupling at the other. These lines come in 50- to 100-foot lengths. One-inch jacketed hose lines lie flat when empty and are generally preconnected with the nozzle attached, or rolled up and stored in a compartment on the apparatus (Figure 4-27).

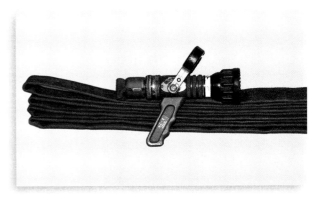

FIGURE 4-27 One-inch, single-jacketed hose lines lie flat when loaded and are preconnected with the nozzle attached. They are also referred to as *trash lines.*

Hose-Handling Techniques and Hose Tools

General Hose-Handling Techniques

There are a few general hose-handling tasks that are common to most types and configurations of fire hose. These techniques will help you safely and efficiently handle a fire hose as you work with it both at the actual fire emergency and during routine maintenance and handling operations.

Because small attack lines are flat when empty, they are prone to severe water flow restrictions when the hose is kinked under pressure (Figure 4-28). *Never walk by a kink in any hose line without straightening it.* Every kink is a danger to the crew on the nozzle and will greatly reduce the effectiveness of the fire stream.

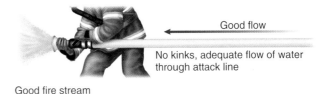

Good flow

No kinks, adequate flow of water through attack line

Good fire stream

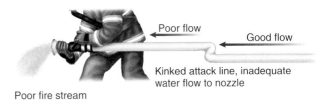

Poor flow

Good flow

Kinked attack line, inadequate water flow to nozzle

Poor fire stream

FIGURE 4-28 The effects of a kinked hose line.

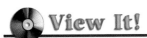 **View It!**

Go to the DVD, navigate to Chapter 4, and select *Connecting Hose Sections.*

Practice It!

Connecting Hose Sections

Use the following procedure to connect two sections of fire hose to each other by yourself:

1. Check the female end for the gasket and insert the male end, lining up the Higbee indicators. Rotate the female coupling clockwise while holding the male coupling in your other hand (Figure 4-29).

FIGURE 4-29

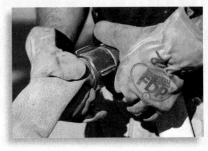

—Continued

2. If you are having trouble holding the male end as you connect the sections, simply step just behind the male end, which will turn it upward and hold it in place as you tighten the female coupling (Figure 4-30).

FIGURE 4-30

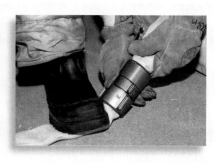

3. Tighten the hose couplings until they are hand-tight. Move on to the next section to be joined.

Use the following method if you have someone to help you connect the hose sections:

1. One person grasps the male end and holds it stationary at waist level.

2. The second person checks for a gasket, attaches the female coupling to the male coupling, and then turns the swivel, screwing the two sections together hand-tight (Figure 4-31). *Tip:* The person holding the male coupling should look away while the person holding the female side does the work. Doing so will prevent the two people from moving the couplings independently, which will cause the couplings to misalign.

FIGURE 4-31

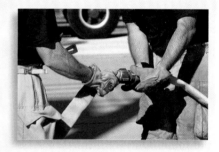

Hose Tools

There are many types and styles of hose tools available today. These devices are specialized tools that are used for various purposes with fire hose and include spanner wrenches, hose straps, and hose clamps. Each has its purpose and use.

Spanner Wrenches

Spanner wrenches are used to tighten and loosen hose couplings. On most hose fittings, there is a flange or lug on the outside of the couplings. The spanner has an indented grip to grasp the pin or lug for turning the coupling end (Figure 4-32). Firefighters should always grab two wrenches because they will need to grasp both hose couplings with the tools to tighten or loosen them.

Do not use spanners to overtighten couplings—doing so will only damage the gasket and make it hard to uncouple the hose later.

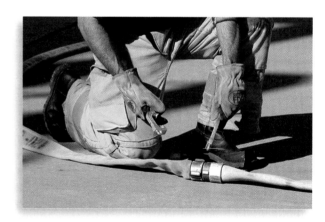

FIGURE 4-32 Always be ready with two spanner wrenches to tighten and loosen couplings—one for each hose coupling. Do not overtighten the couplings.

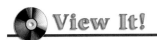 **View It!**

Go to the DVD, navigate to Chapter 4, and select *Using Spanner Wrenches.*

Practice It!

Using Spanner Wrenches

Use the following procedure when tightening or loosening hose couplings with spanner wrenches:

1. Place one spanner wrench so that it fits the lug and will turn the coupling in the desired direction.

FIGURE 4-33

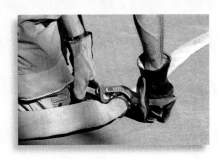

2. Place the second spanner wrench so that it holds the opposite coupling in place as you turn the coupling (Figure 4-33).

3. Loosen the couplings as shown (Figure 4-34).

FIGURE 4-34

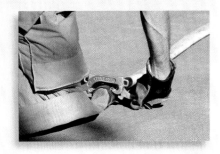

4. If tightening couplings, always remember that they will eventually need to be uncoupled, so only tighten them hand-tight.

Hose Straps

Hose straps are tools that provide firefighters with a handhold on a hose line. They are also excellent for securing hose lines to railings or ladders when needed. Hose straps consist of a metal handle attached to a heavy, webbed strap material. On one end, an open-clasp hook, designed to attach back onto the strap itself, allows the tool to be attached quickly (Figure 4-35).

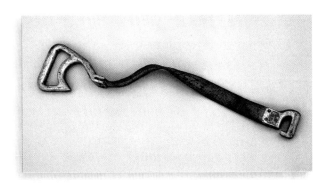

FIGURE 4-35 Hose strap.

View It!

Go to the DVD, navigate to Chapter 4, and select *Using Hose Straps.*

Practice It!

Using Hose Straps

The following method outlines the steps for and benefits of using hose straps:

1. Wrap the hose with the webbing of the strap and hook it back onto itself as shown in Figure 4-36.

FIGURE 4-36

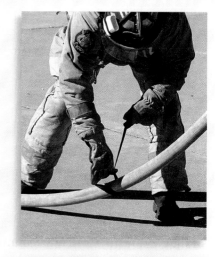

2. The firefighter can now handle the charged hose effectively, using the handle of the strap as a good grip (Figure 4-37).

FIGURE 4-37

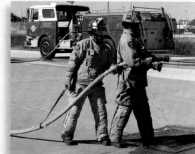

3. In addition, the strap can be used to hook the charged hose to a ladder rung or railing. Doing so is a quick method of securing the charged hose to these areas (Figure 4-38).

FIGURE 4-38

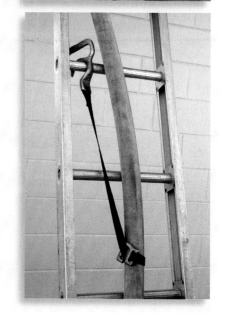

Hose Appliances

Any device through which water passes that is not a handheld nozzle is considered a hose appliance. These appliances include master stream devices, hose coupling adapters, reducers, and devices to connect three or more hoses together.

Coupling Adapters

Coupling adapters are appliances used to connect male to male or female to female. Coupling adapters come in two main configurations: double male and double female adapters (Figure 4-39). The double male adapter consists of one sleeve with threads on the outside of each end. The double female adapter is made up of one sleeve with a threaded swivel at each end. Adapters are used to change the end of a hose section to a male or female end.

Reducers

Reducers are specialized hose coupling adapters that change the size of the end coupling. They are usually constructed of one piece. They feature a female end that is the size of the male end of the hose and a male end that is the smaller size of the hose or nozzle the coupling is hooked into (Figure 4-40).

Gate Valves

Gate valves are hose appliances that are hooked into the supply- and attack-line water systems to control the flow of water through those systems. For small attack lines, they are made up of the valve body and various configurations of gates. These valves can take an incoming water stream and divide it into two or more water streams, each with its own gate.

Two examples of gates used with small attack lines are the gated wye and the water thief. The gated wye usually takes in water from a larger supply, like a 2½-inch or 3-inch supply, and then divides it into two 1½-inch or 1¾-inch lines, each with its own gate valve (Figure 4-41). The water thief has a similar configuration except that the larger supply stream travels through the main gated valve assembly and discharges the same size stream. There are small attack-line gates on either side of the main gate valve assembly.

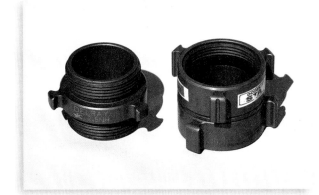

FIGURE 4-39 Double male and double female coupling adapters.

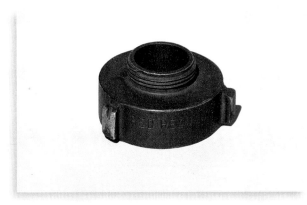

FIGURE 4-40 Reducer coupling on an attack line.

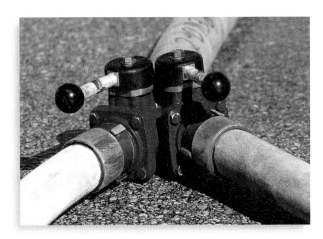

FIGURE 4-41 Gated wye valve.

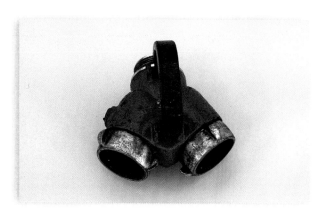

FIGURE 4-42 Siamese device.

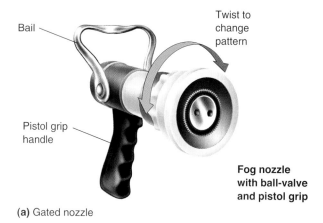

(a) Gated nozzle

Bail

Twist to change pattern

Pistol grip handle

Fog nozzle with ball-valve and pistol grip

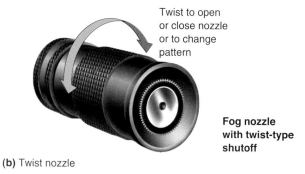

(b) Twist nozzle

Twist to open or close nozzle or to change pattern

Fog nozzle with twist-type shutoff

FIGURE 4-43 Fog nozzles: (a) gated nozzle and (b) twist nozzle.

Siamese Devices

Siamese devices take two or more supply lines and join them into one supply line (Figure 4-42). These devices typically have a flapper valve inside each intake opening that shuts off if only one line connected to the device is flowing water. A Siamese allows two lines to be combined with one line to increase pressure and flow.

Nozzles

General Nozzle Operations

Handheld fire nozzles will open in one of two ways: (1) with an operating valve handle (often called the bale or gate valve) on top of the nozzle body or (2) by twisting on the nozzle (Figure 4-43). In addition, handheld fire nozzles may or may not have a grip handle on the bottom.

Fire nozzles should always be opened and closed slowly to prevent a **water hammer** (Figure 4-44). A water hammer is a reaction to the sudden starting or stopping of water flow through hoses and pipes. This hammer effect can cause damage to the hose, pipes, and fittings.

■ KEY WORD ■

water hammer A reaction to the sudden starting or stopping of water flow through hoses and pipes that momentarily increases the pressure to sometimes dangerous levels in all directions on the line and pump.

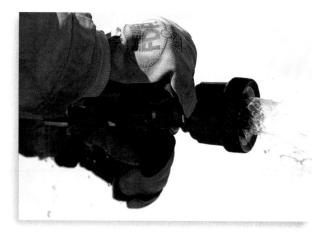

FIGURE 4-44 Open and close the fire nozzle slowly to prevent a water hammer effect.

Types of Nozzles

There are two general types of nozzle designs: fog and solid bore (Figure 4-45). Fog nozzles allow the water pattern to be adjusted, usually by turning the tip end of the nozzle. The pattern of spray can be adjusted from a wide to a narrow pattern, depending on the effect desired from the stream coming from the nozzle.

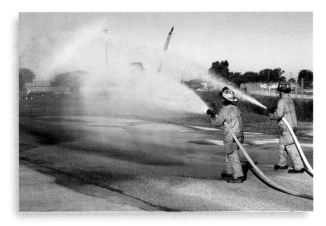

FIGURE 4-45 A comparison of fog and solid bore nozzle streams.

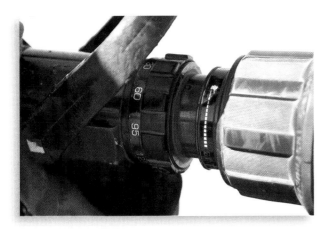

FIGURE 4-46 Some fog nozzles have adjustment rings that the firefighter can use to change the flow of water from the nozzle.

A solid bore nozzle has a gate valve for turning the water on and off. It also features an opening through which the water exits the nozzle, with no adjustment ring. Solid bore nozzles are good for providing a longer or more solid stream of water from the nozzle than is usually accomplished with a fog nozzle.

Adjusting Nozzles

Nozzles come in various designs and capabilities. Some nozzles will allow an adjustment to the pattern of the water stream coming from the tip of the nozzle, as in fog nozzles. Some also have an additional adjustment ring that allows the firefighter to adjust the flow of water (measured in gpm). This additional adjustment ring lets the firefighter change the flow to suit his or her needs (Figure 4-46). Additionally, you can reduce the flow coming out of the nozzle by slightly closing the gate valve. This is an easy way to adjust

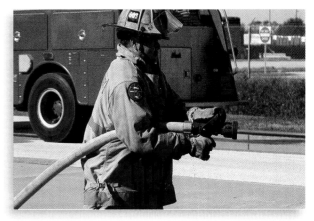

FIGURE 4-47 Proper hand grip and positioning with a small attack line.

the gpm flow if there is no regular adjustment ring on the nozzle.

Holding Nozzles

Hold the nozzle waist-high at your side, with the hose under your arm and one hand either on the body of the nozzle (for nozzles without a pistol grip) or on the pistol grip; your other hand should be on the gate valve control (the bale) or the twist valve, depending on the style nozzle you are using (Figure 4-47). The hose should trail out behind you. Be ready to shut off the nozzle, especially if you trip and fall. Make sure the nozzle is closed before you pass the hose to another person or lay it down.

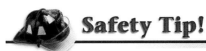 **Safety Tip!**

Hose lines can burst while under pressure, a coupling can fail, or a nozzle is left in an open position and then the line is charged. Each of these can result in an out-of-control hose line, often called a "wild line." An out-of-control hose line is a lethal weapon. The only safe way to control a wild line is to shut it off at the pump panel.

Hose Rolls

When a fire hose is going to be stored for later use or transported to another location, it is best to roll the hose into a small bundle. We are going to describe three methods to roll fire hoses: (1) the straight roll, (2) the donut roll, and (3) the double donut roll.

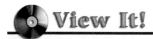
Go to the DVD, navigate to Chapter 4, and select *Straight Roll.*

➥ Practice It!

The Straight Roll

The most common method of rolling a fire hose is the straight roll. The straight roll is an easy method to roll up fire hose as well as protect the male threaded end of the hose.

Use the following technique to roll a fire hose in a straight roll:

1. Stretch the hose sections out flat. Then start at the male end, folding the male end into the hose and rolling it away from you as you proceed (Figure 4-48).

FIGURE 4-48

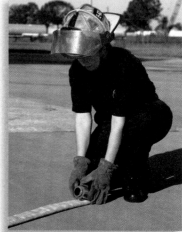

2. Continue rolling the hose until it is completely rolled up (Figure 4-49).

FIGURE 4-49

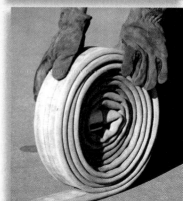

3. Grasp the hose at the top of the roll or tuck it under your arm to carry it (Figure 4-50).

FIGURE 4-50

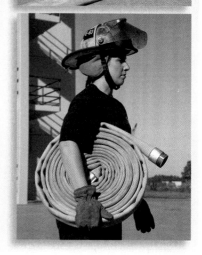

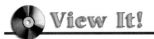

 View It!

Go to DVD, navigate to Chapter 4, and select *Donut Roll*.

Practice It!

The Donut Roll

The donut roll technique provides a single roll with both the female and male ends of the hose on the outside of the finished roll. This roll allows the firefighter to access both ends of the hose at the same time.

Use the following technique to perform a donut roll:

1. Lay the hose out flat, bringing the two couplings evenly alongside of each other (Figure 4-51).

FIGURE 4-51

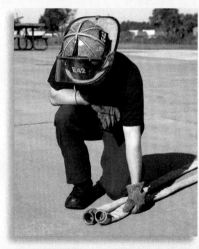

2. Return to the fold in the hose, straightening the hose as you go. With one foot at the fold, kneel and at the point where your knee touches the ground, grasp the part of the hose with the male coupling and begin to roll the hose. The hose will feed itself into one roll as you go along (Figure 4-52).

FIGURE 4-52

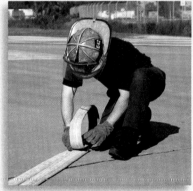

3. Finish by straightening the roll. The male end will be protected by the overlap of the female side of the hose (Figure 4-53).

FIGURE 4-53

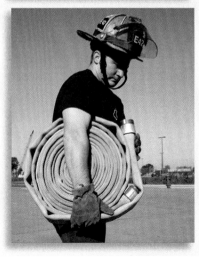

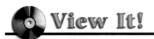

View It!

Go to the DVD, navigate to Chapter 4, and select *Double Donut Roll.*

Practice It!

The Double Donut Roll

A good way to roll a hose and provide a smaller profile with a rolled hose is the double donut roll. This roll is easy to do and results in both ends of the hose on the outside of the roll.

Use the following technique to create a double donut roll:

1. Lay the hose out flat, bringing the two couplings evenly alongside of each other (Figure 4-54).

FIGURE 4-54

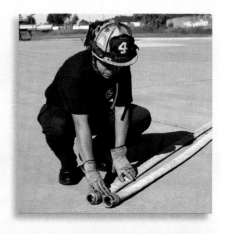

2. Return to the folded end of the two sides and fold the middle, rolling two rolls at the same time (Figure 4-55). Continue rolling the hose over a loop of webbing or rope that can serve as a hand grip later.

FIGURE 4-55

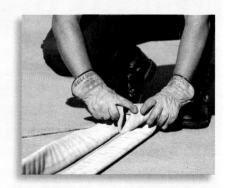

3. Finish rolling the hose and you will have a lower-profile, twin donut roll that is easy to roll out and provides both ends of the hose to the firefighter (Figure 4-56).

FIGURE 4-56

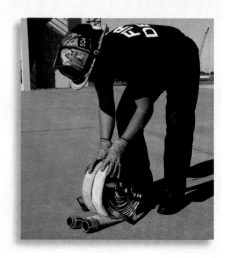

—Continued

A second method, the self-locking double donut roll, is accomplished with the following steps:

1. Lay the hose out flat, bringing the two couplings evenly alongside of each other, with two loops folded at the beginning of the roll (Figure 4-57).

FIGURE 4-57

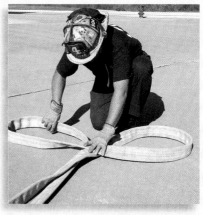

2. After the hose is rolled up, pass one loop into the other to create a convenient carry loop (Figure 4-58).

FIGURE 4-58

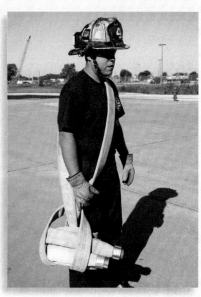

Hose Carry

The usual method for quickly and safely gathering an uncharged (unfilled) fire hose and moving it into the fire scene is the shoulder carry. Dragging couplings across the ground will cause undue wear and will likely cause damage to the couplings. Don't do it.

 View It!

Go to the DVD, navigate to Chapter 4, and select *Hose Carry Technique*.

 Practice It!

Hose Carry Technique

Use the following method to quickly gather and carry a fire hose:

1. Begin at one coupling of a section of fire hose, placing a loop of the hose over your shoulder with the coupling in front (Figure 4-59).

FIGURE 4-59

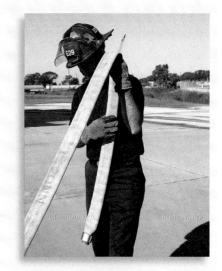

2. Continue looping the hose until all sections of it are draped over your shoulder and the end coupling is off the ground.

3. You are now ready to move the hose to the desired location (Figure 4-60).

FIGURE 4-60

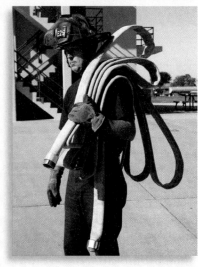

—Continued

An alternative method to carry empty hose is accomplished with the following steps:

1. Place the hose on its edge on the ground (Figure 4-61).

FIGURE 4-61

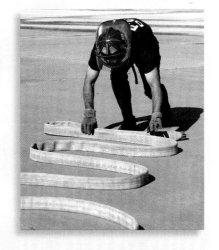

2. Bunch the hose together in the middle of the loops (Figure 4-62).

FIGURE 4-62

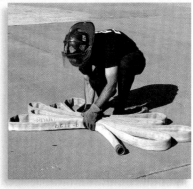

3. Lift and place the hose on your hip or shoulder and carry it to the desired location (Figure 4-63).

FIGURE 4-63

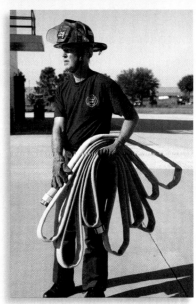

General Care of Fire Hose

The first step in picking up or putting away fire hose is to bleed the water pressure from the hose after the line has been shut off at the fire apparatus. Next, disconnect the nozzle. Then disconnect the hose sections. Finally, walk along the hose, placing it over your shoulder or raising it to your waist, helping the water drain as you walk the line.

Depending upon the practices of your department, the hose is then either placed back on the unit as a hose load, or rolled and returned to the station for storage or cleaning prior to being loaded on the apparatus. Follow the manufacturer's directions and department procedures for washing the fire hose.

After the hose is cleaned and rinsed, it can be placed on its side and allowed to dry. Some facilities may have hose-drying towers or hose-drying machines on which to place wet hose for drying. Make sure to check the hose and couplings for any obvious damage as you wash and maintain it. Look for frayed jacket material and other damage like burns and holes in the jacket of the hose. Check couplings for damaged threads, deformed or damaged sleeves and swivels, and missing gaskets.

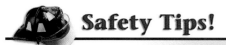 Safety Tips!

Follow these safety tips when working with a charged and flowing fire attack line:

- It is safest to shut off the flow of water before repositioning a line. However, if you must move and flow water at the same time, be ready to shut down the line quickly at the nozzle if you fall or direct the flow into other firefighters. Keep your hand on the bale.
- Hoses flow a large volume of water at high pressures. Directing this flow at fellow firefighters can cause serious injuries, especially from straight streams of water flowing from the nozzle.
- It is preferable to have a second firefighter backing up and assisting the firefighter on the nozzle.
- When you shut down your attack line, be sure to notify your supervisor that you have done so. Your supervisor will notify the driver of the apparatus.

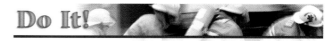 Do It!

Hose Work

Hose work is a fundamental part of firefighting. Although you won't be advancing a line for an interior attack at this point in your training, you may be asked to deploy a line to the edge of the safe zone while the interior firefighters prepare for entry. You may also be ordered to operate an exterior hose stream. Like most fundamentals in the Fire Service, there are a few hose fundamentals that must be followed to ensure the safety and welfare of everyone involved. First, never pass a kink in a hose without straightening it. Second, when on the nozzle, keep your hand on the shutoff bale and be ready to immediately close or open the flow when asked. Third, open and close all valves slowly and deliberately to avoid water hammers.

Prove It

Knowledge Assessment

Signed Documentation Tear-Out Sheet

Exterior Operations Level Firefighter—Chapter 4

Name: _____

Fill out the ten-question quiz below, the Knowledge Assessment Sheet, by circling the correct answer for each question. When finished, sign it and give to your instructor/Company Officer for his or her signature. Turn in this Knowledge Assessment Sheet to the proper person as part of the documentation that you have completed your training for this chapter.

1. The fire attack hose line system begins at the _____ and ends when the stream of water coming from the end of the nozzle effectively reaches the base of the fire.
   a. nozzle
   b. apparatus pump panel
   c. fire hydrant
   d. base of the fire

2. The size of the fittings, couplings, and hose appliances that water passes through can _____ the volume of water and pressure of the stream as it flows out of the nozzle.
   a. increase
   b. have no affect on
   c. reduce
   d. eliminate

3. The inside diameter of small attack lines is _____ .
   a. ¾ inch to 2 inches
   b. 2 to 3 inches
   c. ¾ to 1¾ inches
   d. 1 to 3 inches

4. Booster hose couplings usually require a special type of spanner wrench called a Barway spanner wrench for disconnecting and connecting the couplings.
   a. True
   b. False

5. Most couplings are designed to screw together in a _____ direction. They should be tightened hand-tight.
   a. Clockwise
   b. Counterclockwise

6. Unlike booster lines, the 1-inch jacketed line needs to be _____ before it is loaded.
   a. disconnected
   b. flowed
   c. rolled
   d. drained

7. _____ are used to tighten and loosen hose couplings.

   a. Hose adapters

   b. Water thieves

   c. Spanner wrenches

   d. Gate valves

8. The _____ usually takes in water from a larger supply, like a 2½-inch or 3-inch supply, and then divides it into two smaller hose lines.

   a. gated nozzle

   b. hose adapter

   c. gated wye

   d. hose divider

9. Nozzles should be held waist-high at one's side, under the arm, with one hand either on the body of the nozzle (for nozzles without a hand grip) or on the hand grip; the other hand should be on the valve.

   a. True

   b. False

10. The first step in putting away fire hose is to _____ .

   a. disconnect the nozzle

   b. disconnect the hose sections

   c. bleed off excess water pressure

   d. drain the hose

Student Signature and Date _____   Instructor/Company Officer Signature and Date _____

104

Prove It

Skills Assessment
Exterior Operations Level Firefighter—Chapter 4

Name: _____

Fill out the Skills Assessment Sheet below. Have your instructor/Company Officer check off and initial each skill you demonstrate. When finished, sign it and give to your instructor/Company Officer for his or her signature. Turn in this Skills Assessment Sheet to the proper person as part of the documentation that you have completed your training for this chapter.

Skill	Completed	Initials
1. Describe the components of a fire attack hose line system.	_____	_____
2. Demonstrate how to connect and disconnect hose lines.	_____	_____
3. Describe the application of different hose tools and accessories used with attack lines.	_____	_____
4. Demonstrate methods for rolling and carrying fire hose.	_____	_____
5. Explain good techniques for hose maintenance and care.	_____	_____
6. Explain and demonstrate how fire nozzles operate.	_____	_____
7. Demonstrate how to deploy and load booster lines.	_____	_____
8. Demonstrate how to properly hold and use a flowing booster hose.	_____	_____
9. Demonstrate how to deploy and load other jacketed attack lines.	_____	_____
10. Demonstrate how to hold and use a flowing small attack line.	_____	_____

Student Signature and Date _____   Instructor/Company Officer Signature and Date _____

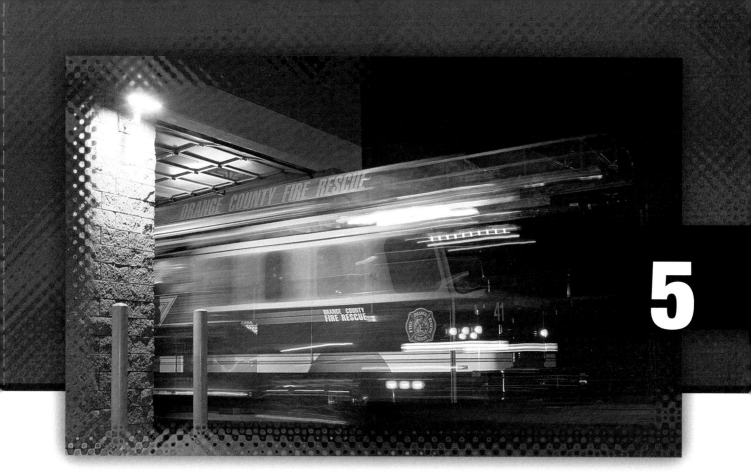

5

Response Safety and Vehicle Crashes

What You Will Learn in This Chapter

In this chapter you will learn actions you can take to help you remain safe while on the roadway, both as a driver and while working at the scene of an emergency. You will learn your responsibilities for responding to the fire station, riding in an emergency vehicle, and safely setting up a proper traffic safety system. We will also cover some of the primary elements of an Emergency Vehicle Operator's Course (EVOC).

What You Will Be Able to Do

After reading this chapter and practicing the skills in a classroom setting, you will be able to

1. Respond safely to the fire station in your personally owned vehicle (POV).

2. Demonstrate how to safely get on the fire apparatus and the use of seatbelts.

3. Demonstrate safely getting off the fire apparatus and awaiting instructions from the Company Officer.

4. Demonstrate proper personal protective clothing for daytime and nighttime traffic control operations.

5. Demonstrate how to safely deploy traffic cones to establish traffic safety lanes for the fire apparatus and emergency workers.

6. Describe the different benchmarks to be encountered on a typical vehicle crash scene in which there is no entrapment.

7. Assist in identifying and handling hazards typically present on a vehicle crash scene.

8. Identify hot, warm, and cold zones of operation on a vehicle crash scene.

Reality!

Wear Your Seatbelt!

Firefighter safety and health is the cornerstone of everything we do. If you are to continue assisting people at the myriad of emergencies that you will encounter, you must maintain a safe and healthy attitude for every alarm.

Safety Lesson

A NIOSH Report

On January 21, 2002, a 26-year-old firefighter was fatally ejected from his personal vehicle, which he crashed while responding to a house fire. The 8-year veteran firefighter served in a volunteer fire department with 22 firefighters serving a population of approximately 5000 in an area of about 35 square miles.

According to the state police report, the firefighter was ejected through the sunroof of his SUV during one of three complete rollovers. The police report indicates that the victim was not wearing his seatbelt at the time of the crash and that an "unsafe speed" was a contributing factor to his death.

Follow-Up

The NIOSH Investigative Report (#F2002-04) recommended: "The fire department shall develop standard operating procedures for safely driving fire department vehicles during nonemergency travel and emergency response and shall include specific criteria for vehicle speed, crossing intersections, traversing railroad grade crossings, and the use of emergency warning devices. Such procedures for emergency response shall emphasize that the safe arrival of fire department vehicle at the emergency is the first priority." The report went on to recommend that fire departments ensure that all personnel responding in privately owned vehicles follow the same practices.

Driving Safety

After heart-related fatalities, vehicle accidents involving firefighters are the second leading cause of firefighter deaths. Vehicle crashes in both personally owned vehicles (POVs) and emergency appa-

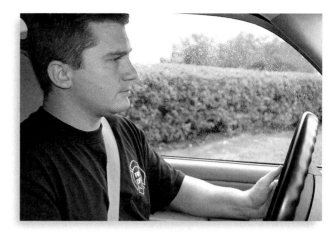

FIGURE 5-1 Whether driving to the fire station to work or responding to an emergency call, always drive responsibly and safely.

ratus happen far too often and must be reduced through proper driver training for members of the Fire Department.

Responding to an Emergency Call in Your Privately Owned Vehicle

As a firefighter, perhaps one of the most dangerous things you will do on a regular basis is to drive to the emergency. In many jurisdictions, especially in volunteer fire departments, firefighters respond in their POVs to the fire station in order to take emergency apparatus to an emergency. They may be required to respond directly to the emergency scene in their private vehicles (Figure 5-1). Even if you are going to and from the station, you still need to be careful. Whatever your destination, you need to be aware of the potential dangers and how to minimize those dangers.

Defensive Driving

We recommend all new recruits attend a **defensive driving** course and eventually an **Emergency Vehicle Operator's Course (EVOC)** before driving any fire or rescue apparatus. A defensive driving course, which also instructs course attendees about departmental, local, and state-level laws and regulations related to private vehicle response, should be given to new firefighters as soon as possible. The basic rules of the road and the laws of physics apply to POVs as well as to fire apparatus. Later in this chapter we'll discuss these components while explaining an EVOC training program.

Defining a True Emergency

Before talking about the causes of many fatal vehicle crashes for firefighters, we need to talk briefly about what defines a true emergency. Many emergency driving rules and regulations assume that the responder is responding to a true emergency. Unfortunately, many firefighters respond to the fire station for incidents that are not true emergencies and, in the process, expose themselves and the public to unnecessary risks.

The Emergency Vehicle Operator's Course developed by the U.S. Department of Transportation (DOT) defines a true emergency as *a situation in which there is a high probability of death or serious injury to an individual or significant property loss, and action by an emergency vehicle operator may reduce the seriousness of the situation.* The majority of fire department call-outs are not true emergencies, and firefighters who drive to the fire station or the emergency scene in their POVs usually do not need to drive as if it were a true emergency.

In today's world, many firefighters are liable for and are charged with negligence if they are involved in a vehicle crash. In simple terms, negligence is either the act of doing something that a reasonable or prudent person would not do, or not doing something that such a person would do in a given situation. The bottom line is that driving to an emergency does not make you immune from being prosecuted if you fail to follow traffic laws.

Causes of Fatal Vehicle Crashes

Statistics show that the main causes of fatal vehicle crashes in which firefighters use their private vehicles are driving too fast, not using seatbelts, rollover crashes, crashes at intersections, the use of alcohol, and head-on crashes (Figure 5-2).

Excessive Speed

Almost every crash studied involved some level of speeding. Firefighters should not exceed the speed

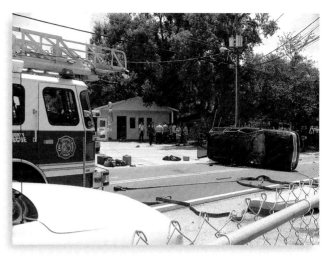

FIGURE 5-2 Firefighter deaths in crashes are caused mainly by driving too fast, not using seatbelts, rollovers, crashes at intersections, the use of alcohol, and head-on collisions.

limit when responding in their private vehicles. Time can be gained by using safe, efficient routes and practicing safe driving habits. Speedy, careless driving risks lives and should always be avoided.

Lack of Seatbelt Use

Not using a seatbelt has contributed to many fatalities. Firefighters should set an example for the community by following the law and wearing their seatbelts at all times (Figure 5-3). It is a proven fact that seatbelt use reduces injury and death in traffic crashes, and basically eliminates the chance of ejection from a vehicle.

Rollover Crashes

Firefighters must maintain control of their vehicles. No one driving any type of vehicle should drive at speeds that cause the vehicle to overturn. Because they are tall, many types of fire apparatus are top-heavy and tend to tip over if driven too fast through a curve. This is especially true of tanker/tenders. In addition, because all kinds of fire apparatus are heavy, a contributing factor to many rollover crashes is simply running off the pavement onto a soft shoulder of the road, where the tires dig in and make the truck flip, or the driver overcorrects and causes the vehicle to roll over.

Crashes at Intersections

Many crashes occur at intersections. During a response, firefighters must recognize the dangers of passing through an intersection. When driving with

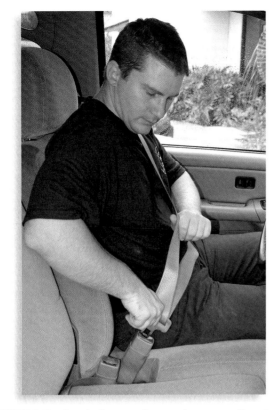

FIGURE 5-3 Seatbelts save lives—always use them!

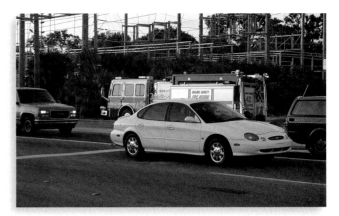

FIGURE 5-4 Taking a right-of-way that is not yours can result in head-on collisions that have deadly results.

your sirens and lights flashing, you are merely asking the public to allow you to proceed. However, if they do not yield to you, you do not have the right to claim the right-of-way. Before entering the intersection, you must stop with the signal, whether it is a yield sign, a stop sign, or a stop light. This driving rule must be followed with no exceptions, whether you are in a POV or a fire apparatus with lights and sirens in use. Always follow local, state, and fire department regulations when driving your POV to the fire station or the emergency scene. *No* emergency is worth the death of or injury to firefighters or innocent civilians in the community. Also use extreme care at railroad crossings. Remember: Trains don't stop on a dime and they can't yield to you.

Alcohol Use

Firefighters are not available for service if they have consumed any alcohol within eight hours prior to an alarm. Any violation of this rule is a clear and serious act of negligence.

Head-On Crashes

Head-on crashes between vehicles can occur when firefighters take a right-of-way that is not theirs (Figure 5-4). Again, firefighters must wait for the public to yield the right-of-way. Driving into oncoming traffic

is extremely dangerous to firefighters and the public and is not allowable under any circumstances.

Private Vehicle Use

Firefighters who receive alarms off duty and have family members with them in their private vehicle are not available to respond to the calls. Family members have been injured in crashes involving firefighters responding to the fire station or the emergency scene with family members in their POVs.

Your fire department will have an established policy regarding private vehicle use. This standard guideline includes information about when and how to respond safely. The policy also includes response requirements under different conditions and techniques. These requirements include speed limits, proper intersection clearance, the use of warning devices and safety devices, seatbelts, and driving practices in bad weather or limited visibility. If safe driving guidelines are not followed, the department should impose severe consequences.

Safe Driving Attitude

A safe driving attitude is an important part of driving safely. It is also crucial to prospective firefighters. Firefighters who are good drivers have the following qualities:

- They respect the danger involved in driving any vehicle.
- They respect other drivers on the roadway and follow all traffic laws, including speed limits, road sign directions, and signals.
- They always have all safety equipment and seatbelts in use while driving.
- They follow fire department rules and regulations regarding driving.

Driver Training

As a firefighter applicant, your driving record will be a factor in your membership in the Fire Department. Many younger drivers have not been driving long enough to gain good experience and respect for the road. This lack of experience can be compensated for with proper and extensive driver training, including an Emergency Vehicle Operator's Course and Collision Avoidance Training.

Emergency Vehicle Operator's Course (EVOC)

One of the first things you will want to do after you have completed your recruit training is to drive and operate various fire department apparatus (Figure 5-5). It is the nature of the business, the need to bring staffing and equipment to the emergency scene, that dictates that driving apparatus is such a high priority. Before driving any fire apparatus, you should receive training in defensive driving and you should also take a course in emergency vehicle operations. You must be certified not only to drive emergency vehicles, but to be physically and mentally ready to operate them.

Fire and rescue apparatus are bigger, heavier, and much more complex than regular automobiles, SUVs, or pickup trucks. Because of their weight, they take much more time and effort to stop. Most modern fire apparatus have antilock braking systems that help you maintain control of the truck during emergency braking.

Using a safe following distance is a key driving safety technique. There are two methods for calculating a safe following distance. The first method is the 3-second rule. This rule requires that you pick a marker—perhaps a tree or a post on the side of the roadway—and begin a count of three ("1001, 1002, 1003") when the vehicle in front of you passes the marker; you should not pass the marker before having reached the third count. If you are responding to an emergency, this distance (the traveling time) should be increased to allow you more reaction time. The second method is to estimate apparatus lengths. Estimate one apparatus length between your vehicle and the vehicle in front of you for every 10 miles per hour that you are traveling.

Fire apparatus need regular maintenance and inspection (Figure 5-6). Their fuel levels must be maintained at the ready, which means approximately three-quarters full or more at all times. EVOC training will also teach you how to perform a routine safety check of the fire apparatus, including inspection pro-

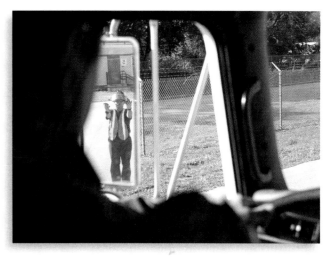

FIGURE 5-5 Driving any fire apparatus requires training and physical and mental ability.

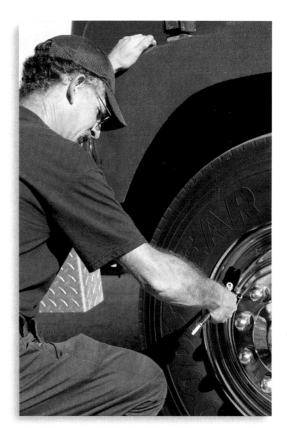

FIGURE 5-6 An EVOC course will teach you vehicle safety inspection as well as safe driving skills.

cedures for things such as mirrors, windshield wipers, emergency brakes, signaling devices, and specific machinery and equipment. Vehicle problems must be repaired as soon as possible and should always be reported to the appropriate officer as soon as they are discovered. You must document any vehicle problems quickly and accurately.

Safety Tip!

Never operate a Fire Department vehicle unless you have received the proper training and have had sufficient time to become familiar with driving that vehicle. You should be certified by your department as having passed all required training and orientation before driving any vehicles.

Classroom Training

EVOC training includes a classroom portion in which students learn about many aspects of driving that they had perhaps never thought of previously. Students learn about the attitudes and experience necessary to operate an emergency vehicle. Driving skills that are adequate with a POV are not sufficient with fire apparatus. You need to be much more careful and learn to anticipate potential road dangers while responding. Your number one priority is your safety and the safety of the crew on the apparatus. You are also responsible for the safety of the general public. The driver of the fire apparatus is the person ultimately responsible for its safe operation.

Legal Requirements

Operators of emergency vehicles are subject to all traffic laws unless they are specially exempted from certain laws while responding to an emergency (Figure 5-7). Even with those exemptions, they are still accountable for their driving decisions and actions. As noted earlier, a red light and a siren only "ask" others to allow you to go against traffic signals. They do not give you the right-of-way or permission to break traffic rules such as speed limits.

Operators need to comply with state, local, and Fire Department requirements for training and licensing. These requirements can include defensive driver and EVOC training, a valid driver's license, minimum age requirements, and a good driving record.

Physical Forces

Many forces act upon an emergency vehicle as it speeds down the roadway to the emergency scene. How these various physical forces affect the apparatus are addressed in the EVOC classroom. These forces include velocity, friction, inertia and momentum, and centrifugal force.

Velocity   Velocity is the speed of an apparatus. The faster a unit travels, the more force is needed to slow it down and stop it. The total **stopping distance** of an apparatus is the reaction time plus the braking distance (Figure 5-8).

■ KEY WORD ■

stopping distance   The total distance needed to stop a vehicle. This distance is calculated by adding the reaction time plus the braking distance.

Friction   The term *friction* applies to the brakes used to stop the apparatus and the grip of the wheels to the surface of the roadway. Fire truck brake components are much more substantial than those of regular ve-

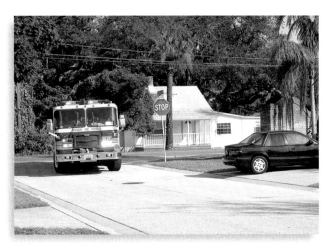

FIGURE 5-7   When driving to an emergency, even though you may be exempt from certain driving regulations, you are still accountable for your driving decisions and actions.

Reaction Time + Braking Distance =

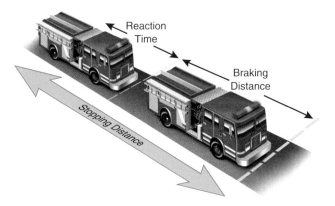

FIGURE 5-8   Reaction time is the time it takes to put your foot on the brake. Braking distance is the time it takes the brakes to stop the truck. The total of the two is the stopping distance for a vehicle.

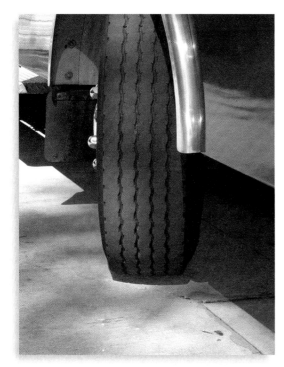

FIGURE 5-9   Fire apparatus tires and wheels are big. Their large size provides more surface contact with the roadway than the tires and wheels of smaller vehicles.

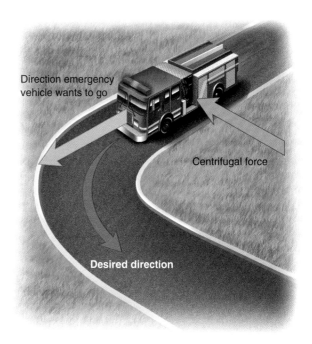

FIGURE 5-10   You must slow down when driving in a curve so that centrifugal force doesn't "push" the vehicle you're driving off the roadway.

hicles. Their tires and wheels are also bigger in order to provide more surface contact with the roadway (Figure 5-9).

Momentum and Inertia   **Momentum** is to the force that builds in an object in motion that tends to keep it in motion. This law applies to moving vehicles such as fire apparatus. The term **inertia** refers to how a moving fire apparatus tends to keep moving when started and to stay still when stopped. Fire apparatus have more momentum than lighter and smaller vehicles. It takes more force to stop them, and they hit with more force than smaller vehicles when involved in a collision.

■ KEY WORDS ■

momentum   The law of nature that describes the force that builds in an object in motion that keeps it moving. The more velocity an object has, the more momentum it has and thus the more force it will take to slow down that object and stop it.

inertia   The law of nature that states that objects set into motion tend to remain in motion and objects that are stationary tend to remain stationary unless acted upon by another object.

Centrifugal Force   **Centrifugal force** the force that affects an object traveling in an arc or circle, such as a vehicle driving on a curve in the roadway. As the vehicle goes around the curve, centrifugal force acting on the vehicle tends to make the vehicle move outside the edge of the curve (Figure 5-10).

■ KEY WORD ■

centrifugal force   The force that acts upon an object traveling in an arc or circle that pushes the object away from the center of the arc or circle.

Practical Driver Training

Practical driver training includes driving a road course and being tested on the operation of equipment specific to the fire apparatus (Figure 5-11).

Safety rules that you must follow when driving any fire apparatus on a practice driving course include the following:

- When on the driving course, you should always have someone with you.
- A common signal term like *stop* or *halt,* agreed to beforehand, should be used to stop the driving operation if a safety concern develops.

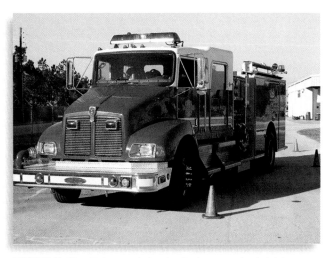

FIGURE 5-11 Driver training includes practical driving as well as the operation of the equipment on that specific apparatus.

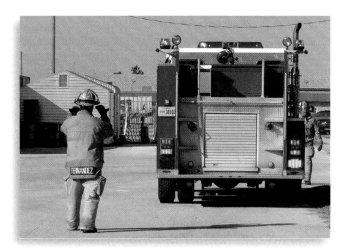

FIGURE 5-12 When backing up the apparatus, always have a second person at the rear of the apparatus to watch for hazards and safety concerns.

- When backing up the apparatus, always have a second person at the rear of the apparatus to watch for hazards and safety concerns (Figure 5-12).
- Practice when road surface conditions are good, never speed, and follow the manufacturer's recommendations for driving the particular fire apparatus.

You will need to complete a timed and graded driving test that includes the following exercises and maneuvers:

- A serpentine exercise
- An alley dock maneuver
- The opposite alley exercise
- A diminishing clearance exercise
- A straight line exercise
- A turnaround maneuver
- A lane change exercise

Other driving exercises may be added to the driving course, depending on the requirements of your fire department and the specific fire apparatus for which you are being trained.

Collision Avoidance Training (CAT)

Another driver training course that you may be required to take is **Collision Avoidance Training (CAT)**. This course teaches you how to react when you lose control of your vehicle. It also teaches safe driving habits, especially under inclement roadway conditions such as ice and rain. This course is taught mainly to law enforcement officers, but your department may require you to attend such a course.

KEY WORD

Collision Avoidance Training (CAT) Driver training that specializes in gaining control of vehicles under different adverse situations and roadway conditions.

Riding Safety

Responding to emergency calls is one of the most common things you will do as a firefighter (Figure 5-13). When the alarm is received and the firefighting crew assembles around the apparatus, many things happen simultaneously.

The driver quickly scans the apparatus as he approaches it. He looks for any obstructions near the vehicle, checking that all auxiliary plugs and hoses are detached and the wheel chocks have been pulled out of place. He also checks for people in and around the vehicle, as well as for any equipment that is out of place and compartment doors that are open.

The Company Officer checks to see if the crew is getting ready and listens for additional information on the call. She begins formulating the response route and a plan of action to handle the potential emergency situation.

The firefighters don their PPE and prepare to board the apparatus. It is important that you don your basic protective clothing *before* you board the truck, with two exceptions: (1) you are the driver, or (2) the bulky clothing will impede the proper wearing of your seatbelt. In these cases, don the equipment immediately after arriving on the scene.

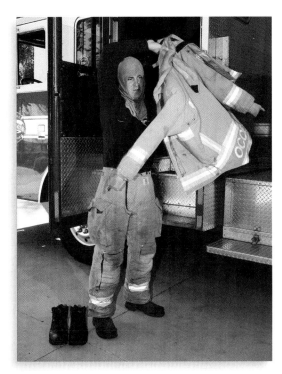

FIGURE 5-13 Safely responding to emergencies on the fire apparatus is one of the fun points of being a firefighter.

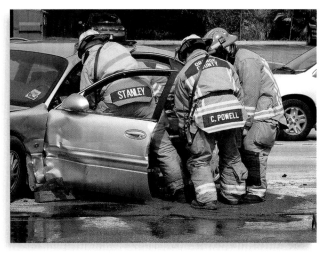

FIGURE 5-14 PPE for vehicle crash incidents should start with protection similar to the gear used for structural firefighting. This gear includes head, eye, hand, body, and foot protection.

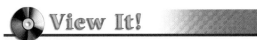

Go to the DVD, navigate to Chapter 5, and select *Working Around Large Vehicles Safely.*

Personal Protective Equipment and Clothing

The level of protective clothing will be dictated by the type of the incident. In general, PPE for vehicle crash incidents should start with protection similar to the gear used for structural firefighting. This gear includes head, eye, hand, body, and foot protection. It is also important to maintain body protection. Many agencies allow the use of full-length, long-sleeve jumpsuits with some degree of fire resistance. If the situation is more hazardous, firefighters may need full PPE for structural firefighting, including an SCBA. Remember that you should wear a bright, reflective traffic vest whenever you are working near traffic (Figure 5-14).

Hearing Protection

A component of your PPE that is specific to responding is hearing protection. Hearing loss is a very common risk in loud work environments. Most modern fire apparatus have an intercom system that provides a protective headset. This headset allows you to hear radio traffic as well as talk among the members in the cab of the truck while responding. The headset eliminates the extra noise associated with sirens and loud horns. Make sure to put on the headset as soon as your seatbelt is buckled.

Working Around Large Vehicles Safely

Fire apparatus present several blind spots to the driver that aren't always obvious to individuals working near them. It is important that you respect these blind spots. Never turn your back on a moving vehicle, especially when it is moving in a tight area, such as when backing into a firehouse (Figure 5-15). You will notice that most fire trucks have a backup alarm that sounds whenever the truck is in reverse. While this signal is a clear warning of potential danger, many firefighters become complacent and are subsequently injured.

Never try to grab or get on or get off of a moving fire truck (Figure 5-16). This may sound obvious, but several firefighters have been injured or even killed while trying to board a truck as it was rolling out of the station.

Never ride on the tailboard or running boards of a fire truck. Although it is no longer a common practice to ride on the tailboard, it is often tempting to step up on it when the truck is backing up a long way or moving a short distance on the scene. *DON'T DO IT!*

A common type of accident involving fire trucks occurs while the truck is being backed up. Most departments require a backup spotter to help avoid these incidents. If you are the spotter, it is important that you remain visible and in a safe position while directing the driver. Wear your Class III reflective

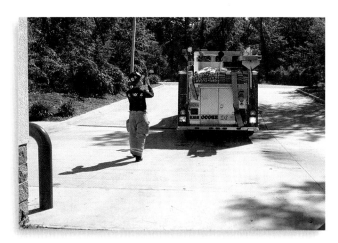

FIGURE 5-15 Fire apparatus have blind spots to the driver that aren't always obvious to individuals working near them. It is important that you respect these blind spots. Never turn your back on a moving vehicle, especially when it is moving in a tight area.

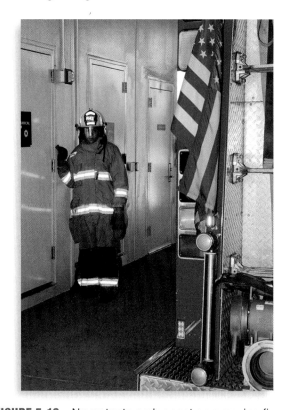

FIGURE 5-16 Never try to grab or get on a moving fire truck. Several firefighters have been injured or even killed while trying to board the truck as it is rolling out of the station.

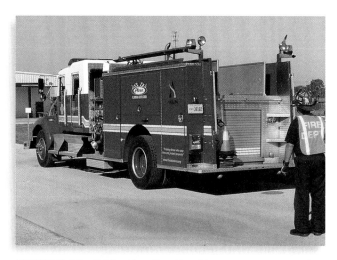

FIGURE 5-17 While directing the driver, you must remain visible and in a safe position. You must wear your Class III reflective traffic vest and a helmet, and you should stand so that you can see the driver in the outside rearview mirror.

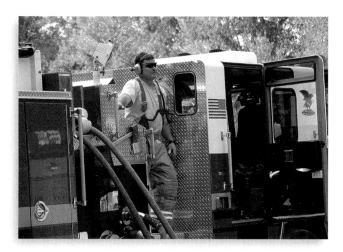

FIGURE 5-18 Wear hearing protection if you are going to be working near a pumping truck for an extended period of time.

traffic vest and a helmet and stand so that you can see the driver in the outside rearview mirror (Figure 5-17). Never cross behind a moving truck. If you must cross over to the other side of the vehicle to check clearance, signal the driver to stop and then walk to the other side. When possible, use a portable radio for better communication with the driver.

When the fire truck is in the pumping mode, the engine runs at high revolutions, causing a lot of noise. Make sure to wear hearing protection if you are going to be working near the truck for an extended period of time (Figure 5-18).

Response Safety

Response safety involves many factors. As a firefighter, you will need to know how to work safely when responding to calls as well as when assisting at vehicle crash scenes.

Responding to Calls Safely

As a firefighter, you need to check your side of the apparatus as you quickly put on your protective clothing. Follow these steps to respond safely to calls:

1. Before you leave for the call, close any open compartments and check for any obstructions under and near the unit (Figure 5-19).

   FIGURE 5-19

   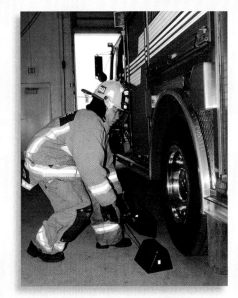

2. Prior to leaving, make sure any onlookers stand clear of the apparatus.

3. The extent and type of protective clothing you need depends on the type of emergency and the policy of your Company Officer and your department.

4. Safely climb onto the apparatus and sit down in your designated position. You will have a personal accountability system (PAS) tag. Hand this tag to your Company Officer as soon as you get onto the fire apparatus (Figure 5-20).

   FIGURE 5-20

   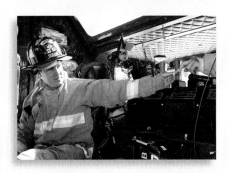

5. Put on your seatbelt and check the area around you for any loose tools or unsecured equipment (Figure 5-21).

   FIGURE 5-21

   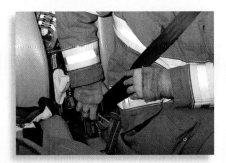

6. Signal to the driver and the Company Officer up front that you are belted in and ready to go. The apparatus will leave the station. It is extremely important that you remain seated and with your seatbelt in place during the entire response.

Safety Tips!

Follow these safety rules when responding to emergencies:

- Never disconnect your seatbelt while the vehicle is in motion, even to put on additional gear such as air packs.
- Never stand while riding on a fire apparatus. If you arrive too late to sit in an approved seat, then dismount and get on the next apparatus ready to respond.
- Wear hearing protection or communication devices while responding (Figure 5-22).
- Responding to an emergency is not a time for "horseplay." Not behaving professionally will cause undue distraction for the Company Officer and the driver.
- Never dismount the apparatus without checking with your Company Officer.
- When dismounting from the apparatus, always check in all directions. Look for traffic and obstructions or hazards on the ground below (Figure 5-23). Carefully step off the apparatus, using the handholds provided to steady yourself.

Assisting at Vehicle Crash Scenes

One of the most hazardous areas in which an emergency worker can work is on or near a roadway. Working around a vehicle crash scene is dangerous, regardless of the size of the incident. Moving traffic always poses a threat to emergency workers working in the roadway. The crashed vehicles present several threats to your

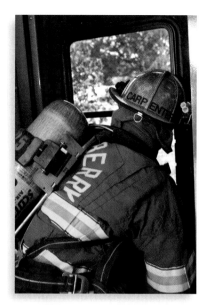

FIGURE 5-23 Always look in all directions before dismounting from the apparatus. Look for traffic and obstructions or hazards on the ground below. Carefully step off the apparatus, using the handholds provided.

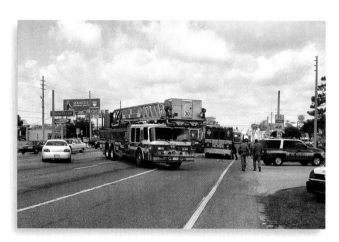

FIGURE 5-24 Many firefighters and rescue workers are injured or killed by being struck by other vehicles while they are off the apparatus and working in the streets.

safety, including the unstable vehicles themselves, dangerous fluids on the ground, and many other hazards. To organize the activities around the crash scene, we generally establish two types of work zones: the traffic control zone and the work safety zone.

Traffic Control

An important reality of firefighting is that you will probably respond to more incidents involving motor vehicle crashes and roadway emergencies than you will to structure fires. Annually, many firefighters and rescue workers are injured or killed by vehicles while they are off the apparatus and working in the streets (Figure 5-24).

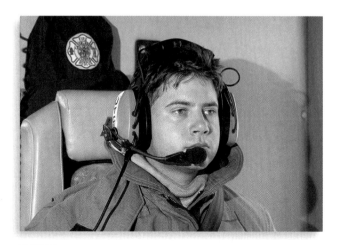

FIGURE 5-22 When responding to an emergency, wear hearing protection or communication devices.

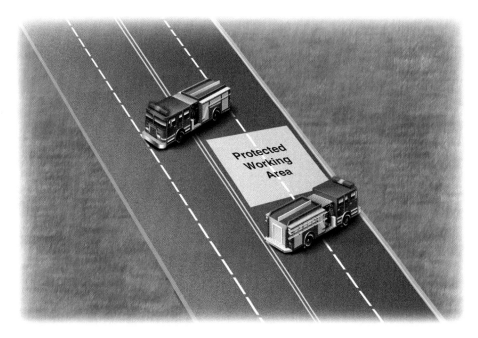

FIGURE 5-25 The apparatus should be parked so that it serves as a shield to protect everyone from flowing traffic.

The driver of the fire apparatus and your Company Officer will already know how to properly position the apparatus in a **fend-off position** (Figure 5-25). This position is used to protect the emergency scene on the roadway. A good driver will park the unit safely, always applying the emergency brake and using proper emergency lights as a warning to all directions of traffic.

■ KEY WORD

fend-off position The positioning of emergency apparatus on a roadway in order to protect the temporary work area in the street by blocking it with apparatus.

The most dangerous aspect of a traffic crash scene is that traffic is still flowing around the general area. Night operations compound this situation immensely. It is essential to everyone's safety that the firefighters take immediate steps to establish a traffic control zone around the entire crash area. The first step is to park the apparatus in a fend-off position. The traffic control zone can then be established by identifying and marking it with reflective traffic cones, road flares, or other traffic control devices. It is always preferable to turn traffic control over to law enforcement as soon as possible (Figure 5-26). Doing so allows a better-qualified person to direct traffic and allows rescue team members to assist with the rescue.

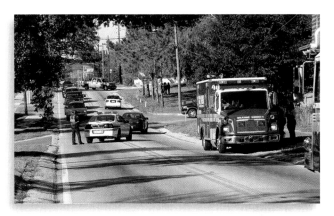

FIGURE 5-26 Turning traffic control over to law enforcement as soon as possible allows a better-qualified person to direct traffic. It also releases rescue team members to assist with the rescue.

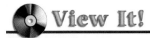 **View It!**

Go to the DVD, navigate to Chapter 5, and select *Traffic Control Safety*.

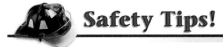 **Safety Tips!**

Traffic Control Safety When working in traffic, you should wear the appropriate protective clothing and a reflective vest.

- You should wear full protective clothing and/or a Class III vest when working near traffic. Your department will have established guidelines for you to follow that describe the minimum personal protective clothing required (Figure 5-27).
- To be seen at night, use flashlights and light the scene with portable lighting (Figure 5-28).
- Road flares can be used only when there are no flammable materials or vapors present. Do not strike a road flare without full protective clothing and eye protection in place. Make sure to get permission from your Company Officer.

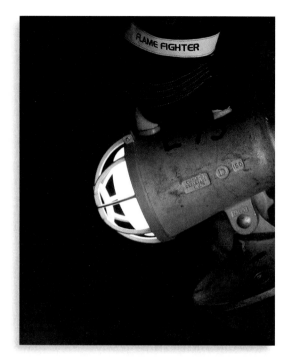

FIGURE 5-28 To be seen at night, use flashlights and light the scene with portable lighting.

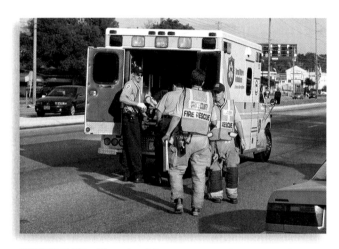

FIGURE 5-27 You should wear appropriate protective clothing and a Class III vest when working near traffic.

➡ Practice It!

Traffic Control Safety

Whenever possible, traffic control should be performed by law enforcement officers. However, in their absence, this job usually falls to firefighters. After making sure that you are wearing the appropriate protective clothing, assist in setting up traffic cones. Place them toward the traffic approaching the rear of the fire apparatus in the fend-off (blocking) position. Cones with reflective collars are recommended for night use.

1. Work in pairs where possible, especially if traffic from one direction must be stopped to allow traffic from the other direction to pass through (Figure 5-29). Communicate with your partner, preferably visually as well as by radio. Be prepared to warn the other firefighter directing traffic if a vehicle unexpectedly continues against the oncoming traffic.

FIGURE 5-29

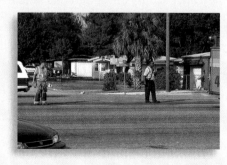

—Continued

2. Place a tapering pattern of 5 cones in a stretch of roadway at a distance of about 75 feet from the rear of the apparatus. This placement provides a transition for traffic from the present pattern to the new lane pattern established by your apparatus placement and the placement of cones (Figures 5-30 and 5-31). As an added precaution, the NFPA suggests that a DOT-approved reflective sign stating "Emergency Scene" be used for additional warning.

FIGURE 5-30

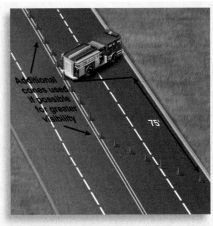

3. For multilane, large-volume traffic and limited-access freeways, place the cones farther apart, perhaps doubling the distance to 150 feet from the rear of the apparatus to the tapered end of the pattern. This placement of cones will allow motorists time to react to the lane changes and the slower speeds near the crash emergency scene (Figure 5-32).

FIGURE 5-31

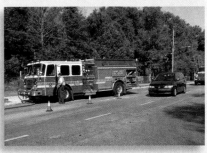

FIGURE 5-32

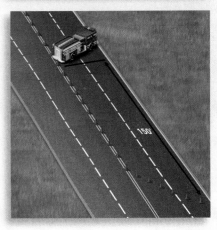

4. If conditions permit, road flares may be placed next to cones to gain motorists' attention as they approach. Road flares can help create a temporary, safe control zone in which to respond to the emergency.

5. Make sure that oncoming traffic is completely stopped before allowing the other direction of traffic to proceed.

 Safety Tips!

Use the following precautions when placing cones and controlling traffic:

- Never assume that the driver of a vehicle sees you or understands the traffic pattern requirements. Remember that many drivers are distracted, perhaps under the influence, or just don't understand the situation.
- Never stand in the traffic lanes, and be ready at all times to step out of the way of traffic.
- Keep your eye on the traffic and never turn your back on it. Face traffic when placing cones and be ready to warn others if a vehicle breaks through your blocking cones and heads for the fire apparatus (Figure 5-33).
- When walking around the corner of a unit near traffic lanes, always stop and carefully lean and look around the corner of the unit for oncoming traffic (Figure 5-34).
- Your fire department will most likely have standard guidelines for working and controlling traffic. Make sure to go over these guidelines as soon as possible when you report for you first duty.

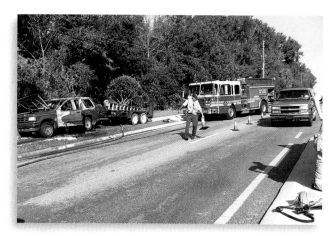

FIGURE 5-33 Face traffic when placing cones.

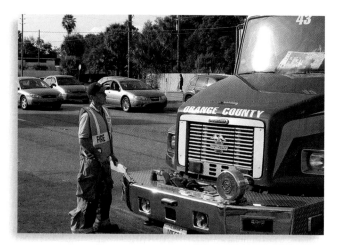

FIGURE 5-34 When walking around the corner of a unit near traffic lanes, always stop and carefully lean and look around the corner of the unit for oncoming traffic.

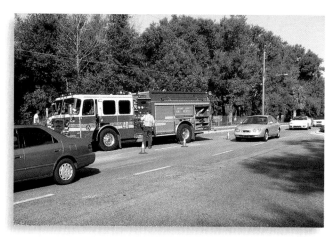

FIGURE 5-35 After safely responding to the emergency call, arriving on the scene, and setting up traffic control, the next step will be to set up a safety zone around the crash scene.

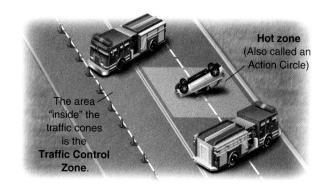

FIGURE 5-36 Safety zones include the hot zone, which immediately surrounds the crash, and the traffic control zone, which covers the area protected by traffic control devices.

Safety Zones

After safely responding to the emergency call, arriving on the scene, and setting up traffic control, you must attend to the actual vehicle crash (Figure 5-35). Your next step will be to set up a safety zone around the crash scene. At this stage in your training, we will discuss a crash emergency with injuries and no entrapment.

Establish a safe area that extends completely around the vehicles and the hazards involved. This safe area is divided into **safety zones** designated as *hot, warm,* and *cool* zones, which extend out in all directions (Figure 5-36). The extent of each zone depends on the hazards presented. Generally, the **hot zone** includes those areas immediately inside and adjacent to the involved vehicles and wreckage. The **warm zone** extends 10 to 15 feet from the vehicles and wreckage, and is commonly referred to as the **action circle.** The **cool zone** extends out from the warm zone as needed for crowd and traffic control. This zone is where tools, equipment, and extra personnel are staged until needed in the hot and warm zones.

KEY WORDS

safety zones Areas established on any emergency scene that designate the areas of operation and the level of hazard or control required. Examples of safety control zones include traffic control zones as well as *hot, warm,* and *cool* zones.

hot zone The area immediately adjacent to the patient or hazard on a crash scene.

warm zone The work area that extends 10 to 15 feet away from the crashed vehicle(s).

action circle The area encompassed by the warm zone and including the hot zone where the actual rescue activities take place.

cool zone The area beyond the warm zone on a crash scene (beyond 10 to 15 feet). Tools, equipment, and extra personnel are staged in this zone until they are needed in the hot and warm zones.

With an emphasis on personal safety, in your firefighter training you will get the skills needed to establish and maintain safety zones. These skills include scene assessment, hazard control, stabilizing heavy objects, accessing the patient, creating a path of egress for the patient, treating and removing the patient, and securing the scene afterward.

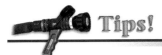 Tips!

Crash Scene Benchmarks

Crash scenes can be better understood by viewing them in stages or benchmarks:

1. *Scene size-up.* The main goal is to look for immediate hazards and the number and severity of injured patients (Figure 5-37).

FIGURE 5-37

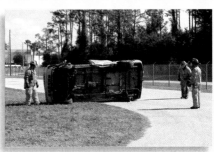

2. *Traffic control.* A traffic control zone is used to detour traffic away from the crash scene. Tools should be staged inside the protected traffic control zone (Figure 5-38).

3. *Work zones.* Work zones usually include hot, warm, and cool zones and often are marked with yellow caution tape. All firefighters who enter the hot or warm safety zones must wear appropriate PPE and must evacuate all bystanders from this area (Figure 5-39).

FIGURE 5-38

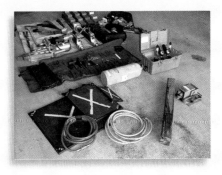

4. *Task assignments.* The Company Officer will establish a quick plan of action, advising the firefighters of his or her plan and giving work assignments.

FIGURE 5-39

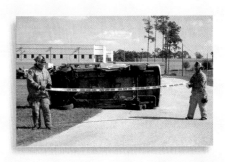

—Continued

5. *Hazard control.* Hazards are controlled as they are encountered. Vehicles carry flammable fuel and oils, and hot radiator fluids, and can also have damaged batteries that release battery acids. In addition, undeployed air bags may discharge unexpectedly (Figure 5-40). Many scene hazards, such as destabilized heavy vehicles or objects or downed power lines, can pose a serious threat to firefighters (Figure 5-41). Firefighters must therefore be aware of scene elements at all times.

FIGURE 5-40

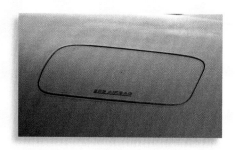

FIGURE 5-41

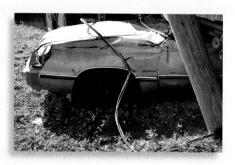

FIGURE 5-42

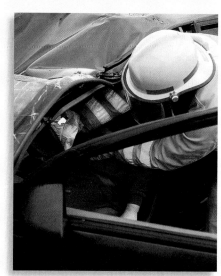

6. *Gaining access and delivering patient care.* Firefighters will gain access and provide first aid to injured individuals as soon as they can (Figure 5-42). Your job will probably involve assisting firefighters with more advanced emergency medical training or other medical personnel with packaging and removing the patients. Remember to use proper body positioning when helping to move patients, especially those who are on backboards (Figure 5-43).

FIGURE 5-43

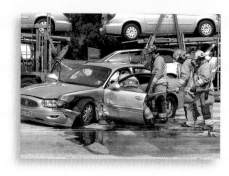

7. *Securing the scene.* Once patients have been transported to emergency facilities, secure all tools and equipment. Traffic control equipment will be returned to the fire apparatus *after* the scene is turned over to law enforcement.

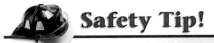

Safety Tip!

Depending on the extent of the crash and the units necessary to manage it, personnel accountability systems may be used at vehicle crash scenes to keep track of firefighters (Figure 5-44).

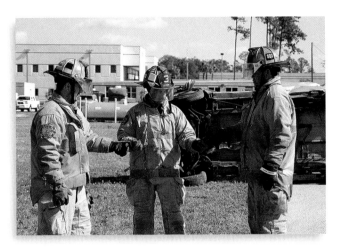

FIGURE 5-44 Personnel accountability systems are used for tracking firefighters on larger or more complicated incidents.

Do It!

Driving Safety

After actual firefighting activities, driving is the next most dangerous thing you will do as a firefighter. For this reason, we stress the importance of good driving habits. You must respond to the station or emergency in a safe manner and, above all, protect yourself, your fellow firefighters, and the community. Additional resources that are sent out to take care of a firefighter involved in a collision while responding to a call detracts from the initial emergency at hand.

Think about the importance of returning home to your family. Slow down! Stop at all signals! Wear your seatbelt! If you cannot drive safely and responsibly, then do not become a firefighter.

Knowledge Assessment

Signed Documentation Tear-Out Sheet

Exterior Operations Level Firefighter—Chapter 5

Name: _____

Fill out the ten-question quiz below, the Knowledge Assessment Sheet, by circling the correct answer for each question. When finished, sign it and give to your instructor/Company Officer for his or her signature. Turn in the Knowledge Assessment Sheet to the proper person as part of the documentation that you have completed your training for this chapter.

1. A defensive driving course for firefighters covers the state and local requirements and regulations for POV responses.
   a. True
   b. False

2. The U.S. DOT defines a _____ as a situation in which there is a high probability of death or serious injury to an individual or significant property loss, and action by an emergency vehicle operator may reduce the seriousness of the situation.
   a. fire emergency
   b. true emergency
   c. rescue incident
   d. true rescue scene

3. _____ is the omission of doing something that a reasonable, prudent person would ordinarily do, or doing something that such a person would not do.
   a. A true emergency
   b. Diligence
   c. Negativity
   d. Negligence

4. Lack of _____ has contributed to many fatalities.
   a. intelligence
   b. seatbelt use
   c. a rear view mirror
   d. speed

5. The extent and type of protective clothing you need depends on the _____ as well as the policy of your Company Officer and your department.
   a. type of fire apparatus
   b. type of weather
   c. type of emergency
   d. response route

6. When getting off the apparatus, always check _____.

   a. for your gloves

   b. in all directions for traffic and hazards

   c. the rear of the apparatus only

   d. the front of the apparatus only

7. When placing traffic cones on a typical two-lane roadway, how many, at a minimum, should you place within 75 feet of the rear of the fire apparatus?

   a. 10

   b. 6

   c. 12

   d. 5

8. The safety rule to use when placing traffic cones is to _____.

   a. always walk toward traffic

   b. always turn your back to traffic

   c. never turn your back to traffic

   d. always walk away from traffic

9. The _____ is the reaction time plus the braking distance.

   a. total stopping distance

   b. total braking distance

   c. total inertia distance

   d. total velocity distance

10. The two methods for determining a safe following distance when operating a fire apparatus are the _____ rule and estimating _____.

   a. 3-minute; one apparatus length

   b. 3-second; one apparatus length

   c. 1-second; two apparatus lengths

   d. 5-second; one apparatus length

Student Signature and Date _____   Instructor/Company Officer Signature and Date _____

Skills Assessment
Signed Documentation Tear-Out Sheet
Exterior Operations Level Firefighter—Chapter 5

Name: _____

Fill out the Skills Assessment Sheet below. Have your instructor/Company Officer check off and initial each skill you demonstrate. When finished, sign it and give to your instructor/Company Officer for his or her signature. Turn in this Skills Assessment Sheet to the proper person as part of the documentation that you have completed your training for this chapter.

Skill	Completed	Initials
1. Provide proof of completion of an approved defensive driving course.	_____	_____
2. Demonstrate safe mounting of the fire apparatus, handing over the PAS tag, applying hearing-protection headsets, and the use of seatbelts.	_____	_____
3. Demonstrate safe dismounting of the fire apparatus and waiting for instructions from the Company Officer.	_____	_____
4. Demonstrate proper personal protective clothing for daylight traffic control.	_____	_____
5. Demonstrate proper personal protective clothing for nighttime traffic control.	_____	_____
6. Safely deploy traffic cones in a transition area behind a fire apparatus on a simulated two-lane roadway.	_____	_____
7. Safely deploy traffic cones in a transition area behind a fire apparatus on a simulated multilane, high-speed, limited-access highway.	_____	_____
8. Demonstrate how to direct traffic in two directions with only one lane open.	_____	_____
9. Participating as a team member, demonstrate how to safely assess a vehicle crash scene.	_____	_____

Student Signature and Date _____   Instructor/Company Officer Signature and Date _____

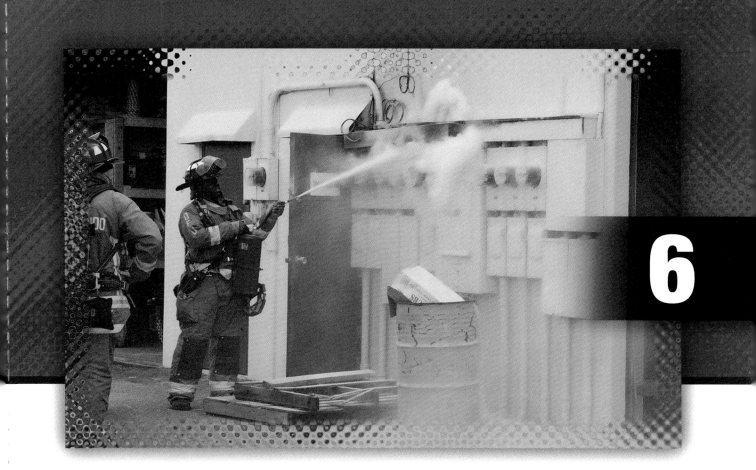

Extinguishing Small Fires

What You Will Learn in This Chapter

In this chapter we will discuss what makes a fire burn and how the material that is burning affects the way we extinguish the fire. You will learn how to select the proper fire extinguisher for different types of fires and how to use it on a small fire. Finally, you will learn how to use two of the small fire attack hose lines on your engine to extinguish slightly larger fires.

What You Will Be Able to Do

After reading this chapter and participating in the practical skill sessions, you will be able to

1. Explain the three phases of an unconfined fire.
2. Explain how heat from a fire causes the fire to spread to other combustible materials.
3. Explain the fire classification system and how it affects the selection of a fire extinguisher.
4. Employ the proper fire extinguisher to extinguish a small fire.
5. Describe the elements of the fire tetrahedron.

Reality!

Small Fires Are Dangerous!

It is very easy to become complacent when working around small fires. At first glance, a small trash fire burning in a vacant lot doesn't look much different from a campfire. A small fire in a cooking pot on top of a stove can easily be extinguished by simply placing the lid back on the pot. A fire burning in a steel refuse dumpster located away from any exposures looks simple enough to extinguish. However, it is not the size of the fire that is of concern—it is the content of the fire that can make it dangerous.

Consider a trash fire. Burning lawn waste and household papers produce smoke that is irritating to the eyes, but as long as you remain upwind it doesn't pose a problem for you. But what happens when that simple trash fire contains an aerosol can, such as a hairspray or spray paint can? Both will rupture from the heat of the fire, often producing a large fireball that can engulf someone standing nearby. The can of spray paint may also contain a steel agitator ball that immediately becomes a flying projectile that can be lethal. The potential for injury at a trash fire is compounded at a dumpster fire because most dumpsters are unsecured and can contain almost any hazardous material dumped by unauthorized individuals.

Because of these issues, practice the following safety recommendations when working around small fires:

- Wear your protective clothing, including using your helmet and visor, whenever you are working near a fire of any size.
- Use your SCBA whenever working near a dumpster fire.
- If possible, know what is burning and use the appropriate extinguisher or extinguishing agent for the type of fire.

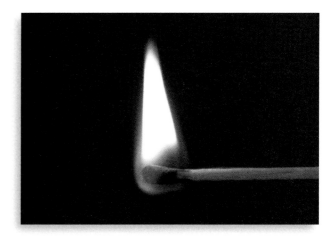

FIGURE 6-1 Evidence that the combustion process is happening? A flame.

Fire Characteristics and Classifications

Have you ever seen a fire? Of course you have. Fires are common. However, starting with this chapter you will look at fire in a different way for the rest of your life. We won't be delving into the intricacies of fire chemistry and behavior, but we will study what makes a fire burn, what makes it spread, and how fires are classified by what is burning. These few simple concepts lay the foundation for every fire-extinguishing method we use.

What Makes a Fire Burn

An open flame is evidence that the process of combustion is occurring (Figure 6-1). Four things need to come together for combustion to occur: fuel, heat, oxygen, and the chemical reaction that keeps the flame burning. These four elements of combustion are often depicted as the **fire tetrahedron** (Figure 6-2). Take away any of the four elements of the fire tetrahedron and fire is not possible. For example, if a piece of paper is burning and you spray it with water, you are rapidly cooling the fuel to below the temperature at which paper burns and are therefore taking away the element of heat. If you place a heavy blanket over the burning piece of paper instead of spraying it with water, you smother the fire, which means you remove the element of oxygen. The same result is achieved, whichever element of combustion is removed.

▰ KEY WORD ▰▰▰▰▰▰▰▰

fire tetrahedron A depiction of the four elements required for combustion to occur: fuel, heat, oxygen,

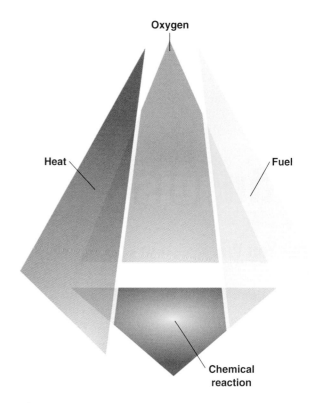

FIGURE 6-2 The fire tetrahedron.

and the chemical chain reaction that keeps the flame burning.

Why Fires Grow

A normal fire in an unconfined area goes through three phases after it is ignited: (1) the growth phase, (2) the fully developed phase, in which all of the material is involved in the fire, and (3) the decay phase, in which the amount of available fuel is reduced as the fire consumes the material. This is true for most fires that burn in an outdoor area that is free of any confinement.

Because the smoke and flammable gasses that are generated by the burning process are confined, fires that start in a confined area, such as a building, go through an additional phase called *flashover*. During flashover, the smoke and heated gasses combine with the right amount of heat and oxygen to ignite suddenly. This is the reason the best course of action for anyone who is inexperienced and ill-equipped to fight an interior fire is to evacuate the area immediately. Interior firefighting is for firefighters who have been trained to Level 1 and above.

Fires grow based on the amount of fuel available to burn. Flames can easily spread to other combustible materials near the original fire through heat transfer; therefore, knowing how flames spread can help you contain a fire. Heat transfers by three primary means: (1) **conduction**, (2) **convection**, and (3) **radiation.**

An example of conducted heat occurs when a fire is on one side of a steel wall. The fire is consuming the fuel, yet the heat penetrates the steel wall, which in turn heats up. Through conduction, the steel wall ignites any combustible material that is touching the other side of the wall (Figure 6-3).

Convection occurs when the fire heats the air near it. When fire is within a building, hot air rises and dissipates if it isn't confined, for example, by the ceiling. Therefore, in most circumstances, any combustible materials that are above a fire are at the most risk of burning due to convection (Figure 6-4).

When we talk about radiation, we aren't referring to nuclear reactive materials. Radiation is the means by which we receive our heat from the sun. Radiation related to fire involves heat transfer from normal, combustible materials that are burning. Open flames emit heat from the light of the flames by the process of radiation. Radiant heat transfer doesn't depend on air currents or direct contact with the flame to spread a fire. For example, a large fire burning outside a building can ignite the curtains inside the building when some of the energy of the original fire radiates through a glass window (Figure 6-5).

KEY WORDS

conduction   A type of heat transfer in which the hot flame or fire-heated object is in direct contact with another, cooler object and heats it up.

convection   A type of heat transfer that occurs when the fire heats the air near it, causing the heated air to rise.

radiation   A transfer of heat through light waves. We receive our heat from the sun through radiation.

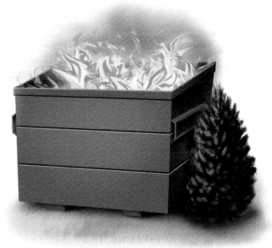
Fire burns in a metal dumpster, heating the sidewall.

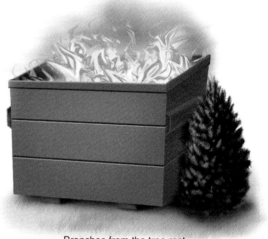
Branches from the tree rest against the hot sidewall of the dumpster.

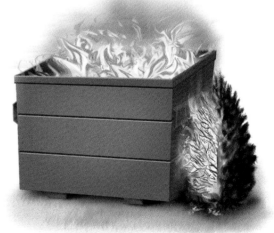
The tree branches catch fire.

FIGURE 6-3   Conducted heat transfer.

② Air heated from the fire rises and heats boxes until they burn.
① Fire burns below a shelf with boxes.

FIGURE 6-4 Convection heat transfer.

① Fire burns in a car next to a house.
② Heat radiates to the house, igniting it.

FIGURE 6-5 Radiant heat transfer.

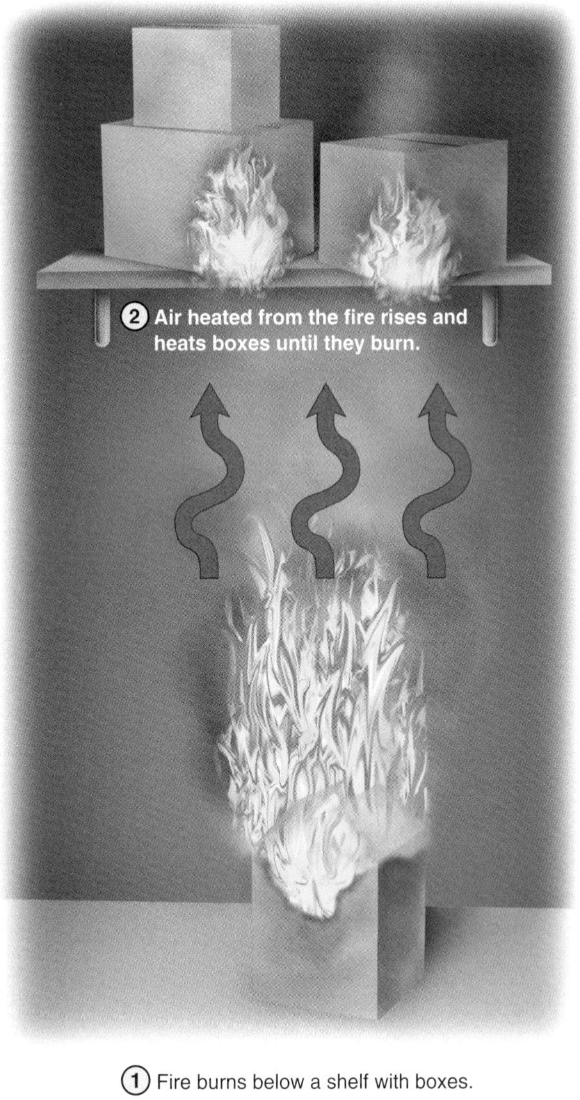

The Fire Classification System

Generally speaking, there are five classes of materials that burn (Figure 6-6). This classification was established to help fire departments and the community select the proper fire extinguishers to use in putting out fires. Table 6-1 shows this classification.

Portable fire extinguishers have labels indicating the types of fires they are designed to extinguish. An extinguisher containing only water is usually effective only for a Class A fire (Figure 6-7). An extinguisher containing a basic dry chemical usually extinguishes Class B fires, so it is referred to as a Class B extinguisher (Figure 6-8). If the extinguisher contains an extinguishing agent that is dry and nonconductive, then it might be useful in extinguishing both Class B and Class C types of fires, so it is referred to as a Class BC extinguisher. Most dry chemical extinguishers contain a multipurpose chemical that is effective against the first three types of fires, so these are referred to as Class ABC extinguishers.

Class D fires, which involve flammable metals, require a fuel-specific extinguishing agent, so specialized dry powder extinguishers rated for Class D fires are used. Because burning metal is a rare event and is thought of as a hazardous materials type of fire, we will not be discussing Class D fires in detail at this point in your training.

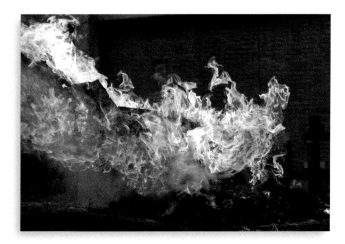

FIGURE 6-6

TABLE 6-1 The Fire Classification System

Class A:	Normal, ordinary combustibles in their solid form, such as wood, paper, and cloth
Class B:	Flammable liquids, such as oil, gasoline, and kerosene
Class C:	Any fire involving energized electricity
Class D:	Flammable metal fires
Class K:	Cooking oils and fats

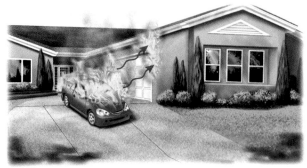

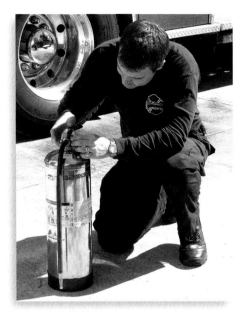

FIGURE 6-7 Water pressure fire extinguisher.

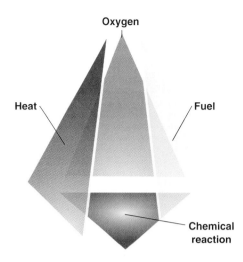

Removal of any side of the fire tetrahedron, that is: fuel, heat, oxygen or the chain reaction, results in extinguishment of the fire.

FIGURE 6-9 The fire tetrahedron and fire extinguishment.

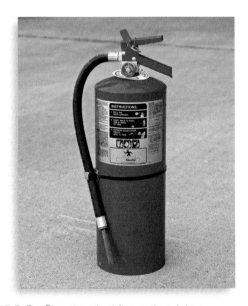

FIGURE 6-8 Dry chemical fire extinguisher.

Only recently has the Fire Service started looking at cooking oils and fats as a separate class of fire. Most problems encountered with Class K fires are handled on a small scale with a Class B extinguishing agent. Class K agents are usually found in large cooking facilities with automatic extinguishing systems and not in small, portable fire extinguishers.

Fire Classification and the Fire Tetrahedron

The fire classification system is directly related to the fire tetrahedron. A Class A fire is usually extinguished by cooling the burning material, so it is best fought by cooling the fuel below its ignition temperature. A Class B fire is usually extinguished by isolating the fuel from the oxygen source or smothering it with a chemical or foam, so Class B fires are best fought by removing the source of oxygen. Class C fires involve energized electrical energy. The electricity usually is not the only element burning; however, everything will continue to burn as long as the electrical current applies energy to the fire. Therefore, the best way to extinguish a Class C fire is to stop the flow of electricity, which removes the heat source. Once the heat source has been removed from an electrical fire, any remaining fire involves either Class A or Class B combustible materials and should be extinguished accordingly (Figure 6-9).

The fact that we classify fires by the material that is burning also indicates where our firefighting efforts for small fires should be focused—on the burning material and not on the flames. Regardless of the classification of fire, the extinguishing agent should be applied at the base of the flames and on the material that is burning.

As we stated in the introduction to this text and in previous chapters, we are going to introduce you to the various tools, equipment, and operations in context. We start with simple scenarios and provide direction about the applications of the different tools, equipment, and techniques utilized to control a fire emergency in the scenario presented. Because each scenario builds upon the previous one, as you progress through the content and advance in your training, it is extremely important that you read the fire emergency scenarios in order.

Types of Small Fires

Small fires include trash fires, burning liquids, electrical fires, and dumpster fires. Each type of fire requires a different method of extinguishment.

Trash Fires

Trash fires typically involve Class A materials. The extinguishing agent best suited for these materials are water or Class A foam extinguishing agents. We will discuss Class A foam in a later chapter, so for now we'll concentrate on water from a water extinguisher and hose lines.

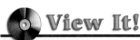

Go to the DVD, navigate to Chapter 6, and select *Class A Trash Fire, Water Extinguisher.*

Using a Water-Type Fire Extinguisher

To extinguish a simple trash fire involving mainly Class A materials, a firefighter may first use a water fire extinguisher, following these basic steps:

1. Pull the extinguisher off its mounting and pull the safety pin located in the operating handle (Figure 6-10).

FIGURE 6-10

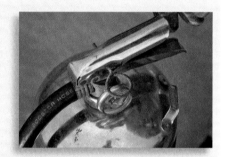

2. Approach the fire from a safe position with the wind to your back (Figure 6-11). *Never* let the fire get between you and your exit point.

FIGURE 6-11

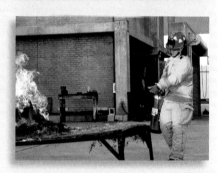

3. Point the nozzle at the base of the fire and depress the operating handle. Direct the water onto the burning materials until the fire is extinguished (Figure 6-12). Use your finger over the nozzle to break up the stream slightly. This will help avoid spreading the fuel around and will allow the water to better absorb the heat.

FIGURE 6-12

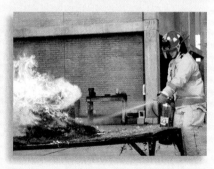

—Continued

4. After use, the water extinguisher should be marked as "empty" so others will know it is not ready to be used again. Then at the fire station, the water extinguisher should be refilled and recharged (Figure 6-13). Your department will have specific procedures for indicating that an extinguisher is empty and for refilling a discharged water pressure fire extinguisher.

FIGURE 6-13

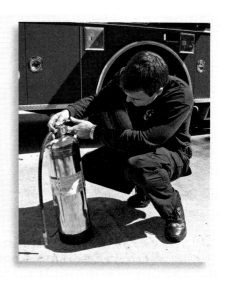

The General Care and Maintenance of Fire Extinguishers

The general care and maintenance of all fire extinguishers can be accomplished by visually inspecting them using the following steps:

1. Inspect the operating handles and cylinders of the fire extinguisher for physical damage (Figure 6-14). Damaged fire extinguishers should be immediately removed from service and documented. You should also notify your Company Officer.

FIGURE 6-14

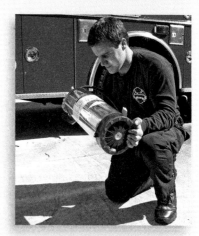

2. Check the hydrostatic date that is stamped on the shell of a carbon dioxide extinguisher and report any out-of-date extinguisher to your Company Officer (Figure 6-15).

FIGURE 6-15

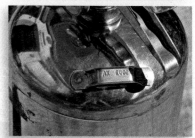

3. Look for an inspection tag (except on water pressure fire extinguishers). (Figure 6-16.) Make sure that it is up to date. Out-of-date fire extinguishers should be immediately reported to your Company Officer.

FIGURE 6-16

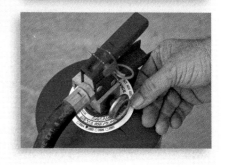

—Continued

4. Make sure that the extinguisher is properly mounted, whether in the fire station or on the fire apparatus (Figures 6-17 and 6-18).

FIGURE 6-17

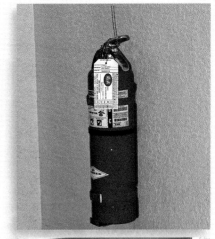

FIGURE 6-18

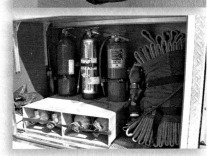

Practice It!

Extinguishing a Trash Fire with a Small Attack Line

One-inch attack lines used to extinguish trash fires include booster lines and single-jacketed lines. Use these steps to extinguish a trash fire with a small attack line:

1. Grab the nozzle and advance the line toward the fire. If someone else is advancing with the nozzle, grab the hose about 25 feet behind him or her and help pull the line (Figure 6-19).

FIGURE 6-19

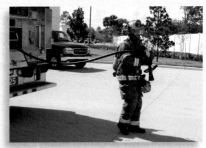

2. Point the nozzle at the ground, slowly open it, and adjust the spray pattern (Figure 6-20). Bleeding the nozzle ensures that you have water at the nozzle before approaching the fire.

FIGURE 6-20

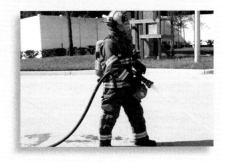

—Continued

3. Shut off the flow of water at the nozzle, hold the line and nozzle under your arm with both hands, and approach the fire (Figure 6-21).

FIGURE 6-21

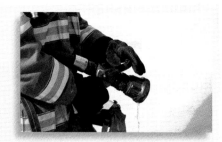

4. Flow water onto the base of the trash fire, which will quickly extinguish the fire. For a trash fire, start with a straight stream and continue cooling it with a wide-pattern fog stream (Figure 6-22).

FIGURE 6-22

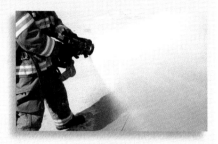

5. Flow water until the fire is completely extinguished (Figure 6-23). With some trash fires, the debris will need to be turned in order for the water to reach hidden fires.

FIGURE 6-23

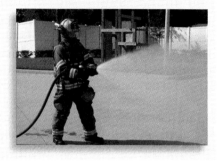

Burning Liquids

The extinguishing agents best suited for small fires involving flammable liquids work by smothering the flames. Common examples of small, burning liquid fires include cooking oil fires and fires involving spilled gasoline around lawn mowers (Figure 6-24). Anything larger than these types of fires is beyond the capabilities of most portable fire extinguishers. Class B fire extinguishers include a carbon dioxide (CO_2) extinguisher and a dry chemical extinguisher. Most dry chemical extinguishers are useful for both Class A and Class B fires.

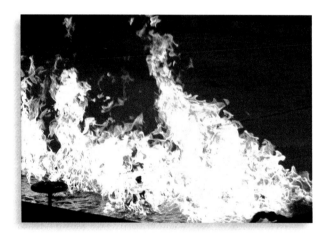

FIGURE 6-24 Class B fire extinguishers can be used on small, burning liquid fires.

When the burning liquid has spread out on level ground and the fuel that is burning is only a millimeter or so deep, the fire will usually go out and stay out when you apply the extinguishing agent as long as the extinguishing agent stays in place until the fuel cools down.

When the fire involves a liquid that is deeper than a millimeter or so, applying the extinguishing agent with too much force can make the liquid spread or splash out of its container. Burning liquids can be spread when the nozzle from the fire extinguisher is too close to the burning liquid. Another problem with burning liquids is that they are affected by gravity. Until the source of a burning liquid is either controlled or exhausted, the fire will flow downhill. Running liquid fires are much larger than can be handled with portable fire extinguishers, so if the fire moves, evacuate the area and don't try to fight it.

The most important principle to follow when extinguishing a liquid fire is to approach it from the upwind and/or uphill side. Start at one side of the fire and allow the extinguishing agent to push its way across the surface of the fire (Figure 6-25).

Carbon Dioxide Fire Extinguisher

As its name implies, a carbon dioxide (CO_2) fire extinguisher is filled with pressurized carbon dioxide. When applied to a burning liquid, it smothers the flames by dispersing the available oxygen, replacing it with carbon dioxide, which does not support combustion. The large horn at the end of the hose best differentiates a CO_2 extinguisher from a typical dry chemical extinguisher. This horn allows the carbon dioxide gas to expand slightly as it directs the gas to the flames (Figure 6-26). Because the carbon dioxide gas is under pressure, you must take care to avoid blowing the burning fuel out of its container, thus spreading the fire.

Because a CO_2 extinguisher uses a gas as the primary extinguishing agent, it leaves no contaminating residue to be cleaned up. However, this feature of a CO_2 extinguisher provides both an advantage and a disadvantage. CO_2 dissipates rapidly and doesn't require clean up, but it often dissipates before the flammable liquid is allowed to cool; therefore, the liquid often re-ignites.

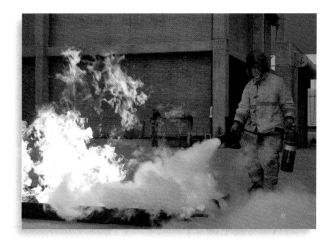

FIGURE 6-25 When extinguishing a liquid fire, approach it from the upwind and uphill side. Start at one side of the fire, allowing the extinguishing agent to push its way across the surface of the fire.

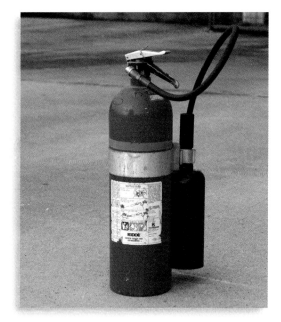

FIGURE 6-26 Carbon dioxide fire extinguisher.

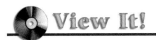

View It!

Go to the DVD, navigate to Chapter 6, and select *Carbon Dioxide Fire Extinguisher.*

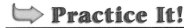

Practice It!

Using a Carbon Dioxide Fire Extinguisher

To extinguish a small fire involving Class B materials, a firefighter can use a carbon dioxide extinguisher, following these basic steps:

1. Pull the extinguisher off its mounting and pull the safety pin located in the operating handle (Figure 6-27).

FIGURE 6-27

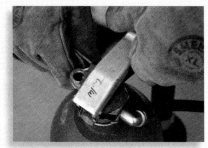

2. Approach the fire from a safe position with the wind to your back (Figure 6-28). *Never* let the fire get between you and your exit point.

FIGURE 6-28

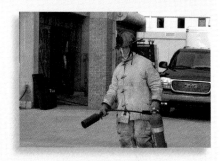

3. Point the nozzle at the base of the fire and depress the operating handle. Direct the agent onto the burning materials until the fire is extinguished (Figure 6-29).

FIGURE 6-29

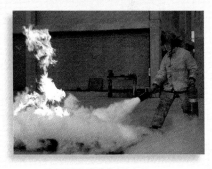

Dry Chemical Extinguisher

Dry chemical extinguishers contain a nonflammable, powdered chemical that is expelled by a harmless gas when you squeeze the trigger of the extinguisher. The chemical coats the surface area of the burning material to break the connection between the fuel and heat. This type of extinguisher works on the chemical reaction side of the fire tetrahedron (Figure 6-30). Because the extinguishing agent is expelled under pressure, a dry chemical extinguisher can spread a fire involving a puddle of a burning liquid if you aren't careful when you operate the device.

As with the other portable extinguishers we have discussed, approach the fire from an upwind, safe area and start applying the dry chemical from a safe distance, moving in on the fire as the flames subside.

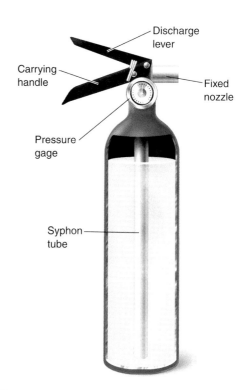

FIGURE 6-30 Dry chemical fire extinguisher.

 View It!

Go to the DVD, navigate to Chapter 6, and select *Dry Chemical Fire Extinguisher.*

Practice It!

Using a Dry Chemical Fire Extinguisher

To extinguish a small fire involving Class A, B, or C materials using a dry chemical extinguisher, following these basic steps:

1. Pull the extinguisher off its mounting and pull the safety pin located in the operating handle (Figure 6-31).

FIGURE 6-31

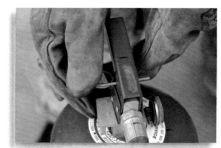

2. Approach the fire from a safe position with the wind to your back (Figure 6-32). *Never* let the fire get between you and your exit point.

FIGURE 6-32

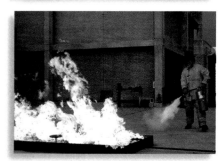

—Continued

3. Point the nozzle at the base of the fire and depress the operating handle. Direct the agent onto the burning materials until the fire is extinguished (Figure 6-33).

FIGURE 6-33

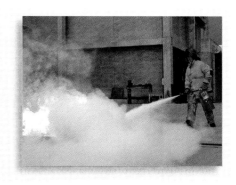

Electrical Fires

Although many types of fire extinguishers are rated for Class C fires involving energized electrical equipment, the best approach to an electrical fire is from the heat side of the fire tetrahedron. An energized electrical fire receives its main heat source from electricity and not from what is burning. For example, if a small electrical appliance is on fire, switching off the electrical source at the circuit breaker will usually stop the fire or at least decrease the fire from a Class C fire to a lower-grade fire. By stopping the electrical current, the fire can be switched from a Class C to a Class A or Class B fire, depending on the material that is left burning. In addition to extinguishing the fire, your concern is for individuals' safety from the hazard that the electrical current presents. Therefore, isolating the electrical source is an important measure.

Isolating the electrical source from a small appliance is simple enough when you can safely unplug the cord or switch off a circuit breaker (Figure 6-34). However, if the electrical fire involves anything more than a small appliance (for example, a downed power line), then controlling the electricity should be left to the power company. You need to secure the area and stay away!

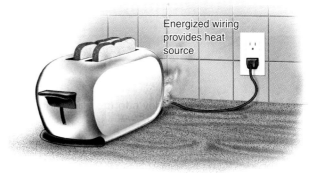

Energized wiring provides heat source

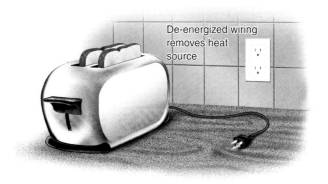

De-energized wiring removes heat source

FIGURE 6-34 Turn off the electricity!

Dumpster Fires

There are many types of trash containers that you will encounter in responding to trash fires. The most common trash containers at commercial businesses and construction sites are dumpsters. Dumpsters are commonly metal containers of various sizes that have a metal or plastic lid. They may or may not be locked and might be situated next to a large trash compactor.

You will use the same tools and techniques on a dumpster fire as you will with any trash fire, with few exceptions. Be ready to place a small ladder to get access to the top of the dumpster. You may need to force entry to any locked access doors. You may also need a larger flow of water through large hose lines and nozzles due to the increased amount of the material inside the dumpster.

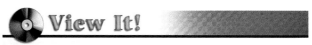

Go to the DVD, navigate to Chapter 6, and select *Dumpster Fires.*

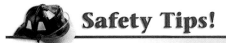

Use the following precautions when extinguishing a dumpster fire:

- Always wear full PPE, including an SCBA (Figure 6-35).

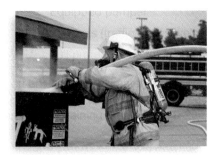

FIGURE 6-35

- Fires in metal dumpsters are hot, so remember not to touch the metal surfaces.
- Always approach a dumpster fire with caution, because you do not know what is burning in the dumpster. Stay protected and have a good water supply (Figure 6-36).

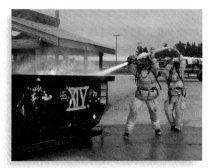

FIGURE 6-36

- Large, roll-off type dumpsters with trash compactors have other hazards, including pressurized hydraulic lines and electrical hazards. Consider these to be large machinery fires that present additional hazards not expected at a normal dumpster fire.
- Never climb inside a dumpster!

Do It!

Extinguishing Small Fires Safely

As a firefighter, you need to know how fire burns and how the materials burning affect the way you extinguish the fire. You should know how to use a fire extinguisher or a small attack line to extinguish a trash fire and a dumpster fire. You should also remember the characteristics of burning liquid and electrical fires. Always remember that whatever the size of the fire or the materials burning, all fires can be dangerous. Wear appropriate personal protective equipment at all times when working to control these incidents.

Prove It

Knowledge Assessment

Signed Documentation Tear-Out Sheet

Exterior Operations Level Firefighter—Chapter 6

Name: _____

Fill out the ten-question quiz below, the Knowledge Assessment Sheet, by circling the correct answer for each question. When finished, sign it and give to your instructor/Company Officer for his or her signature. Turn in this Knowledge Assessment Sheet to the proper person as part of the documentation that you have completed your training for this chapter.

1. Four things need to come together for combustion to occur: fuel, heat, _____ , and the chemical reaction.
   a. carbon dioxide
   b. water
   c. oxygen
   d. nitrogen

2. A fire grows in size based on the amount of _____ there is to burn.
   a. oxygen
   b. nitrogen
   c. fuel
   d. air

3. _____ doesn't depend on air currents or direct contact with flames to spread a fire.
   a. Radiation
   b. Convection
   c. Conduction
   d. Fire spread

4. A water extinguisher would work best on a _____ fire.
   a. Class A
   b. Class B
   c. Class C
   d. Class K

5. An example of a small, burning liquid fire would be _____ .
   a. a spill and fire at an oil refinery
   b. a burning gasoline tanker on a highway
   c. spilled gasoline around a lawn mower
   d. magnesium metal shavings burning outside a machinist shop

6. In most small fires, the extinguishing agent should usually be applied to the _____ of the fire.
   a. top
   b. back
   c. front
   d. base

7. Energized electrical fires receive their main heat source from _____ .

   a. oxygen

   b. electricity

   c. nitrogen

   d. radiation

8. Fire extinguishers rated for use on Class B fires include carbon dioxide and _____ extinguishers.

   a. water

   b. dry chemical

   c. light water

   d. heavy chemical

9. Dumpsters are the most common type of trash containers located outside of commercial businesses.

   a. True

   b. False

10. Full PPE is NOT required for dumpster fires because they are so small.

   a. True

   b. False

Student Signature and Date _____   Instructor/Company Officer Signature and Date _____

146

Prove It

Skills Assessment

Exterior Operations Level Firefighter—Chapter 6

Name: _____

Fill out the Skills Assessment Sheet below. Have your instructor/Company Officer check off and initial each skill you demonstrate. When finished, sign it and give to your instructor/Company Officer for his or her signature. Turn in this Skills Assessment Sheet to the proper person as part of the documentation that you have completed your training for this chapter.

Skill	Completed	Initials
1. Employ a pressurized water extinguisher.	_____	_____
2. Employ a carbon dioxide water extinguisher.	_____	_____
3. Employ a dry chemical fire extinguisher.	_____	_____
4. Deploy and use a booster line.	_____	_____

Student Signature and Date _____   Instructor/Company Officer Signature and Date _____

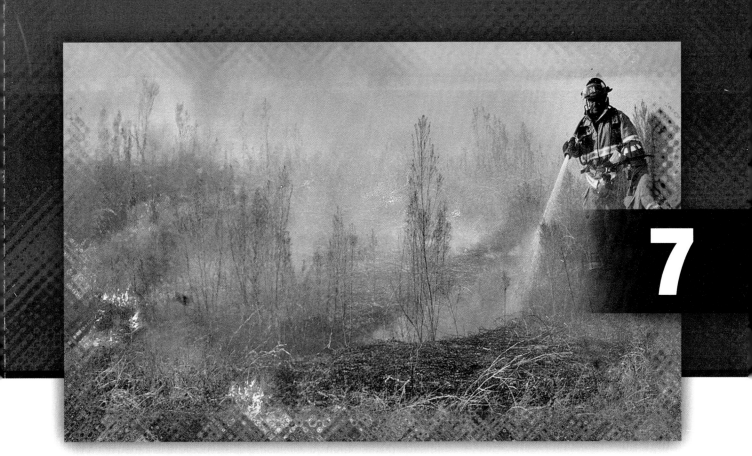

Ground Cover Fires

What You Will Learn in This Chapter

In this chapter we will discuss ground cover firefighting and introduce you to basic aspects of wildland or brush fires. We will explain some of the terminology that is unique to these types of fire operations. You will learn about ground cover fire movement and behavior along with some extinguishing methods. You will also learn about the black-line approach, protective clothing, and personnel accountability systems used at a typical brush fire operation. Finally, you will learn about tools, equipment, and brush truck operations.

What You Will Be Able to Do

After reading this chapter, you will be asked to tour the fire station so that you know where to find items that are important to your safety. After reading the chapter and taking the tour, you will be able to

1. Define basic terms used at brush fire incidents.
2. Describe the basic parts of a typical brush fire.
3. Explain how to safely approach a brush fire.
4. Explain your part in a brush fire accountability system.
5. Demonstrate the proper donning of the brush fire protective clothing your agency uses.
6. Explain the "black-line" firefighting approach.
7. Demonstrate the use of various hand tools associated with brush fire operations.
8. Describe the fire movement and assessment safety issues that pertain to brush fires.
9. Given the brush fire apparatus your agency uses, demonstrate how to safely ride on it, deploy and extend hose lines, and utilize tools and equipment carried on the apparatus for fighting a small brush fire.

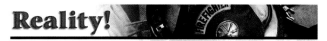

Reality!

Safety Lesson: A NIOSH Report

Wear Your Gear, Even on Small Fires!

On August 1, 2002, a firefighter in South Dakota was severely burned while fighting a fire that was consuming a wheat field. He had responded directly to the fire in his personal vehicle (POV) where he met up with another firefighter whose POV, a pickup truck, was equipped with a 75-gallon water tank and a gasoline-driven pump. According to the NIOSH report, although numerous firefighters responded to the scene, there was no Incident Command System established. The firefighters on the scene dispersed on their own as they arrived on the scene. The victim and the firefighter with the pickup truck talked on the scene and agreed that the victim would spray water from the bed of the truck while the other firefighter drove.

The two firefighters proceeded through a gate and into the field near the encroaching head of the fire. While fighting the fire, the victim was wearing tennis shoes, denim jeans, a T-shirt, and a baseball cap. A sudden gust of wind blew fire and smoke over the truck. The driver immediately pulled the truck forward and to the right. It is unknown if the victim fell from the truck as a result of being overcome by the fire and smoke or from the sudden forward movement of the truck. He ran about 200 yards, where he encountered a barbed wire fence and became entangled in the barbed wire. Other firefighters rushed to his aid, and the victim was evacuated by a medical helicopter to the burn center, where he died 5 days later from his injuries.

Follow-Up

NIOSH Report #F2002-37

After this incident was reviewed and evaluated, the NIOSH investigative report recommended that the following practices be implemented:

- Ensure that firefighters follow established procedures for combating ground cover fires.
- Develop and implement an Incident Command System.
- Provide firefighters with personal protective equipment (PPE) that is appropriate for wildland fires and is also NFPA 1977 compliant.
- Provide firefighters with appropriate wildland firefighter training.

Small Ground Cover Fires

Firefighters are called upon to perform many different jobs, including extinguishing **ground cover fires.** Ground cover fires occur in grassy vacant lots, rural wooded areas, parks, and even in the median areas on roadways (Figure 7-1). These fires are quite different from building fires. Ground cover fires are more like large Class A trash fires in that the fuel is spread out over a wider area. The tactics that firefighters use to extinguish these fires must take into consideration such elements as weather conditions, the humidity level, the type and arrangement of foliage, natural and manmade **firebreaks,** and the direction the fire travels as it burns.

In the United States, urban and suburban areas have been encroaching more and more on the wildland areas surrounding them. This spread is referred to as the **wildland/urban interface.** In this interface there is little or no separation between homes and even commercial buildings and the heavily wooded areas they are near. Property loss often results when large wildfires occur.

At this point in your training, we are going to limit our discussion to small ground cover fires. Even though we see and hear about the massive fires that occur in vast wildland areas, most ground cover fires are less than an acre in size and are controlled by a small crew

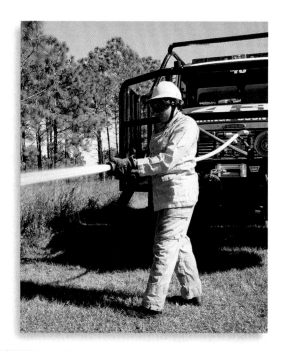

FIGURE 7-1 Ground cover fires are very common, even in urban areas. Most are small enough to be extinguished with a small hose line.

of firefighters. These smaller fires occur everywhere—in big cities and in small, rural communities.

Wildfires

Firefighters who work routinely on **wildfires** in wildland areas receive additional training specific to these very different and much larger fire incidents. The operations for wildfires involve an extensive Incident Management System (IMS) and different firefighting apparatus, such as air **tankers** and fire-line tractors. These fires are major events and require some prequalification training in order to understand their scope and to understand and participate in tactical operations (Figure 7-2). This special training can result in certification and becoming a "red-card" status **wildland firefighter.** Though structural firefighters will respond to and assist in these events, you will be assigned duties within your scope of training and your capabilities, as established by your agency.

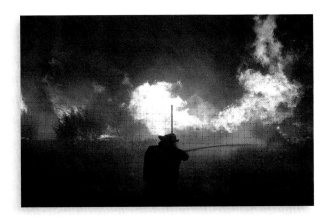

FIGURE 7-2   Large brush fires require extensive training and are coordinated through an Incident Management System.

Fire Movement and Behavior

Ground cover fires involve natural plant growth fuels burning in an open area. These fuels can be grass, brush, and even trees, as well as combinations of these items. These fires are usually handled by one or two firefighting crews.

Depending on wind direction, the topography of the landscape, and the dryness and arrangement of the ground cover growth involved, the fire tends to spread outward. As it burns, it moves in the direction of the wind. In hilly or mountainous areas, the fire tends to burn up a slope toward the unburned area until it is affected by winds at the top of the hill or mountain (Figure 7-3).

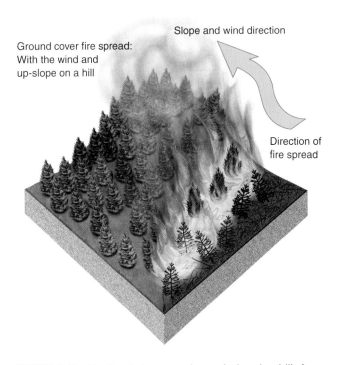

Slope and wind direction

Ground cover fire spread: With the wind and up-slope on a hill

Direction of fire spread

FIGURE 7-3   Fire tends to move downwind and uphill. A fire burning up the side of a hill will move until it is affected by winds at the top of the hill.

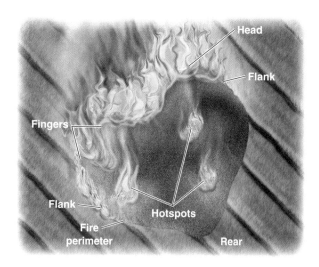

FIGURE 7-4 Parts of a ground cover fire. The fastest moving part of a brush fire is called the head, the sides are the flanks, and the point opposite the head is the rear.

Common Fire Terms

There is usually a concentrated, heavy involvement at the leading edge of a fire. This part of the fire is known as the **head** of the fire and is the most rapidly moving area of the fire. The parts of the fire on either side of the head are known as the **flanks** of the fire. The edge of the burned fire area opposite the head is known as the **rear** (Figure 7-4). The area around the edge of the entire fire area, including both the burned and the still burning areas, is known as the **fire perimeter.** As the fire burns, involved areas can extend beyond the main perimeter in narrow burning areas called **fingers**. The ground cover fire may also feature an area called a **hotspot** that is located inside the burned area. The hotspot may continue to burn because it has more fuel than the surrounding brush. Hotspots can also be located outside the original fire area due to hot embers falling from the main body of the fire. Finally, a rapidly spreading ground cover fire with a well-defined head is said to be **running.**

■■■ KEY WORDS ■■■■■■■

fingers   Small extensions of fire growth that protrude from the main body of a ground cover fire.

fire perimeter   The outside edge of the entire ground cover fire. The inside of the fire perimeter contains the burned area while the area outside the perimeter is unburned.

flanks   The smaller fire-involved areas on either side of the head of a ground cover fire.

head   The main burning area of a brush fire that occurs on the perimeter of the fire. It is located on the side in the direction in which the fire is moving and will have the most intense fire characteristics.

hotspot   An area of burning located either within the burned perimeter of a brush fire or outside the fire perimeter where fire has jumped over from the main body of fire. A hotspot continues to burn inside a burned-out area of a ground cover fire. Hotspots can also develop from hot ashes and burning embers that drop from the fire, landing outside the fire area and starting a small fire or hotspot.

rear   The edge of the burned fire area opposite the head.

running   Rapid movement of a ground cover fire.

Extinguishing Ground Cover Fires

Extinguishment Methods

Ground cover fires can be extinguished in three main ways: (1) with water and other extinguishing agents, (2) with firebreaks, and (3) with a combination of these items. Whatever method is used, the head and flanks of the fire should always be extinguished from the burned side of the fire. Because ground cover fires can suddenly change intensity and direction, approaching them from the burned side reduces exposure to an uncontrolled and often deadly onrush of fire. This approach should be used even on small grass fires that are extinguished with a small booster line connected to a pumper.

Water and Other Extinguishing Agents

If the fire is small enough and a water supply is available, the fire can be extinguished directly with the application of water or another extinguishing agent like a Class A foam. Class A foams are usually added to the attack-line water supply. Because these types of foam agents allow the water to be more easily absorbed by the natural wood and brush materials, they provide more extinguishing capability to the water as it is applied. Water can be applied with a booster line or a trash-line hose connected to a standard fire pumper, a **brush truck,** or a **tender (water tanker)** (Figure 7-5).

KEY WORDS

brush truck   A specialized piece of fire apparatus designed to deliver tools, manpower, and some water to the scene of a ground cover fire. It may or may not have off-road capability and can be used to extinguish smaller fires as well as to protect equipment, personnel, and fire lines on larger wildland fire operations.

tender   A piece of specialized firefighting apparatus designed to deliver large amounts of water to a fire scene where a water supply is not readily available. Under the National Incident Management System, wheeled apparatus that had previously been called a tanker is now called a tender. The term *tanker* is now used to refer to an airplane that delivers water or other extinguishing agents via an air drop.

water tanker   Under the National Incident Management System, this apparatus is now called a *tender*.

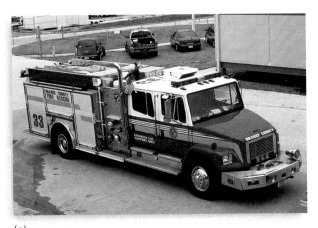

(a)

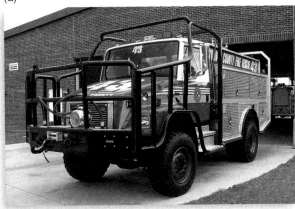

(b)

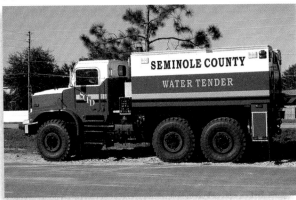

(c)

FIGURE 7-5   (a) Engine, (b) brush truck, and (c) tender.

Firebreaks

Ground cover fires can be extinguished by preparing the unburned area as the fire burns, steering the fire by the use of firebreaks, both manmade and natural. Examples of natural firebreaks include rivers, lakes, streams, and sparsely vegetated areas. Examples of manmade firebreaks include roadways, parking lots, and farmlands. Manmade firebreaks also include trenches made by teams of fire crews using hand tools or specially designed forestry tractors in areas well ahead of the fire. Foliage can also be cleared utilizing a backfire technique. It involves intentionally but carefully setting fire to foliage ahead of the running head of a fire to slow its progress. This technique requires special training and must be performed by qualified personnel.

Firebreaks can also be prepared by applying fire retardant agents delivered by air drop or sprayed by hose lines. The fire burns up to the firebreak, stops, and burns the remaining fuel inside the perimeter. The work area around the fire that is prepared as a firebreak is known as the **fire line** (Figure 7-6). After

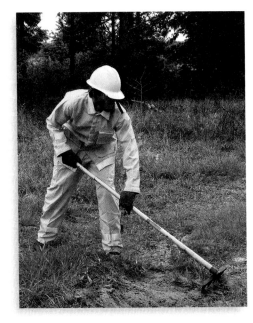

FIGURE 7-6   A firebreak can be created by scraping away any flammable ground cover until mineral soil is exposed.

creating firebreaks, firefighters then monitor them and quickly extinguish any small spot fires that may spread beyond the firebreaks.

Combination Method

The third method of extinguishing ground cover fires is a combination of the previous two methods—stabilizing the firebreaks and extinguishing the head and flanks of the fire with water or other extinguishing agents (Figure 7-7). Even a small ground cover fire can be dangerous. The combination method of extinguishing a ground cover fire is considered an advanced method and should not be attempted without proper supervision and support from experienced crews.

The Black-Line Approach

If left unchecked, most ground cover fires burn until they run out of readily consumable fuel. The **black-line approach** is a method of controlling ground cover fires by allowing the fire to burn to a natural or manmade firebreak where it runs out of fuel. Typically, a fire that is running through light fuels, such as tall grass or knee-high vegetation, burns until it reaches an open field of grass, a plowed field, or a road, where it slows down or self-extinguishes (Figure 7-8). Use this dynamic to your advantage by approaching the fire from the burned side or by letting the fire burn across open areas until it reaches a road or plowed firebreak. When the fire reaches short grass, the intensity diminishes and a simple dousing with water takes care of the fire at that point. This isn't to say that a wildfire won't jump a firebreak or road, but remember, for our purposes we are concerned with fires in light fuels, such as knee-high grass, weeds, or crops. Any fires that start outside the fire area due to hot ashes and burning firebrands dropping down result in spot-over fires. Spot-over fires are handled quickly with available water.

Protective Clothing: Wildland Gear

Protective clothing for structural firefighting is often sufficient for the short term in ground cover firefighting operations. In some areas of the country,

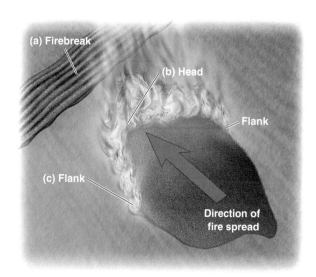

FIGURE 7-7 Firebreaks, head, and flank of a groundcover fire. (a) Firebreak, (b) head, and (c) flank.

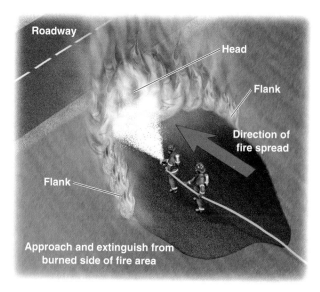

FIGURE 7-8 The black-line approach takes advantage of natural breaks, such as roadways, to allow the intensity of the fire to diminish naturally.

structural firefighters may be assigned wildland fire-fighting protective clothing. This clothing is lighter weight and is designed for longer-term firefighting operations at wildland fires. Be sure to wear the appropriate gear as designated by your agency's policy and your Company Officer.

A typical wildland firefighter's personal protective clothing includes the following items (Figure 7-9):

- Head protection, provided by an approved light-weight helmet
- Eye protection, provided by approved goggles and a face shield
- Additional head protection, provided by a face and neck shroud (such as fire-resistant material attached to the helmet)
- A face protector, independent of the helmet
- Body protection, provided by an approved two-piece garment (pants and coat) or an approved one-piece jumpsuit
- Hand protection, provided by approved gloves
- Approved footwear

Accessories may also be used, including belts, clips, and small tools. Small, personal, fireproof enclosures called fire shelters may also be included. If you are issued protective clothing, become familiar with properly donning it for ground cover fire operations.

Tools and Equipment

In fighting ground cover fires, it is important to establish a small firebreak around the perimeter of the fire to help ensure that a rekindling does not occur. To establish a firebreak, you can use several common ground cover firefighting tools:

- *Shovel.* Used to clear an area of vegetation around the fire perimeter (Figure 7-10).
- **Council rake.** Used for clearing vegetation and debris (Figure 7-11).
- **Brush axe.** Used to cut down small bushes and shrubs that may provide fuel for a rekindling (Figure 7-12). It is important that you carry any axe

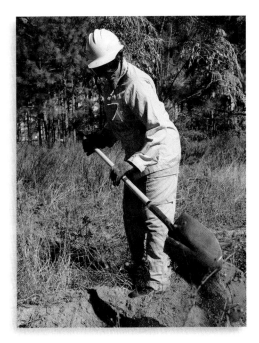

FIGURE 7-10   Shovel.

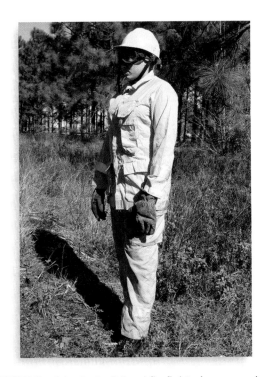

FIGURE 7-9   A typical wildland firefighter's personal protective clothing: (a) head protection, (b) eye protection, (c) face and neck shroud, (d) face protector, (e) body protection, (f) hand protection, and (g) foot protection.

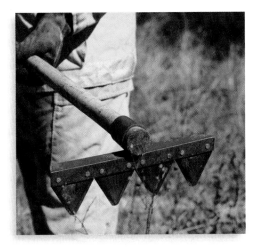

FIGURE 7-11   Council rake.

safely. Carry it with the point down and throw the tool clear if you stumble or fall.

- *Backpack-style water extinguisher.* A backpack that holds up to 5 gallons of water that is sprayed with a hand-operated pump sprayer (Figure 7-13). It is a good tool to handle small spot-fires and to overhaul small areas.

▨ KEY WORDS ▨

council rake   A specialized tool used by firefighters to clear undergrowth and debris in order to create a fire-break at a ground cover fire.

brush axe   A brush-clearing tool used by firefighters in preparing firebreaks.

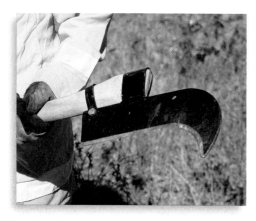

FIGURE 7-12   Brush axe.

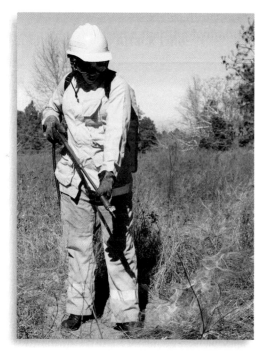

FIGURE 7-13   Backpack-style water extinguisher.

Ground Cover Fire Operations

Alarm Response

When you receive an alarm to respond to a ground cover fire, your response and arrival are no different than for any other type of fire. You may be responding on a regular structural fire pumper, a tender, or even a specially designed brush truck. Regardless of the type of apparatus, the safety rules are the same: you should wear your seatbelt, sit in a designated seat, and put on your gear either before leaving the station or after arriving on the scene.

If you are responding to the ground cover incident in your private vehicle, make sure to park it where you can leave the area quickly if necessary. Also, carry your keys in your pocket or consider leaving them in your car. Be aware of the firefighting operations and be ready to move your vehicle if necessary.

Scene Arrival and Assessment

When your unit arrives on the scene, your Company Officer will perform a rapid size-up of the fire-involved area, looking for the extent of the involvement, the type of ground cover burning, and how fast and in which direction it is spreading (Figure 7-14). Any exposures to the fire as well as safety hazards are noted as the assessment progresses. Your Company Officer will then develop a plan and advise dispatch of both the situation and the initial actions your crew will be taking and establish Incident Command.

The personnel accountability systems used in ground cover fires are similar those used in structural fire operations. If the incident is large and requires multiple units and agencies, the PAS tags are given to the Incident Commander so that the locations of

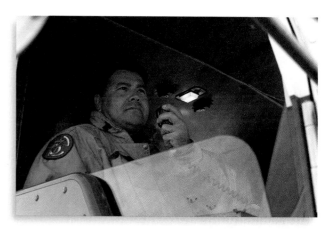

FIGURE 7-14   The first step to developing a plan is to size up the situation.

the firefighters are monitored according to wildland firefighting procedures.

Extending Hose Lines and Fire Extinguishment

The most important thing to remember when extending a line to extinguish a brush fire is to remain constantly aware of your surroundings. Be aware of the limited extinguishing capabilities of a small fire attack line and nozzle. Stay out of brush and ground cover that is higher than your knees. The fuel in higher brush and in trees exceeds the extinguishing capabilities of the line.

Enter the fire area from the burned side and knock down the head first, especially if the fire is spreading rapidly (Figure 7-15). Watch for trip hazards as you extend the line through the ground cover. Continue applying water down one flank and then down the other.

Next, extinguish the fire along the rest of the perimeter. Make sure the fire perimeter has been completely extinguished and then wet down the unburned area adjacent to the perimeter and completely around the fire area (Figure 7-16).

Finish with the interior of the fire perimeter, extinguishing any hotspots in the burned area (Figure 7-17).

Brush Truck Operations

Some fire apparatus is designed especially for fighting ground cover fires (Figure 7-18). These units are usually designed with a small amount of water on

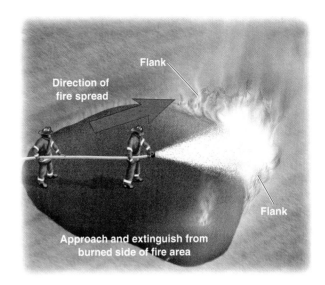

FIGURE 7-16 Extinguish the flanks to stop the spread of the fire.

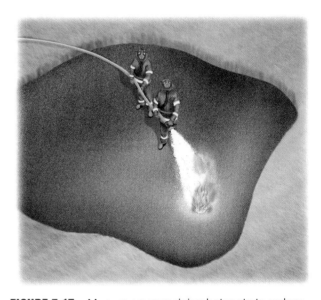

FIGURE 7-17 Mop up any remaining hotspots to reduce the chance of another fire.

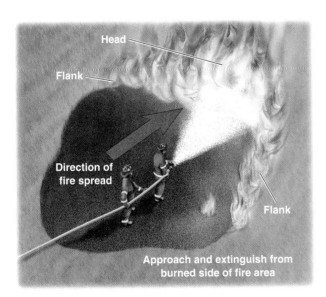

FIGURE 7-15 Knock down the fire at the head first to stop the fire's travel.

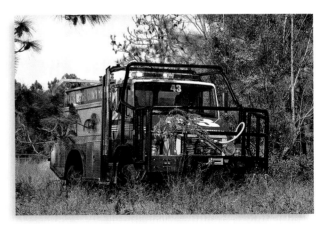

FIGURE 7-18 Brush trucks are specifically designed for off-road work.

board; they are also designed for off-road capability. They contain pumps and hose lines for attacking ground cover fires that are easily accessible and deployable. Brush trucks also have an array of brush firefighting tools, a first aid kit, and perhaps some drinking water.

As we stated before, you should respond on these units in a safe and designated seat, with your seatbelt in place. Whether these units are traveling on or off the roadway, we do not recommend riding on the front or the rear. Doing so is unsafe.

The unit will respond to the brush fire. You will deploy a small attack hose line and extinguish the fire as you would any ground cover fire. If the unit goes into the fire perimeter, it will approach it from the burned side, away from the direction the head of the fire is traveling in. The brush truck should never be positioned in front of the head of the fire (Figure 7-19).

In larger wildland incidents, brush trucks are used to protect exposures, monitor the perimeter of the fire and the fire-line area, extinguish spot-over fires, and protect other fire equipment (Figure 7-20).

The water tanks of brush trucks are refilled similarly to those on regular fire pumpers, with a fill hose at a fire hydrant. If the ground cover fire is in a remote area, the brush truck may need to be refilled by tenders. Again, the refilling procedure is basically the same, except that you will connect the brush truck refill hose into the discharge port of a tender's pump. The tender driver will then coordinate with the brush truck driver to discharge and refill the brush truck's water tank (Figure 7-21).

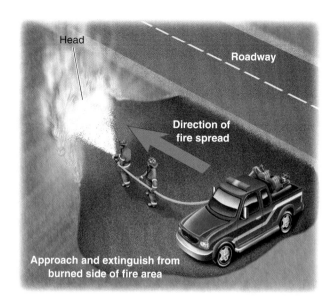

FIGURE 7-19 On small, low, ground cover fires, a brush truck may be positioned so that you can work inside the blackened area.

Brush trucks are very effective for the rapid knockdown and extinguishment of ground cover fires and can be a great asset for protection on larger wildland fires. Always be extremely careful when working around these vehicles as they travel in and around the fire area. If you are on foot, the driver may not be able to see you; therefore, stay clear of these units while they are moving (Figure 7-22).

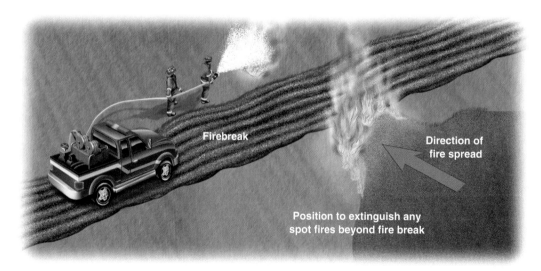

FIGURE 7-20 On larger fires, the brush truck may be positioned at a fire break to be ready to extinguish spot fires ahead of the blaze.

Evolution 7-1

Extinguishing a Ground Cover Fire

Training Area: Open area, preferably with trees and other obstacles

Equipment: Pumper or brush truck with small-diameter hose line

At least 10 targets (traffic cones or 2-liter plastic soda bottles filled with water)

PPE: Head, eye, hand, and foot protection is suggested, but follow your department's policy. ***This is not a live-fire drill.***

1. Mark off a perimeter approximately 50 feet in diameter. Arrange the targets around the perimeter, grouping 4 together at the far end of the circle to simulate the head of the fire, 2 on each flank, and setting 2 targets about 10 feet apart to simulate the rear. It is preferable if there are some trees or bushes inside the "burn area" that will offer obstacles to the hose team. If more targets are available, set them in clumps 15 or 20 feet outside the circle to simulate fingers burning outside the perimeter of a fire.

2. Each member of the crew takes a turn pulling the hose line, snaking it into the burn area from the rear. The object is to knock over all the targets at the head, then at the flanks, and then to extinguish any remaining hotspots along the entire perimeter of the fire area. Guard against horseplay and running with the hose line over uneven ground. The object of this practice drill is to teach, not to injure.

It is important that the crewmembers function as a team during this drill and follow these drill components:

- Crew members should practice spacing evenly along the hose line as it is deployed.

- A firefighter should take a position at each obstacle to keep the line moving and to prevent kinks in the hose.

- Each firefighter should rotate through all the positions in the line.

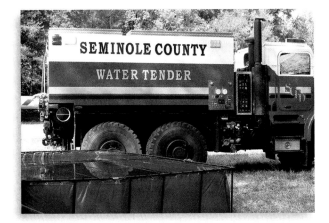

FIGURE 7-21 Tenders are usually positioned in safe areas where the brush trucks can return for more water when needed.

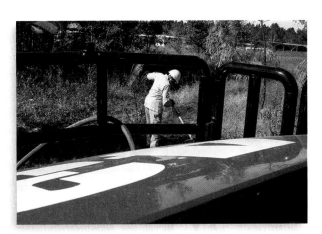

FIGURE 7-22 Because they are large, some brush trucks and tenders prevent the driver from seeing the area close to the unit. For your safety, stay clear of moving apparatus.

Evolution 7-2

Making a Firebreak

Training Area: Open area, preferably with trees and other obstacles

Equipment: Necessary tools may include a shovel, a council rake, and some sort of axe

PPE: Head, eye, hand, and foot protection is suggested, but follow your department's policy. ***This is* not *a live-fire drill.***

1. Firebreak tools are assigned to clear away the ground cover in order to establish a firebreak around the perimeter of a ground cover fire.

2. Discuss the various methods and techniques for using each tool to rake back the ground cover in order to expose mineral soil around the entire perimeter of a burn area. If the area can be cleared, demonstrate the techniques for clearing a firebreak. If the training area is in an open area where damage to the landscape is a concern, do not perform the exercise but simply discuss the tools and tactics you will use.

3. Demonstrate and explain overhauling the burn area.

4. Finally, after the fire is declared under control and has been put out, replace your tools and equipment on the unit and return to the fire station.

5. Some agencies may require checking the fire a few times after the incident, looking for any rekindling of the fire. This practice is particularly important during hot and dry weather conditions when blowing embers can quickly start a spot fire outside the fire perimeter (Figure 7-23).

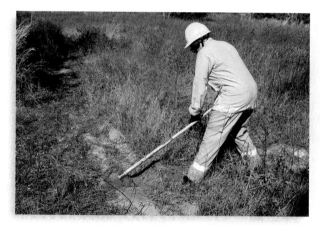

FIGURE 7-23 It is important to check for any rekindling of a fire, especially during hot and dry weather conditions.

Do It!

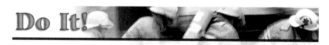

Respecting Ground Cover Fires

Brush fire operations involve their own set of extinguishing tactics and practices. These firefighting skills are just as dangerous as any other firefighting skill you will learn. Having a serious respect for ground cover fires will enhance your safety while operating at these fire incidents.

In this chapter, we discussed ground cover firefighting and introduced wildfire incidents while explaining some of the terminology that is unique to these types of fire operations. We explained ground cover fire movement and behavior along with some extinguishing tactics. You learned about the black-line approach, protective clothing, and the personnel accountability systems used at a typical brush fire operation. You also learned about tools and equipment, and about brush truck operations. You should use everything you learned in this chapter to safely extinguish ground cover fires.

Knowledge Assessment

Signed Documentation Tear-Out Sheet

Exterior Operations Level Firefighter—Chapter 7

Name: _____

Fill out the ten-question quiz below, the Knowledge Assessment Sheet, by circling the correct answer for each question. When finished, sign it and give to your instructor/Company Officer for his or her signature. Turn in this Knowledge Assessment Sheet to the proper person as part of the documentation that you have completed your training for this chapter.

1. The majority of ground cover fires are _____ in size.
   a. more than half of an acre
   b. less than an acre
   c. more than one tenth of an acre
   d. more than an acre

2. In hilly or mountainous areas, a ground cover fire tends to burn _____ .
   a. up the slope
   b. down the slope
   c. at an angle to the slope
   d. in a circular direction on the slope

3. A concentrated area of heavy fire involvement at the leading edge of a ground cover fire is referred to as the _____ .
   a. firebreak
   b. base
   c. flank
   d. head

4. The _____ is the area around the edge of the entire ground cover fire area.
   a. flank
   b. fire perimeter
   c. finger area
   d. fire base

5. A roadway would be an example of a _____ .
   a. natural wind break
   b. wildland fire line
   c. manmade firebreak
   d. poor firebreak

6. In many cases, it is much safer to allow a brush fire to burn to a firebreak, such as a roadway, than to extinguish any spot-over fires.
   a. True
   b. False

7. It is acceptable to put on safety gear while responding on a brush truck to a ground cover fire.

    a. True

    b. False

8. When using small-diameter fire attack lines, stay out of brush _____ .

    a. that is higher than your chest

    b. that is higher than your knees

    c. that is higher than your ankles

    d. at all times

9. A good tool for clearing ground vegetation and debris at a ground cover fire is a _____ .

    a. pike pole

    b. flat-head axe

    c. council rake

    d. Halligan bar

10. Brush trucks enter the fire area and fight the brush fire from the _____ .

    a. burned side of the fire

    b. unburned side of the fire

    c. uphill side of the fire

    d. unburned side of the head of the fire

Student Signature and Date _____   Instructor/Company Officer Signature and Date _____

Prove It

Skills Assessment
Signed Documentation Tear-Out Sheet

Exterior Operations Level Firefighter—Chapter 7

Name: _____

Fill out the Skills Assessment Sheet below. Have your instructor/Company Officer check off and initial each skill you demonstrate. When finished, sign it and give to your instructor/Company Officer for his or her signature. Turn in this Skills Assessment Sheet to the proper person as part of the documentation that you have completed your training for this chapter.

Skill	Completed	Initials
1. Define some basic terms used at brush fire incidents.	_____	_____
2. Describe the basic parts of a typical brush fire.	_____	_____
3. Explain how to safely approach a brush fire.	_____	_____
4. Explain your part in a brush fire accountability system.	_____	_____
5. Demonstrate the proper donning of the protective clothing used by your agency for brush fires.	_____	_____
6. Explain the black-line firefighting approach.	_____	_____
7. Demonstrate the use of various hand tools associated with brush fire operations.	_____	_____
8. Describe fire movement and assessment safety issues as they pertain to brush fires.	_____	_____
9. Demonstrate how to safely ride on the brush fire apparatus used by your agency.	_____	_____
10. Demonstrate how to deploy and extend hose lines on the apparatus for fighting a small brush fire.	_____	_____

Student Signature and Date _____   Instructor/Company Officer Signature and Date _____

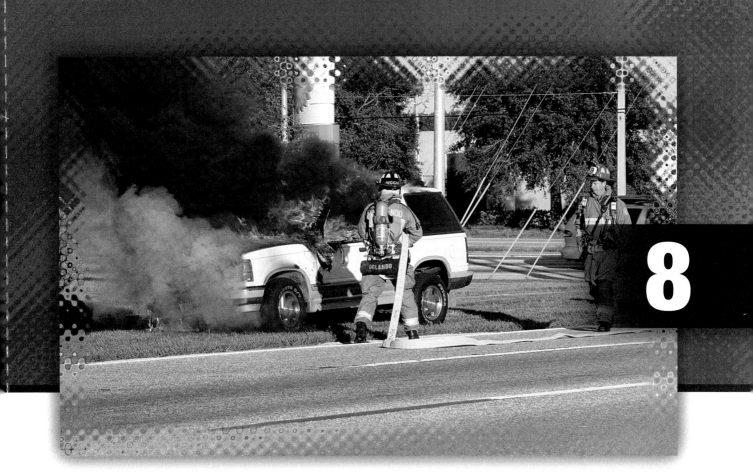

Passenger Vehicle Fires

What You Will Learn in This Chapter

In this chapter we will introduce you to vehicle fire operations, starting with personal protective equipment (PPE) and proper safety zones at vehicle fires. Then we will discuss vehicle design and burn characteristics. We will conclude the chapter with extinguishment techniques for vehicle fires.

We should also mention what you will *not* learn in this chapter. Fighting fires that involve a single automobile or light truck is much different from fighting fires in cargo-type vehicles or large, over-the-road equipment. Large vehicles often carry dangerous cargo and, at the very least, large amounts of flammable fuels that require a skill set that goes beyond the scope of this introductory chapter. For now, we will keep our focus on automobiles and light trucks, such as passenger vans, pickup trucks, and sport utility vehicles (SUVs).

What You Will Be Able to Do

After reading this chapter and participating in the practical skills sessions, you will be able to

1. Participate as a team member in setting up a typical safety zone and the traffic control needed at the scene of a vehicle fire.
2. Demonstrate how to chock the wheels and remove the keys of a vehicle involved in a fire.
3. Explain the safety risks of a vehicle fire and the importance of wearing full PPE and SCBA at a vehicle fire.
4. Describe the burn characteristics of the passenger, engine, and cargo compartment areas of a vehicle.
5. Demonstrate how to safely approach a vehicle fire with a small attack hose line.

6. Demonstrate the methods for safely extinguishing a fire in the passenger compartment of a vehicle.

7. Demonstrate the methods for safely accessing and extinguishing a fire in the engine compartment area of a vehicle.

8. Demonstrate the methods for safely accessing and extinguishing a fire in the cargo compartment of a vehicle.

9. Participate as a member of a two-member team demonstrating proper hose line stretch and control.

10. Participate as a member of a two-member team demonstrating proper charged hose line movement and nozzle control.

11. Demonstrate safely advancing a charged, small attack hose line.

12. Demonstrate safely performing overhaul operations on a vehicle that has been involved in a fire.

Reality!

Putting a Vehicle Fire into Perspective

Most vehicle fires that you will respond to are a lost cause from the very start. Therefore, the risks from aggressive extinguishment are seldom justified by the potential for a favorable outcome. Traffic is usually the most significant danger you will encounter anytime you are working in a street. However, toxic smoke, the potential for exploding car components, and rapidly advancing flames are all very real hazards that must be addressed while fighting a car fire. The reality is that any significant fire in a car or light truck usually results in a total loss of the vehicle. Your efforts should be scaled accordingly.

Although rare, there are occasions when a person is trapped in a burning car. In these instances, your rapid action can make the difference between life and death. However, anyone trapped in a fully involved car fire most likely will not survive. Therefore, firefighters should not take excessive risks in an attempt to rescue the victim. The goal for fighting a well-involved vehicle fire is to overwhelm it early with a large amount of water applied from a safe distance. This action cools the flames to a safe level before you approach the vehicle.

Vehicle Fires

Vehicle fires are common, representing about 200,000 fires (or 17% of the fires) in the United States each year. You will probably respond to more vehicle fires than structural fires. In this chapter, we present a set of new skills that build upon the skills we have already covered.

Safety Zones at Vehicle Fires

Vehicle fires present significant hazards to firefighters, many of which are not obvious at first glance. Although any smoke is hazardous and should not be breathed, the toxic gases created when an automobile burns contain more **hydrogen cyanide** than any other type of fire. Therefore, it is important that you use a self-contained breathing apparatus (SCBA) whenever you are near a burning vehicle (Figure 8-1).

In addition to the **traffic control area,** the hazards associated with a burning vehicle require observation of a wide area as a safety zone around the burning car. The following represent rapidly changing conditions or hazards that can potentially harm anyone within 50 feet of a burning automobile:

- Fuel spills or the potential for a burning or melting fuel tank that will dump highly flammable liquids
- The potential for exploding components such as pressurized cylinders used to assist in opening doors, the hood, and airbags

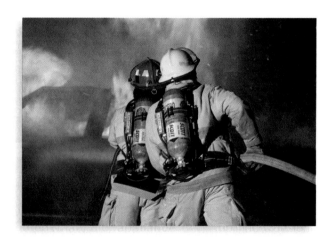

FIGURE 8-1 Because vehicle fires are very hazardous, full PPE, including an SCBA, is the minimum required protection for firefighters.

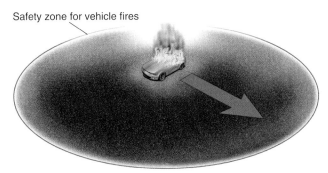

Safety zone for vehicle fires

Initially 50 feet in all directions

FIGURE 8-2 Safety zones for vehicle fires initially extend 50 feet in all directions from the burning vehicle.

Anyone working within 50 feet of a car or light truck that is well-involved in fire must be properly protected with full PPE, including breathing apparatus (Figure 8-2). It is never a good idea to breathe smoke, especially when you consider the products of combustion that are liberated from the burning plastics and other manmade materials in a motor vehicle.

■■■ KEY WORDS ■■■

hydrogen cyanide A highly poisonous gas created when plastic materials burn. This gas is present in the immediate area anytime plastics burn. It mixes with other dangerous gases that are by-products of fires involving flammable liquids and caustics.

traffic control area The area around a vehicle crash or vehicle fire incident in which any traffic passing through is safely directed by personnel or traffic cones away from the safety zone.

Traffic Control

A burning car on the side of a road is particularly distracting to drivers in the area, especially when the brilliant flames light the area on a dark night. Because of this distraction, working near traffic at the scene of a vehicle fire is particularly dangerous. Therefore, controlling the traffic flow should be your first action in stabilizing the scene. Remember, if the vehicle is well-involved in fire and it is obvious that it is unoc-

cupied or the fire is not survivable, then there is need to take a chance of being struck by traffic.

Safe Working Zones

The procedures for establishing a **safe working zone** around a burning vehicle are the same as those presented in Chapter 5, with one exception: The entire roadway or at least the lanes of travel on a divided highway that are within 50 feet of the fire should be totally blocked while the fire is actively burning. The potential is great for projectiles to fly under pressure when components of a burning car explode. The struts from pressurized cylinders used to assist in opening hoods and rear cargo lids, airbags, bumpers, and other objects explode when heated by fire. Equally hazardous is the potential for a pressurized fire from a venting fuel tank. Traffic flow can be released around an established safe working area once the fire has been controlled and the overhaul phase begins.

■■■ KEY WORD ■■■

safe working zone The designated safety area around a burning vehicle that includes the entire roadway or at least the lanes of travel on a divided highway that are within 50 feet of the fire. This area should be totally blocked while the fire is actively burning.

Chocking Wheels and Removing Keys

To protect yourself from being struck by the car, chock the vehicle's wheels as soon as possible and before moving to a position in front of or behind the vehicle. A burning vehicle should not be considered safe from unintentional movement until the electrical system has been neutralized and the wheels chocked.

Another component that will concern you is the burning vehicle itself. It is not unusual for a car engine to start on its own when the electrical system has been compromised by fire. Shorted wires can also short-circuit any vehicle safety systems that prevent the car from starting while in gear, so don't take a chance on having the car lurch forward or backward, striking you during the firefight. If the passenger compartment is not involved in fire, confirm that the ignition switch is in the *off* position and the keys are removed.

Methods of Chocking Wheels and Removing Keys at a Vehicle Fire

Use the following steps to chock the wheels and remove keys from a vehicle that is or has been involved in fire:

1. Position a 4 x 4 inch piece of cribbing in front of and behind one wheel of the vehicle.
2. Safely access the interior of the vehicle. The method of access depends on the extent of fire involvement and the resulting damage.
3. Reach in and turn off the ignition, if needed, and then remove the keys.
4. Place the keys in your pocket or hand them to your Company Officer.

Vehicle Design and Burn Characteristics

Passenger cars, vans, SUVs, and light trucks can be divided into two or three distinct segments: the engine and the passenger and cargo compartments. Obviously, any motor vehicle has an engine and passenger compartment, and most passenger cars and pickup trucks have a separation between the passenger compartment and the cargo area. Passenger vans, SUVs, and station wagon style vehicles usually do not have a separation between the passenger and cargo areas. The significance of dividing the vehicle into compartments is that each compartment presents a different set of inherent hazards as well as a different challenge in accessing the seat of the fire.

The Engine Compartment

Most accidental fires involving light vehicles start in the engine compartment area (Figure 8-3). The engine compartment is where all the electronics and fuels come together in a single location; therefore, this can be the most dangerous area when on fire. Most hazards associated with the engine compartment are due to the following four items:

- The deadly smoke liberated by burning plastics
- Exploding batteries, which result in eye and skin injuries
- Melted **radiator** or heater hoses, which cause steam burns
- Projectiles that can fly from heated struts, such as the lift-assist cylinders that help open and close the hood of a car

The main defenses against these hazards are your PPE, copious amounts of flowing water for cooling these items, and a prudent approach to the area.

■■■ KEY WORD ■■■

radiator A part of any water-cooled internal combustion engine that provides a coil and air vents to cool fluids that in turn cool the engine as it operates. In most vehicles, the radiator is located at the front of the engine compartment.

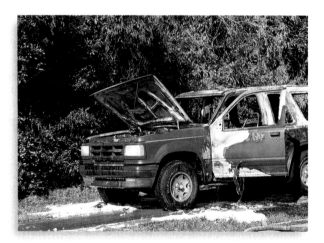

FIGURE 8-3 In light vehicles, the engine compartment is the area most likely area to have an accidental fire. It is also the most dangerous area when it is on fire.

Never Breathe Smoke

The fluids and manmade materials that burn in the engine area liberate thick, black, choking smoke that can incapacitate you with a single breath. Large amounts of deadly gases, including hydrogen cyanide, are present in the immediate area anytime plastics burn. These gases mix with the other dangerous gases that are by-products of fires involving flammable liquids and caustics. Because vehicle fires usually occur outdoors, many firefighters are tempted to simply approach the fire from upwind of the incident, relying on a breeze or wind to blow the smoke away. This approach is extremely dangerous, as a momentary shift of wind or position will expose you to deadly gases. Wear your SCBA with the mask in place whenever you are near a burning or even smoldering vehicle. Proper PPE is essential.

Lead-acid batteries are usually found in the engine area. In some models, this type of battery may be located elsewhere, such as in the rear cargo compartment or even underneath the back seat of some sedans. The plastic case of a lead-acid battery usually burns and melts during a fire, spilling the caustic acid. However, it is not uncommon for a battery to explode when heated or when the wires short out elsewhere during a fire involving the vehicle's electrical system.

If the battery has not been involved in fire and is accessible, it is necessary to disconnect the electrical battery cables. Doing so reduces the chance of a secondary fire from the vehicle's battery power. It also helps to eliminate the possibility of an accidental restart of the vehicle's motor. Disconnecting the electrical battery cables is also the primary step toward preventing the accidental deployment of any nondeployed airbags. Be extremely careful when disconnecting the cables and continue to wear your full PPE during the procedure. Start with the ground (negative) side and then proceed to the positive side of the battery. If you cannot reach the bolts that connect the leads to the battery, use a pair of insulated cable cutters to cut a section out of each wire—again, starting with the negative side first. Making a single cut in each wire is not sufficient because it allows a chance for the wires to accidentally touch and re-energize the circuits. Cutting out at least an inch-long section of wire and covering the exposed ends with electrical tape helps prevent this hazard (Figure 8-4).

Steam and pressurized fluids released from small leaks in the hoses within the engine compartment present an immediate hazard to exposed skin. Many pressurized fluids, such as transmission fluid or engine oil, are highly flammable when atomized under pressure. These fluids present a significant exposure to re-ignition when the atomized, flammable fluids make contact with hot objects in the area. Once again, the best defense against this hazard is full PPE and the application of copious amounts of water to cool the area.

The Passenger Compartment

The hazards associated with the passenger compartment of light vehicles currently manufactured have changed in recent years. As with any other part of the car, burning plastics present the most obvious threat

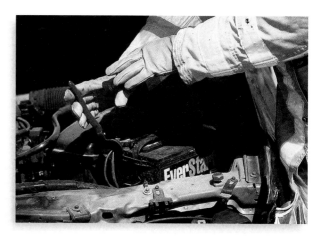

FIGURE 8-4 If cutting battery cables, start with the negative cable and cut out a 1-inch section of the cable, leaving a gap.

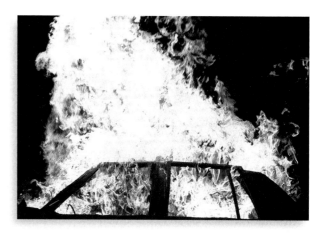

FIGURE 8-5 Burning plastics present the primary respiratory health hazard in the passenger compartment of light vehicles.

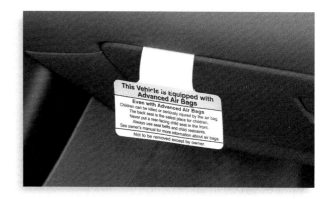

FIGURE 8-6 Airbag systems that deploy during a passenger compartment fire present the main strike hazard for firefighters during a vehicle fire in this area.

to your respiratory system (Figure 8-5). The changes in hazards are due to the potential strike hazards associated with the passive-restraint systems (airbags and **seatbelt pretensioners**) in modern cars and light trucks (Figure 8-6).

The elements that deploy most airbags found in the dash and seatbacks are flammable products that burn rapidly at a relatively low temperature. Side-curtain airbags are usually inflated with an inert gas that is contained in a pressurized cylinder, which can be contained in the A **post,** the C post, or even the roof rail on some model cars. When the vehicle's passenger compartment is well-involved in fire, the airbags often deploy from the heat, sounding like a shotgun blast. In rare cases, these pressure releases have caused either burning materials from the airbag or some small hard components of the assembly to fly out of the passenger compartment, often traveling several feet in the air.

A fire that does not involve the passenger compartment can also cause an unintentional deployment of one or more airbags if the circuits short as wires melt. Therefore, it is extremely important that the electrical system be neutralized anytime a fire occurs in a passenger vehicle that is equipped with passive-restraint systems.

■ KEY WORDS ■

posts The parts of a vehicle's construction that connect the roof of the vehicle to the body. They are constructed of rolled sheet metal and are given alphabetical labels, starting with *A* at the front and continuing with *B* and *C* for each of the next posts on the same side of the vehicle.

seatbelt pretensioner A device designed to automatically retract a seatbelt to better secure the user during a collision.

The Cargo Compartment

A fire that involves the cargo compartment of a car is a very unpredictable event because the material that is burning is an unknown. As an example, picture a fire involving a cargo compartment that contains clothing the driver purchased during a shopping trip to the local mall. Now picture the same car and the same driver as he or she is returning from the local garden center with three bags of fertilizer and a bottle of concentrated pesticide. The types of smoke and vapors liberated from a cotton shirt differ greatly from the smoke and vapors liberated from the pesticide. In the case of fertilizer, the contents can become explosive when mixed with other materials, like a plastic bottle of motor oil that the driver was also carrying and had forgotten about.

The cargo compartment can also become unpredictable because the fuel tank of most cars is near the cargo area. In addition, aftermarket alternative fuels

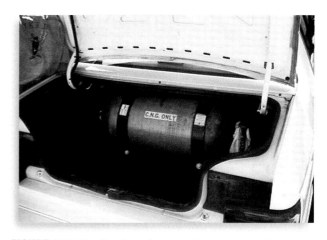

FIGURE 8-7 The fuel tank is normally located under the rear cargo area. Some vehicles are equipped with alternative fuel systems whose fuel tanks are located inside the trunk area.

such as **propane** or **compressed natural gas** might be located in the cargo compartment (Figure 8-7).

Again, the common element to your personal safety with any vehicle fire is exactly like that of any significant fire: Wear your PPE in the proper manner, no exceptions!

■ KEY WORDS ■

compressed natural gas A type of fuel found as a gas in nature that is liquefied and stored in compressed gas cylinders for use. As a gas, it is lighter than air and will rise when released. It can be used as an alternative fuel for a gasoline-powered internal combustion engine.

propane A type of fuel found as a gas in nature that is liquefied and stored in compressed gas cylinders for use. As a gas, it is heavier than air and will seek its lowest level when released. This material can be used as an alternative fuel for a gasoline-powered internal combustion engine.

Hybrid Vehicles

Hybrid vehicles, which use both a conventional gasoline motor and a high-voltage electric motor for propulsion, are becoming more common with each model year. The high-voltage circuits derive their power from banks of dry-cell batteries, very similar to flashlight batteries. However, unlike a flashlight that uses two or three 1.2-volt batteries for power, the rechargeable batteries in a hybrid vehicle are assembled in a series,

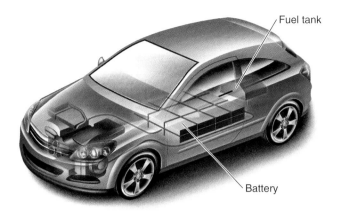

FIGURE 8-8 The battery cell in a hybrid car. Hybrid vehicles have large banks of batteries that deliver high voltages of electricity. These batteries disconnect when the ignition is shut off, the normal engine battery is disconnected, or a fuse is activated.

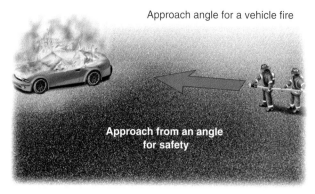

FIGURE 8-9 For safety, approach a vehicle fire at an angle.

which means that their voltage is multiplied. The entire battery cell in a typical hybrid vehicle can deliver more than 400 volts of power (Figure 8-8).

The high-voltage circuit on a hybrid vehicle is protected by fuses that are designed to interrupt power in the event of a short circuit. The high-voltage circuit is also designed to be disconnected when the ignition key is switched off and any time the low-voltage, conventional battery is disconnected. The high-voltage wires on a hybrid vehicle are clearly covered with a bright, orange-colored wrapping. Avoid coming into contact with any of these wires when you are working near a hybrid vehicle. It is also wise to avoid contact with any substance leaking around the batteries in any type of vehicle, including a hybrid.

Extinguishing Vehicle Fires

For your immediate safety, fires of any significance involving a passenger vehicle require a hose line capable of at least a 95-gpm flow and should be backed up with a hose line of equal capacity. Because most light-vehicle fires are quickly extinguished with less than 100 gallons of water, there is usually no reason to connect to a sustained water supply for the operation. However, it is a good idea to locate a water source, just in case something changes during the fire that requires more water than the booster tank carries.

Passenger Compartment Fires

Choose your approach path wisely when deploying the hose line to extinguish a vehicle fire. You should take into consideration three main factors: the wind,

the terrain, and the vehicle. Even when wearing full PPE and breathing fresh air from an SCBA, it is a good idea to approach the burning vehicle from the upwind and uphill side whenever practical. The upwind approach allows the wind to blow the thick smoke away from you, greatly improving your visibility. The uphill approach also helps prevent any flammable runoff from flowing toward you and your apparatus during the approach.

It is most often advisable that you approach the vehicle from an angle rather than moving directly in line with the front or rear of the car, or perpendicular to the side (Figure 8-9). The front or rear approach can put you in line with most of the struts or other components that can eject from the car during a free-burning fire. The perpendicular approach can put you in the path of a fireball as it erupts from a venting gasoline fill spout.

Begin flowing water from at least 30 feet away when approaching a well-involved fire, using a tight pattern to reach the seat of the fire and overwhelming it with force. First direct the stream toward any fire that is near the fuel tank and then concentrate on each of the three compartments as you go. The passenger compartment will emit a large volume of fire that can be knocked down quickly with a tight stream from a relatively safe position. As you approach the car, widen the stream to keep from "overshooting" the blaze. As you approach, play the water in a sweeping motion underneath the car.

Break any glass that prevents you from applying water to the seat of the fire and also to release trapped smoke. A striking tool, like an axe or a Halligan bar, works well for this purpose. If the passenger compartment is well-involved in fire, then a short **ceiling hook** used at a distance of approximately 6 feet can also be used to break the **tempered glass** on the sides and rear of the car from a safer distance than the shorter **Halligan bar** or an axe allows.

A fire in the passenger compartment can be quickly extinguished, but the area underneath the dash will probably continue to burn. This is due to the fuel load (the coatings on wires and plastic components). The area beneath the dash will also burn because any fire in the engine compartment will probably travel through the so-called firewall until it can be controlled.

▰▰ KEY WORDS ▰▰

ceiling hook   A common hand tool used by firefighters to access inside wall and ceiling areas in light vehicles. It has a handle with a specialized head on one end of the handle that is used to puncture and then cut and pull interior ceiling and wall coverings.

Halligan bar   A specialized firefighter's hand tool made up of a handle with a pry fork at one end and a combination adze and pick at the opposite end. This tool was developed to aid in forcing entry into buildings through door and window openings. It has since been adapted for many other uses in the Fire Service.

tempered glass   A type of glass commonly used in the construction of side and rear vehicle windows. This type of glass is heat-treated and tempered, which add strength to the glass. It is broken by applying a small point of contact with a large amount of force, which breaks it into many small pieces.

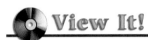 **View It!**

Go to the DVD, navigate to Chapter 8, and select *Extinguishing a Passenger Vehicle Fire.*

Practice It!

Extinguishing a Passenger Compartment Fire

Use the following method to approach and extinguish a fire in the passenger compartment of a vehicle:

1. Approach a burning vehicle from the upwind and uphill side when possible, and begin flowing water from about 30 feet away, using a tight stream pattern (Figure 8-10).

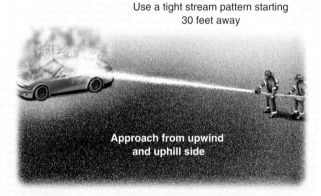

Use a tight stream pattern starting 30 feet away

Approach from upwind and uphill side

FIGURE 8-10

2. With a well-involved vehicle fire, first apply water near the fuel tank area and then to the three compartment areas. Widen the stream pattern as you get closer to the vehicle, using a sweeping motion (Figure 8-11).

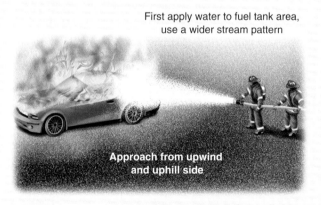

First apply water to fuel tank area, use a wider stream pattern

Approach from upwind and uphill side

FIGURE 8-11

3. If you cannot open the doors of the passenger compartment and all the windows are closed, you can remove the side and rear windows by using a striking tool to break the tempered glass. To break the glass, use a ceiling hook from approximately 6 feet away or a Halligan bar at a closer distance (Figure 8-12).

4. Complete the process by extinguishing the rest of the vehicle as necessary.

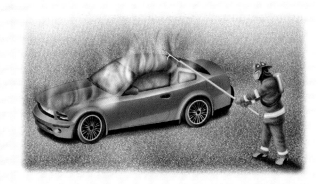

FIGURE 8-12

Engine Compartment Fires

The main obstacle to controlling a fire in the engine compartment is the lack of access to the area. Fires in the engine compartment can be knocked down to some extent by flowing water through the wheel wells. Most passenger vehicles have plastic inner liners placed on their fenders in the engine compartment that usually burn out of the way, making this area a quick path for applying water. Another method, which is less effective, is to train a tight stream through the front grille and radiator area. This method won't extinguish the fire, but it may buy you some time until the hood can be opened.

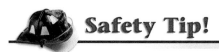 **Safety Tip!**

WARNING: Opening the hood while the engine compartment is burning can cause a rush of fresh air to reach the seat of the fire, producing a rush of heat and flame. You can prepare yourself for this by wearing your full PPE and breathing from your SCBA.

Opening the hood of a burned car can be a frustrating exercise. More often than not, the hood release cable or mechanism has burned away in the passenger compartment near the dash, making the conventional method of "popping the hood" ineffective. Because it will take a few minutes to open the hood, it is usually most effective to simply use a pry bar to pry open a small access point on the side of the hood between the hood and the fender. Once this access point is created, flow plenty of water into the area to cool it (Figure 8-13).

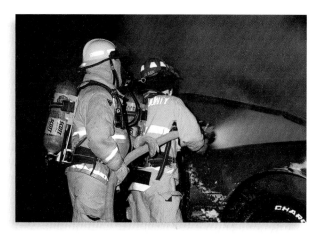

FIGURE 8-13 As an opening is made into the engine compartment, make sure to flow plenty of water into it.

There are a couple of steps you can take to open a hood after most of the operating cable has burned away. First, break away any grille that is in your way and locate the remaining hood release cable, which should be in front of the radiator just behind the grille. A quick tug on this cable usually operates the first position of tho hood latch. If you cannot reach the cable with your gloved hand, use the forked end of a Halligan bar to catch the cable and then twist it, wrapping it around the forked end until the latch operates. The secondary latch operates normally with a gloved hand.

More often than not, the plastic clips that hold the insulation blanket that lines the underside of the hood will have melted away, causing the blanket to drop down over the motor. Be careful when removing the blanket, taking care to wet it first. Use a long-handled tool such as a pike pole to drag the blanket out of the way as another firefighter stands by with a charged hose line to take care of any flare-ups.

Accessing and Controlling an Engine Compartment Fire

Use the following steps to access and control a fire in the engine compartment of a vehicle:

1. As with passenger compartment fires, approach an engine compartment fire at an angle. Use a tight-pattern stream of water and widen it as you get closer.

FIGURE 8-14

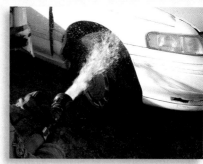

2. When you are at the engine compartment area, apply water into the wheel well or to the front grille (Figure 8-14).

3. To open the front hood, access the cable in the passenger compartment or break out the front grille with a Halligan bar. Locate the latch-operating cable with your gloved hand and pull it outward (Figure 8-15).

FIGURE 8-15

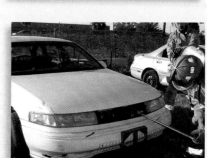
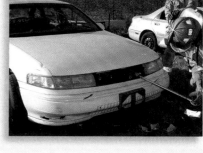

4. An alternative method for operating the cable is to twist the cable with the forked end of the Halligan bar (Figure 8-16).

FIGURE 8-16

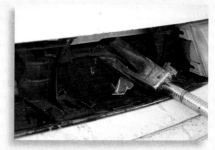

5. Carefully raise the hood and be ready to extinguish any additional fire that develops when more air reaches the engine compartment fire (Figure 8-17).

FIGURE 8-17

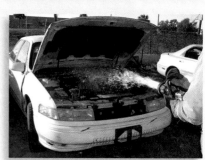

Cargo Compartment Fires

As with engine compartment fires, the main obstacle to controlling a fire in the cargo compartment is the lack of access to the area. In addition, fires in the cargo area will present their own set of access obstacles that will vary, depending on the style and model of vehicle that is burning. Many cars have fold-down rear seats or small access panels that allow long objects to pass into the passenger compartment. These areas make great access points for directing water to the seat of a cargo compartment fire. However, there are some alternative actions you can take if you are unable to readily access the compartment and keys are not available to operate the latch in the conventional manner.

First, cool the cargo area as much as possible by breaking out a taillight assembly and flowing water in. This action usually takes care of any active fire. To force entry to the cargo area, use the pick-end of a Halligan bar to punch out the key cylinder and then use a small tool such as a screwdriver to turn the latch assembly, unlocking the trunk.

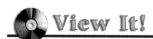

Practice It!

Accessing and Controlling a Cargo Compartment Fire

Use the following steps to access and control a fire in the cargo compartment of a vehicle:

1. Approach the cargo compartment fire from an angle as you would a passenger compartment fire, using a tight-pattern stream until you get closer to the cargo area and then widening the stream pattern.

FIGURE 8-18

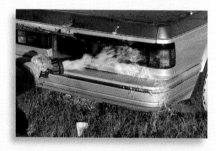

2. Next, cool the cargo area by breaking out a taillight and flowing water in (Figure 8-18).

3. Access the cargo compartment by using the pick-end of a Halligan bar to punch out the key cylinder. Then, using a small tool like a screwdriver, turn the latch assembly, unlocking the trunk lid (Figure 8-19).

FIGURE 8-19

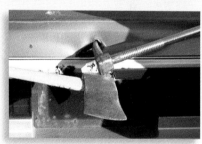

View It!

Go to the DVD, navigate to Chapter 8, and select *Stretching a Dry Hose Line and Nozzle Control.*

Evolution 8-1

Stretching a Dry Hose Line and Nozzle Control

Training Area: Open area; level ground free of trip hazards

Equipment: Equipped pumper

3 targets (traffic cones weighted on the bottom or 2-liter plastic soda bottles filled with water)

PPE: Full protective clothing and SCBA. *This is **not** a live-fire drill.*

1. Mark off an area approximately 150 feet in length. Arrange the targets approximately 50 feet apart at one end of the training area (Figure 8-20).

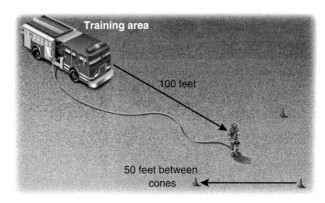

FIGURE 8-20

2. Position the pumper approximately 100 feet from the targets.

3. Working in teams of at least two, the simulated crew takes a turn pulling a preconnected hose line, stretching it to the target area (Figure 8-21). They then signal for the line to be charged. Once the line is stretched, practice flowing it for at least 4 minutes, flowing various patterns. Then use a narrow stream pattern to knock down all 3 targets. The additional team member should be positioned as a backup person, taking much of the load off the nozzle person. Guard against horseplay. The object of all practice drills is to teach, not to injure.

FIGURE 8-21

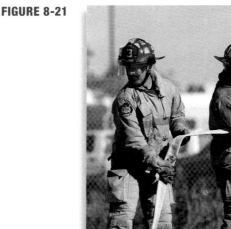

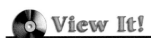 **View It!**

Go to the DVD, navigate to Chapter 8, and select *Advancing a Charged Hose Line and Nozzle Control—2-Person Drill.*

Evolution 8-2

Advancing a Charged Hose Line and Nozzle Control—2-Person Drill

Training Area: Open area; level ground free of trip hazards

Equipment: Equipped pumper

3 targets (traffic cones weighted on the bottom or 2-liter plastic soda bottles filled with water)

PPE: Full protective clothing and SCBA. ***This is not a live-fire drill.***

1. Mark off an area approximately 150 feet in length. Arrange the targets approximately 50 feet apart at one end of the training area.

2. Position the pumper approximately 100 feet from the targets.

3. Working in teams of two, the crew takes a turn pulling a preconnected hose line, stretching it enough to allow the line to be charged and then advancing it at least 75 feet while charged. Once the line is stretched, the team works together to knock down all 3 targets using a narrow stream (Figure 8-22).

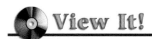

Go to the DVD, navigate to Chapter 8, and select *Advancing a Charged Hose Line and Nozzle Control—1-Person Drill.*

FIGURE 8-22

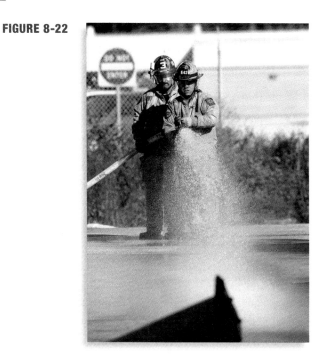

Evolution 8-3

Advancing a Charged Hose Line and Nozzle Control—1-Person Drill

NOTE: This is an optional drill at the Exterior Operations level.

Training Area: Open area; level ground free of trip hazards

Equipment: Equipped pumper

3 targets (traffic cones weighted on the bottom or 2-liter plastic soda bottles filled with water)

PPE: Full protective clothing and SCBA. ***This is <u>not</u> a live-fire drill.***

1. Mark off an area approximately 150 feet in length. Arrange the targets approximately 50 feet apart at one end of the training area.

2. Position the pumper approximately 100 feet from the targets.

3. Each member of the simulated crew takes a turn pulling a preconnected hose line, stretching it enough to allow the line to be charged and then advancing it at least 75 feet while charged. Once the line is stretched, each crew member should take turns knocking down all 3 targets using a narrow stream (Figure 8-23). Guard against horseplay and running with the hose line. The object of this practice drill is to teach, not to injure.

FIGURE 8-23

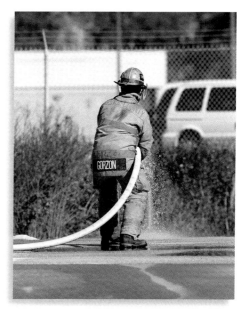

Vehicle Fire Overhaul

Overhaul is the process of systematically looking for any hidden fire or hot areas and taking measures to completely extinguish any of these remaining problems. Overhaul begins once the main body of the fire has been extinguished and continues until there is no chance of an accidental re-ignition. Overhaul is an important process in any fire operation; it is the best defense to prevent a rekindling of the original blaze (Figure 8-24). It is often best to let the vehicle cool down for a few minutes to let any hidden hotspots either die out or re-ignite so that you will know where to look for any hidden fires that remain.

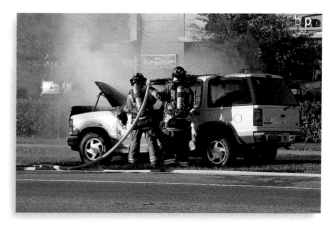

FIGURE 8-24 Proper overhauling prevents rekindling of a vehicle fire.

Because smoke and products of combustion are released until the car is completely cooled, it is important that you keep your air mask on during overhaul. It is also important that your hands are protected by gloves and that all of your remaining PPE remains in place. The metal on the car will be very hot for a few minutes after the fire has been extinguished. Therefore, there is an obvious chance of accidental burns to exposed skin from contact with hot objects.

Overhauling a vehicle fire is usually best accomplished by flowing a lot of water, flushing out any hidden embers. Open every compartment, including the glove box. Because it is common for most drivers to carry important papers such as insurance records and vehicle registration documents in their glove box, open it first and salvage anything you can before flooding that area. If smoke is still issuing from underneath the dashboard area, water can be trained down through the defroster vents. If more room is needed for water flow, the entire glove box can be removed with a little force from a Halligan bar so that water can be applied directly to the fire source or area of smoldering.

Upholstered and padded areas in a car can sometimes smolder for quite a while, so the Company Officer or pump operator may decide to put an additive called **Class A foam** into the water. This additive allows the water to soak into the padded areas to better extinguish any deep-seated fire or embers. You will notice a foamy consistency as it strikes the surface of wherever you are directing the fire stream; however, there is no difference in the way you will handle the nozzle and hose line (Figure 8-25). Just be aware

that when you see the foam, the Class A additive is working.

▰ KEY WORD ▰

Class A foam A fire-extinguishing additive applied to fires involving Class A materials. It provides additional absorption capability to the water to which it is added.

Overhauling a Vehicle Fire

After the vehicle fire has been initially extinguished, use the following steps to extinguish any remaining fires:

1. With PPE and SCBA still in place, open all compartments and look for hidden fires and hotspots. Flow water onto them to extinguish them.
2. If the dashboard is still smoldering, flow water down into the defroster vents or remove the glove box with a Halligan bar.
3. In order to provide better soaking capability to upholstered seats and other areas inside the vehicle, your supervisor may add a Class A fire foam agent to your water supply. Douse the areas the same as you would with plain water.

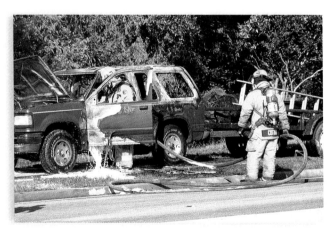

FIGURE 8-25 Applying a Class A foam agent during the overhaul of a passenger compartment can be more effective than simply applying water to smoldering upholstery.

Do It!

Managing Vehicle Fires Safely

Vehicle fires require taking all the safety and protection precautions necessary for any other fire event. The importance of having adequate protection, using proper PPE and SCBA, and controlling traffic cannot be overemphasized. Remember to always have an adequate-size fire attack hose line and water supply. Apply the water from a distance first and approach at an angle as well as from uphill and upwind when possible. Keep in mind the potential dangers involved in vehicle fires, stay alert, and work as an effective firefighting team member.

Prove It

Knowledge Assessment

Exterior Operations Level Firefighter—Chapter 8

Name: _____

Fill out the ten-question quiz below, the Knowledge Assessment Sheet, by circling the correct answer for each question. When finished, sign it and give to your instructor/Company Officer for his or her signature. Turn in this Knowledge Assessment Sheet to the proper person as part of the documentation that you have completed your training for this chapter.

1. Vehicle fires are common, representing about _____ of the fires throughout the United States each year.
   - **a.** 77%
   - **b.** 50%
   - **c.** 25%
   - **d.** 17%

2. Anyone working within _____ feet of a car or light truck that is well-involved in fire must be properly protected with full personal protective equipment, including breathing apparatus.
   - **a.** 150
   - **b.** 50
   - **c.** 100
   - **d.** 30

3. Most accidental fires in light vehicles start in the _____ compartment area.
   - **a.** cargo
   - **b.** rear seat
   - **c.** passenger
   - **d.** engine

4. Large amounts of the deadly gas hydrogen cyanide are present in the immediate area anytime plastics burn and mix with other dangerous gases that are by-products of fires involving flammable liquids and caustics.
   - **a.** True
   - **b.** False

5. When the vehicle's passenger compartment is well-involved in fire, the airbags will often _____ from the heat.
   - **a.** melt
   - **b.** remain unaffected
   - **c.** deploy
   - **d.** shrink

6. Fire in the _____ compartment can be unpredictable because the fuel tank of most cars is near this area.
   - **a.** cargo
   - **b.** passenger
   - **c.** engine
   - **d.** glove

7. The entire battery cell in a typical hybrid vehicle can deliver more than _____ volts of power.

    a. 400

    b. 600

    c. 800

    d. 900

8. Begin flowing water from at least _____ away when approaching a well-involved fire, using a tight pattern to reach the seat of the fire and overwhelming it with force.

    a. 100 feet

    b. 30 feet

    c. 75 feet

    d. 10 feet

9. Fires in the engine compartment can be knocked down to some extent by flowing water through the wheel wells.

    a. True

    b. False

10. _____ begins once the main body of the fire has been extinguished and continues until there is no chance of an accidental re-ignition.

    a. A vehicle fires

    b. The donning of PPE

    c. Flowing water

    d. Overhaul

Student Signature and Date _____   Instructor/Company Officer Signature and Date _____

Prove It

Skills Assessment
Signed Documentation Tear-Out Sheet
Exterior Operations Level Firefighter—Chapter 8

Name: _____

Fill out the Skills Assessment Sheet below. Have your instructor/Company Officer check off and initial each skill you demonstrate. When finished, sign it and give to your instructor/Company Officer for his or her signature. Turn in this Skills Assessment Sheet to the proper person as part of the documentation that you have completed your training for this chapter.

Skill	Completed	Initials
1. Participate as a team member in setting up a typical safety zone and the traffic control needed at the scene of a vehicle fire.	_____	_____
2. Demonstrate how to chock the wheels and remove the keys of a vehicle involved in a fire.	_____	_____
3. Explain the safety risks of a vehicle fire and the importance of wearing full PPE and SCBA at a vehicle fire.	_____	_____
4. Describe the burn characteristics of the passenger, engine, and cargo compartments of a vehicle.	_____	_____
5. Demonstrate how to safely approach a vehicle fire with a small attack hose line.	_____	_____
6. Demonstrate the methods for safely extinguishing a fire in the passenger compartment of a vehicle.	_____	_____
7. Demonstrate the methods for safely accessing and extinguishing a fire in the engine compartment area of a vehicle.	_____	_____
8. Demonstrate the methods for safely accessing and extinguishing a fire in the cargo compartment of a vehicle.	_____	_____
9. Participate as a member of a two-member team demonstrating proper hose line stretch and control.	_____	_____
10. Participate as a member of a two-member team demonstrating proper charged hose line movement and nozzle control.	_____	_____
11. Demonstrate safely advancing a charged, small attack hose line.	_____	_____
12. Demonstrate safely performing overhaul operations on a vehicle that has been involved in a fire.	_____	_____

Student Signature and Date _____   Instructor/Company Officer Signature and Date _____

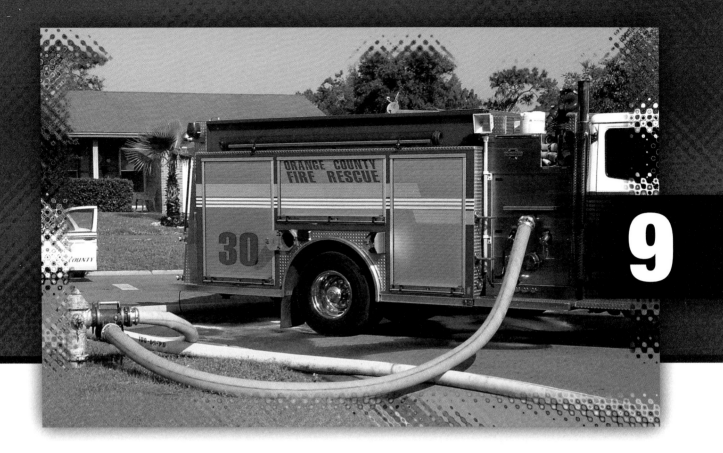

Supply Hose Lines

What You Will Learn in This Chapter

This chapter will introduce you to the elements of a proper water supply for fighting fires. We will explain the initial water supply that is carried to the fire by the apparatus and sustained water supplies. In addition, we will discuss the water supply that is adequate and non-interruptible. You will also learn the methods used to assist with developing and utilizing the different types of water sources.

What You Be Able to Do

After reading this chapter and participating in the practical skills sessions, you will be able to

1. Explain the elements of an initial and a sustained water supply.
2. Help establish a water supply from various static sources, including portable tanks, lakes, and streams.

3. Work safely around a static water supply.
4. Help refill a booster tank and a tanker truck.
5. Operate a fire hydrant.
6. Assist in establishing a drafting operation.
7. Assist in establishing a sustained water supply from a hydrant using various hose configurations and layouts.
8. Explain the differences among hard suction hose, conventional supply hose, and large-diameter supply hose.

Reality!

Water Supply—A Critical Firefighting Factor

When most citizens think of firefighters, they immediately conjure an image of heroic acts in which a greater-than-life hero is walking from a burning inferno carrying a just-rescued child in his or her arms.

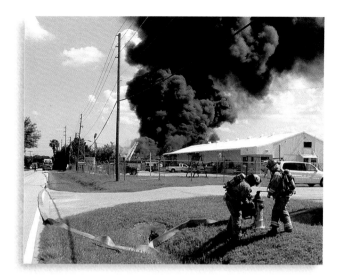

FIGURE 9-1 A good supply of water is essential to any fire operation.

Certainly, there are extraordinary acts of humanity performed daily by firefighters everywhere, but the reality is that fighting fires is *always* a team effort. No single job is more or less important to the safety and efficiency of the mission than others; however, some tasks are absolutely critical to a mission. So while the news cameras are trained on the firefighters who are moving in and out of a burn area, flowing large amounts of water on the blaze, an educated firefighter knows that somewhere in the scheme of things all of that water has come from somewhere. Although one would seldom think it a meritorious act, simply connecting the hose to a fire hydrant and charging the line at the proper time is often critical to the entire operation (Figure 9-1). No positive actions on the fireground will take place very long without an adequate supply of water to flow through the lines.

Water Supplies

Firefighters cannot extinguish fires with their hose lines if they do not have an adequate water supply. This fact has never changed for the Fire Service. The water supply needed can be brought to the scene on the fire apparatus along with the hose and other firefighting tools and personnel. It can arrive on a specialized tender unit that is specially designed to haul large amounts of water to the fire scene. A supply of water can be obtained from a static water supply. Static water supplies are not under pressure. A lake, stream, river, swimming pool, and water storage tank at ground level are good examples of static water sup-

plies. Water can be obtained from a piped-in water main system in which water is under pressure and fire hydrants are attached as access points for use by the Fire Service.

Generally speaking, the water supply on most fire scenes comes from a combination of sources. Most often, water is initially brought to the scene by a fire apparatus. This **initial water supply** is often replaced by a **sustained water supply,** which comes from a more substantial source of water.

KEY WORDS

initial water supply The first supply of water that is accessed for extinguishing a fire. This water supply is usually established prior to a sustained water supply. It is usually carried to the scene by the fire apparatus or specially designed tenders.

sustained water supply The water supply established with a substantial water supply system or source, like a municipal water system or a large static water resource, such as a stream or a lake.

Initial Water Supply

The initial water supply is usually developed from water carried on an engine in its **booster tank** (Figure 9-2). It can also be supplied by a second fire apparatus on the scene through an engine-to-engine water supply operation. Many fires can be adequately handled with an initial water supply. Often a sustained water supply is developed as a safety backup for the initial water supply but is not put into use.

Booster tank location

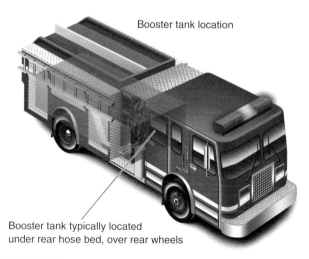

Booster tank typically located under rear hose bed, over rear wheels

FIGURE 9-2 Booster tanks are not visible on most fire apparatus. They can carry between 250 and 1000 gallons of water, depending on their design.

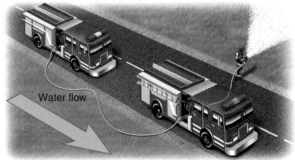

(b) Supply pumper

Water flow

(a) Attack pumper

FIGURE 9-3   (a) Attack pumper and (b) supply pumper.

▓▓ KEY WORD ▓▓▓▓▓▓

booster tank   The onboard water supply tank on a fire apparatus usually used as an initial water supply at a fire scene.

Booster Tanks

A water supply that arrives on a fire apparatus is usually 250 to 1000 gallons, depending on the needs of the fire department and the design of the fire apparatus. If a small fire attack line flows 100 gpm on a fire, then it is easy to estimate that the fire apparatus has about 5 minutes of water supply with one small fire attack line flowing. The water on a fire apparatus can be refilled from any type of water source. This onboard water supply is commonly referred to as the booster tank.

Engine-to-Engine Water Supply

There are instances in which one fire engine uses all of the water in its booster tank on a fire and needs more water supplied from a second fire engine on the scene. The second engine provides water to the first engine by connecting its water tank to the first engine through its pump. In this instance, the first engine, which is supplying water to the nozzles, is called the **attack pumper.** The engine that is delivering its

booster tank of water to the attack pumper is called the **supply pumper** (Figure 9-3).

▓▓ KEY WORDS ▓▓▓▓▓▓

attack pumper   A fire truck located at the fire scene to which water is supplied from a sustained source during the firefighting operation. This fire truck distributes the supplied water to the fire attack hose lines at the fire.

supply pumper   The fire truck that provides water to the attack pumper, either from its own booster tank or by pumping water in water supply hose lines to the attack pumper.

 View It!

Go to the DVD, navigate to Chapter 9, and select *Engine-to-Engine Water Supply.*

 Practice It!

Establishing an Engine-to-Engine Water Supply

When fire engines connect to each other to transfer a booster tank water supply, they usually use a section of a 2½- or 3-inch hose. Use the following procedure to assist in making the connection:

1. Remove a section of supply hose from one of the fire engine hose beds. Connect the female end of the supply hose to a discharge outlet on the fire engine providing the water supply (Figure 9-4).

FIGURE 9-4

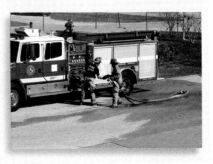

—Continued

2. Connect the male end to an intake outlet on the fire engine that is taking in the water supply (Figure 9-5).

FIGURE 9-5

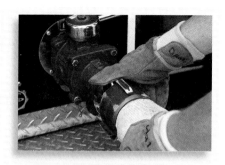

3. Advise both pump operators that the supply line is properly connected to each pumper. Walk the hose line, loosening any kinks in the charged line (Figure 9-6).

FIGURE 9-6

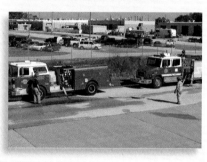

Fire Hydrants

Fire hydrants are simply valves that firefighters open and close to provide the water supply from a water main system for fire department operations (Figure 9-7). A typical fire hydrant has two or three outlet ports. These ports have male thread ends with female caps. The top of the hydrant features an operating nut. The tool used to open the hydrant is called the hydrant wrench. This wrench is adjustable and is designed to open and close the valve inside the fire hydrant. Nearly all fire hydrants open in a counterclockwise direction and close in a clockwise direction. For our purposes, we will assume that the hydrants we use

open and close in this manner. An arrow on or near the operating nut on every hydrant indicates the operating direction (Figure 9-8). Open a hydrant slowly to avoid a water hammer at the other end.

In climates that experience freezing weather, dry-barrel hydrants are used. A dry-barrel hydrant has a long stem that operates a valve well below the freeze line in the ground, so the part of the hydrant that is above the freeze line remains dry. There is a drain valve at the base of the hydrant that remains open unless the hydrant is under pressure. Because it takes pressure to close this valve, the hydrant should be fully opened when used and fully closed when not in use—otherwise the drain valve can leak and cause the ground around the hydrant to erode away. Sus-

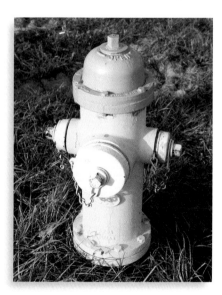

FIGURE 9-7   A typical fire hydrant has two 2½" connections and one 4½" connection.

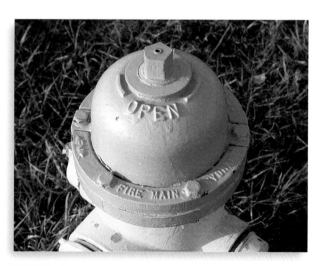

FIGURE 9-8   The operating nut has an arrow that indicates the direction to turn the valve.

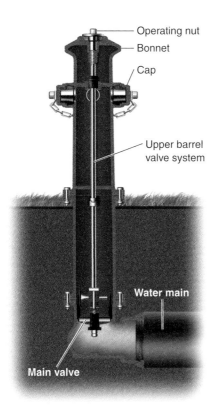

FIGURE 9-9   Dry-barrel hydrant.

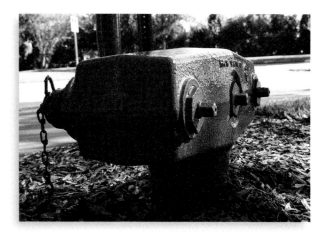

FIGURE 9-10   Wet-barrel hydrant.

pect that the drain valve has a problem anytime you open a port on a dry-barrel hydrant and find water at the cap or when you see a leaking cap on a hydrant that is fully closed off. Report this to your Company Officer so that arrangements can be made to repair the hydrant (Figure 9-9).

■ KEY WORD ■

fire hydrant   A valve opened and closed by a firefighter that provides the water supply from a water main system for fire department operations. A typical fire hydrant has two or three outlet ports that have male thread ends with female caps. An operating nut on top of the hydrant opens and closes the water flow from the appliance.

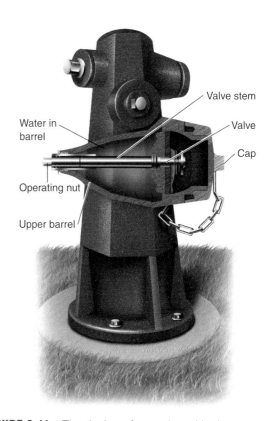

FIGURE 9-11   The design of a wet-barrel hydrant.

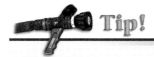

To check the drain valve on a hydrant, cap all but one of the ports and flow some water. When the water is shut down, hold your hand over the uncapped port. You should feel the hydrant "suck" on your hand as the water inside the barrel drains.

Wet-barrel hydrants are typically used only where there is no chance of freezing weather (Figure 9-10). A wet-barrel hydrant remains full of water that is under pressure to a point just behind the port. A wet-barrel hydrant operates by opening a valve directly behind the port (Figure 9-11).

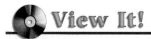 **View It!**

Go to the DVD, navigate to Chapter 9, and select *Fire Hydrants.*

 Practice It!

Opening and Closing a Fire Hydrant

Use the following procedure to open and close a fire hydrant:

1. Remove one of the discharge outlet caps. If needed, use the hydrant wrench to loosen the cap (Figure 9-12).

FIGURE 9-12

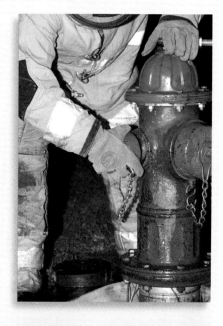

2. Place the hydrant wrench on top of the operating nut of the hydrant and slowly turn it in a counterclockwise direction until water flows out of the open discharge outlet (Figure 9-13).

FIGURE 9-13

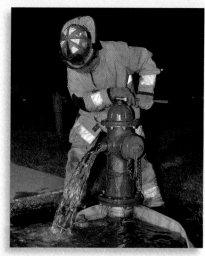

3. Finally, close the hydrant valve with the wrench. Turn the operating nut in a clockwise direction with the hydrant wrench (Figure 9-14).

FIGURE 9-14

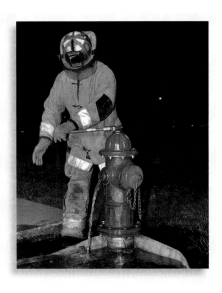

Booster Tank Refill

When you extinguish a fire and utilize water straight from the fire apparatus with no outside water supply, you will need to refill the apparatus with water. For this reason, you need to learn how to use a fire hydrant to refill the booster tank of the fire apparatus.

Usually you will use a 2½- or 3-inch supply hose line to refill the booster tank on a fire apparatus. There may be a short section of this hose on the fire apparatus that is usually used to refill the booster tank. This procedure can also be used for other water supply sources by following Steps 2 through 5 in "Practice It! Refilling a Booster Tank."

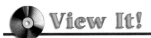

View It!

Go to the DVD, navigate to Chapter 9, and select *Booster Tank Refill.*

Practice It!

Refilling a Booster Tank

Follow these steps to use a fire hydrant to refill the booster tank on a fire apparatus:

1. With the supply hose laid out to the fire apparatus, use the hydrant wrench to remove at least one of the hydrant caps. To clear the waterway of any debris or contaminants in the water as well as to ensure proper operation of the hydrant, open the hydrant slowly and only partially, and flow some water (Figure 9-15). Shut off the hydrant so you can attach the fill hose.

FIGURE 9-15

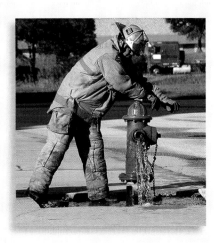

—Continued

2. Attach the supply refill hose to the hydrant discharge using the female end of the coupling (Figure 9-16). Tighten to hand-tight. Attach the male end of the hose to the intake gate on the fire apparatus (Figure 9-17). The intake gates have various designs and are found in various locations, depending on the apparatus design.

FIGURE 9-16

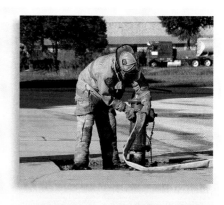

3. The driver will open the tank refill valve on the fire apparatus and signal to you when he or she is ready for you to slowly open the hydrant. When opening the hydrant, use the hydrant wrench to turn the operating nut counterclockwise until it stops turning.

FIGURE 9-17

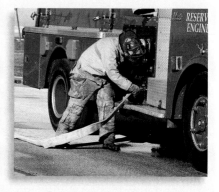

4. Maintain eye contact with the driver at the pump panel. The driver will signal when the tank is full so that you can close the valve (Figure 9-18). To close the valve, turn it clockwise with the hydrant wrench.

FIGURE 9-18

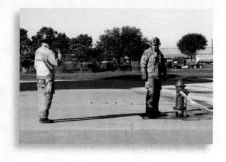

5. Properly detach the hose line, hand-tighten the discharge cap on the hydrant, and roll up the refill supply hose line. Put the hose back onto the fire apparatus and return the hydrant wrench to its correct storage location.

Sustained Water Supply

As the fire progresses, the fire department busily starts setting up and establishing a sustained water supply. The sustained water supply replaces the initial water supply, which ensures that adequate water is available to extinguish the fire.

Tenders (Water Tankers)

Depending on your location, the trucks that bring an additional water supply to the fire are called *tenders* or *water tankers*. The term *tanker* has now been given to airplanes that drop large amounts of water on forest fires. For our use, the terms *tender* and *water tanker*

are interchangeable. Use the term that your instructor says is appropriate for your area.

These apparatus can carry from 1000 to more than 8000 gallons of water. Tenders can be connected into the fire pumper on the scene as a water supply. They can even be used in conjunction with portable water tanks, set up on the scene as water reservoirs. Tenders connected into pumpers can have pumps that supply the water to the pumper or they can allow a gravity-fed supply.

Fire departments utilize several tenders in rotation to supply the fire scene. Refilling a tender is similar to refilling a booster tank on a fire apparatus. Each tender is refilled as the other deploys its load of water, thus establishing a sustained water supply.

This operation is commonly referred to as a **tender water shuttle operation** (Figure 9-19).

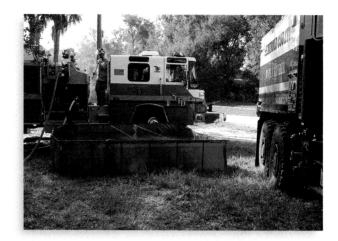

FIGURE 9-19 Multiple tenders can be used to shuttle water from the supply source to the fire scene.

⇨ Practice It!

Hooking into a Tender

When a tender apparatus connects to a pumper to provide a water supply, a section of 2½- or 3-inch hose is usually used. Use the following procedure to assist in making the connection:

1. Remove a section of supply hose from the fire engine or tender apparatus.

2. Connect the female end of the supply hose to a discharge outlet on the tender that is providing the water supply (Figure 9-20).

3. Connect the male end to an intake outlet on the fire engine that is taking in the water supply.

4. Advise both driver-pump operators that the supply line is properly connected to each pumper. Walk the hose line, loosening any kinks in the charged line.

FIGURE 9-20

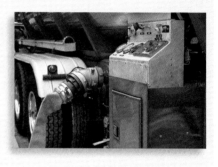

Static Water Supplies

Natural bodies of water, such as streams, rivers, ponds, and lakes, provide substantial water supply resources. Additional static water resources include manmade reservoirs, swimming pools, and above- and below-ground water tanks. An above-ground water tank is considered a static supply when it is at ground level. Anytime the tank is elevated above the ground, it becomes a pressurized water supply. The fire department may also have portable water tanks that are set up for use during a fire. These static water supply resources can be accessed by portable fire pumps placed nearby. They can also be set up before- hand with special hydrants, called **drafting hydrants.** Fire apparatus can also directly access a static water supply with a water drafting operation.

Drafting Water from Natural Sources

Most fire department pumpers can be set up near a natural source of a static water supply. They have a specially designed fire hose referred to as **hard suction hose.** When deployed into a body of water, hard suction hose can draw water into a pumper, providing a sustained water supply for the fire scene (Figure 9-21).

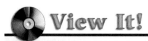

hard suction hose   A specially designed fire hose that is deployed into a body of water to draw water into the fire apparatus pump and provide a sustained water supply for the fire scene.

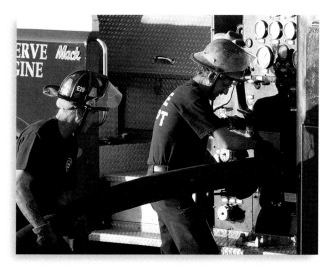

FIGURE 9-21   A drafting operation allows us to take advantage of static water supplies.

View It!

Go to the DVD, navigate to Chapter 9, and select *Drafting Operations.*

Practice It!

Participating in Drafting Operations

Follow the procedure below to assist with setting up a drafting operation:

1. The crew places drafting hose lines (hard suction hose) into the static water supply source with a drafting strainer attached to the end (Figure 9-22). This strainer assures that chunks of debris do not enter the fire pump during drafting operations.

2. The strainer end of the hard suction hose is secured to the pumper with ropes in order to suspend the strainer in the water supply. It is important to maintain a good depth within the water supply. This also keeps the strainer end off the bottom of the water supply and from potential clogging materials that may be sucked into the strainer during drafting operations.

FIGURE 9-22

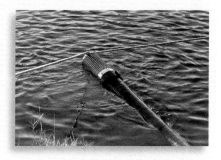

The fire apparatus pump creates a negative pressure in the hard suction hose and water is lifted into the pump. Water is then supplied to the fire scene with a supply hose line or it is directly applied onto the fire through fire attack lines.

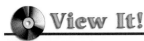
WARNING: Conventional PPE for firefighters is bulky and cumbersome and can be deadly if you accidentally fall into the water. Consider this any time you are working around an open static water source, and avoid wearing full gear around the water whenever possible. Some agencies require that life jackets be worn while working near open water. Follow your agency's protocols.

View It!

Go to the DVD, navigate to Chapter 9, and select *Drafting Hydrants*.

Practice It!

Assisting with Drafting Hydrant Water Supply Operations

Follow the procedure below to assist with setting up a drafting hydrant water supply:

1. With the fire apparatus positioned within reach of the drafting hydrant with hard suction supply hose, the crew removes the hard suction hose from the apparatus (Figure 9-23).

FIGURE 9-23

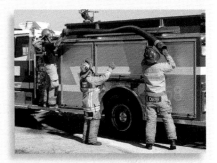

2. Attach the female end of the hard suction hose to the drafting hydrant (Figure 9-24).

FIGURE 9-24

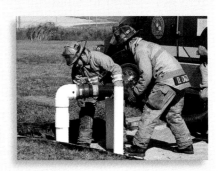

3. Attach the other end of the hard suction hose to the fire apparatus pump. This end of the hard suction hose may have a large male threaded end or it may have a double female adapter if it is being attached to the large port on the pump.

The fire apparatus pump creates a negative pressure in the hard suction hose and water is lifted into the pump. Water is then supplied to the fire scene with a supply hose line or it is directly applied onto the fire through fire attack lines.

Portable Water Tanks

Because they are constantly being refilled by tenders, portable water tanks allow a fire pumper to draw from a steady supply of water. The fire apparatus uses drafting operations to draw the water and develop a sustained water supply through a rotation of units. A sustained water supply can also be created by laying a supply hose line from the portable tank to the apparatus needing water on the fire scene (Figure 9-25).

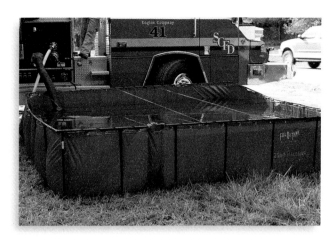

FIGURE 9-25 Portable water tanks provide a reservoir of water for drafting operations where a natural body of water doesn't exist.

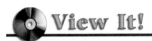 **View It!**

Go to the DVD, navigate to Chapter 9, and select *Portable Water Tank Operations.*

Practice It!

Setting Up a Portable Water Tank

Use the following procedure to assist in setting up a portable water tank:

1. Position a team member at the apparatus carrying the portable water tank. Assist in disconnecting any straps, hooks, or openings on the compartment area.

FIGURE 9-26

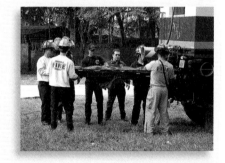

2. Using good body positioning, carefully assist removing the unit from the apparatus (Figure 9-26).

FIGURE 9-27

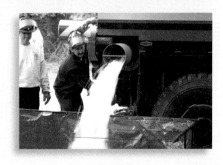

3. Assist in unfolding the unit. Position it on an area that is as level and as safely accessible as possible. Check the water drain, making sure that it is closed. Position the tank so that the drain is at the lowest point to help drain the tank later, when the operation is complete. It is now ready to receive water and act as a water supply source for the fire operation (Figure 9-27).

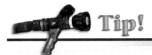
Some departments have found it helpful to place a heavy tarp on the ground to help protect the bottom of the portable tank from sharp objects. This added layer of protection is a good idea if there is any reason to expect that damage can occur.

Portable Fire Pumps

Portable pumps are carried on some fire apparatus and deployed at the water source. They come in two basic styles: land-based and floating. These pumps are usually used to refill tenders or to supply a fire apparatus at a fire scene. If the portable pump is land-based, then a drafting operation is set up using hard suction hose to draw water from a static source into the portable pump. A supply line is then hooked into the portable pump. If the portable pump is a floating type, then it floats on the surface of the water source and supplies water through a supply line to where it is needed.

Portable pumps do not provide a great deal of water but are adequate for filling booster tanks and attacking small fires. The main difference between a land-based portable pump and a float pump is that the float pump has no hard suction hose attached. It simply draws the water from beneath it as it floats on the surface.

Practice It!

Setting Up a Floating Fire Pump

Use the following steps to assist in setting up a float pump:

1. Assemble the crew at the float pump on the fire apparatus. Remember to use good body mechanics and posture when lifting. Float pumps are usually heavy and require two or more people to safely unload and move. Assist in a coordinated lift and removal of the pump (Figure 9-28).

FIGURE 9-28

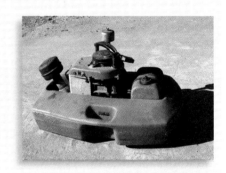

2. Place the pump on a level area at the water's edge. Connect the hose to the pump's outlet and float the pump onto the water (Figure 9-29).

FIGURE 9-29

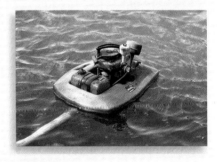

3. The pump operator will start the engine power unit, and the pump will draft water into itself. The pump will discharge water from the outlet side of the pump either to the fire apparatus needing to be refilled or to the fire apparatus on the fire scene (Figure 9-30).

FIGURE 9-30

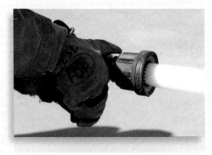

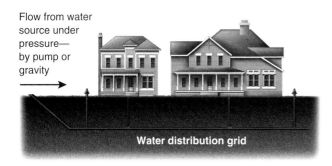

FIGURE 9-31 A typical water main system.

Water Main Systems

One of the best sources of a water supply for fire operations is the water main system. This system is composed of a water source that is placed under pressure by either gravity or pumps. The water is distributed to the community through a system of valves and pipes. The fire department accesses this water source via fire hydrants that are installed at specified intervals throughout the system (Figure 9-31).

Supply Hose

Most fire apparatus designed as the first-in (first-arriving) fire attack units carry water supply fire hose that is loaded so that it is ready for deployment on a fire scene. The sections are connected together in preset lengths, but the hose is not connected to the pump. Perhaps you have seen firefighters laying out their hose as they approach a building fire in a neighborhood. This hose is carried on the hose bed of the fire apparatus and deploys (flakes off) the back of the fire apparatus as it slowly drives from the water supply to the fire (Figure 9-32). Typical supply hose is 2½ to 3 inches in diameter. Hose of this size usually comes in 50-foot lengths. Supply hose that is 2½ to 3 inches in length can also be used as an attack line, which we will discuss in detail in Chapter 10. Large-diameter supply hose, which is between 4 and 6 inches in diameter, is explained later in this chapter in the section "Large-Diameter Supply Hose."

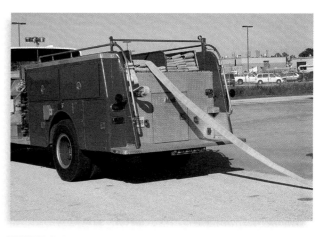

FIGURE 9-32 Because the supply hose is connected together in the hosebed, the pumper can lay the supply hose out as it goes from the water source to the fire.

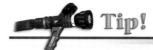 **Tip!**

If you are hooking only one line to a hydrant, take a moment to connect a gate valve to the unused hydrant port before charging the line. By doing so, you can attach another line later without having to shut off the hydrant. Remember, open and close the gate valve slowly to avoid a water hammer.

Gated Manifold Appliances

One supply line can be made into two or more smaller supply lines by using a **gated manifold appliance** (Figure 9-33). Some gated manifold appliances are designed for use with large-diameter supply hose. For example, a 5-inch manifold appliance may branch into two 2½-inch supply lines, each with its own gated valve for operation.

■ KEY WORDS ■

appliance Any Fire Service–related device through which water flows. These devices include manifolds, master stream appliances, adapters, and others.

gated manifold appliance An appliance designed for use with large-diameter supply hose. It allows one

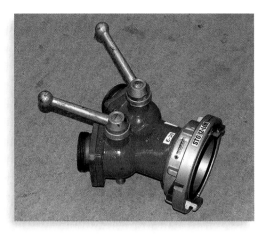

FIGURE 9-33 Gated manifold appliance.

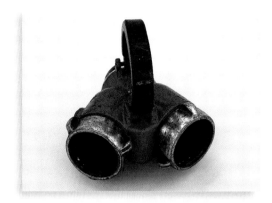

FIGURE 9-34 Siamese appliance.

large supply hose to be branched into two or more smaller supply hose lines. For example, a 5-inch manifold appliance may branch into four 2½-inch supply lines, each with its own gated valve for operation.

Siamese Appliances

Siamese appliances take two or more supply lines and join them into one supply line (Figure 9-34). These appliances typically have a clapper valve inside each intake opening that shuts off if only one line connected to the appliance is flowing water. These appliances allow two or more supply lines to combine to provide more water flow and pressure to one supply line, a fire attack line, or a master stream appliance.

■■■ KEY WORD ■■■■■■

Siamese appliance A hose appliance that combines two or more supply lines into one supply line. Normally, this appliance has a clapper valve inside each intake opening that shuts off if only one line coming into the appliance is flowing water. This appliance allows two or more supply lines to combine to provide more water flow and pressure to one supply line, a fire attack line, or a master stream appliance.

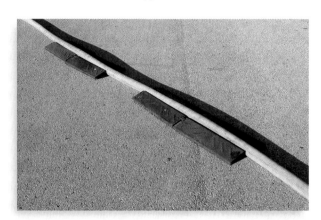

FIGURE 9-35 Never drive directly over an unprotected, charged hose line. Hose bridges allow for traffic to pass slowly over a supply hose.

Hose Bridges

Many times supply hose lines are laid out in neighborhood streets or across highways. Vehicles should never be allowed to drive over charged hose lines. If traffic is going to be allowed to pass over these supply hose lines, specially designed hose bridges should be used (Figure 9-35). These bridges provide protection for the charged supply hose lines.

Supply Hose Loads

A supply hose is usually laid out from a fire apparatus in two primary directions: (1) *to* the fire (a forward lay) or (2) *away from* the fire and toward the water supply (a reverse lay). The supply hose can be loaded on the fire apparatus in several ways. Variations to these basic loads are many and are specific to the needs of your community and the design of the fire apparatus.

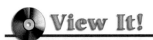

Go to the DVD, navigate to Chapter 9, and select *Loading Supply Hose*.

➡ Practice It!

Loading Supply Hose

Use the following steps to assist in loading supply hose:

1. Drain and lay flat the fire hose section that will be loaded as a supply hose.

FIGURE 9-36

2. Position yourself to assist in the hose load. This positioning will be on the hose bed, on the tailboard of the fire apparatus, or on the ground behind the apparatus (Figure 9-36).

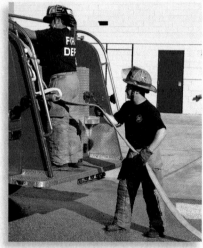

3. As the section is loaded, stop as you get to the end of the section and allow the next section to be connected (Figure 9-37).

4. If the apparatus must be moved, step down from it and remain clear of the apparatus until it is finished being repositioned. Then return to loading the hose.

FIGURE 9-37

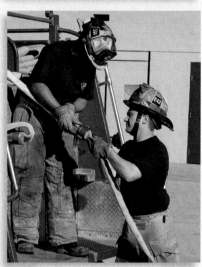

Safety Tip!

One, and only one, person should be designated as the safety person who signals the driver to move the vehicle. That person should remain visible in the driver's rearview mirror at all times. However, anyone near the truck should be aware of the dangers and should yell **Stop!** if necessary.

Large-Diameter Supply Hose

The large-diameter fire hose designed for water supply is typically 4 to 6 inches in diameter (Figure 9-38). This type of hose may have quick-connect couplings. All these couplings are identical—that is, there is no male–female differentiation. In addition, they connect with a quarter turn. Small locking mechanisms on each coupling usually secure the couplings together. A large-diameter fire hose (LDH) usually

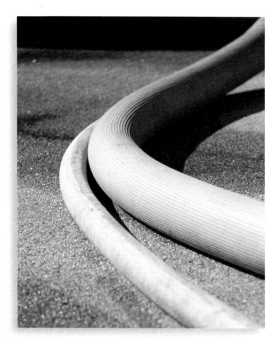

FIGURE 9-38 A large-diameter fire hose.

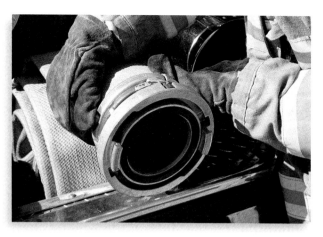

FIGURE 9-39 A typical quick-connect coupling: (a) lugs, (b) gasket, and (c) locking mechanism.

comes in sections that are 50 to 100 feet in length. This type of hose is heavy and sometimes cumbersome, but it can supply large amounts of water to the fire scene very quickly.

Quick-Connect Hose Couplings

Quick-connect couplings attach to each other differently than threaded couplings do. Because the two ends of a quick-connect coupling are identical, there is no need to find matching ends. These couplings are primarily found on large-diameter hose (Figure 9-39). The gaskets in a quick-connect coupling should be lubricated per the manufacturer's instructions so that the coupling works freely. A dried-out gasket makes it very hard to couple or uncouple the fittings.

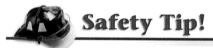

Safety Tip!

It is very important that quick-connect couplings be fully connected and locked in place before pressurizing the hose. You should hear and feel a solid "click" when the coupling is made.

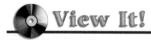

View It!

Go to the DVD, navigate to Chapter 9, and select *Quick-Connect Couplings*.

Practice It!

Coupling and Uncoupling Quick-Connect Hose Couplings

The following procedures can be used to connect and disconnect hose sections. Separate procedures are provided for one firefighter and for two firefighters.

Coupling and uncoupling quick-connect hose couplings with one firefighter:

FIGURE 9-40

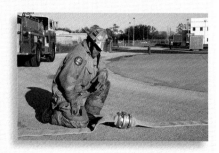

1. Hold one hose section end in place on the ground with your knee and foot (Figure 9-40).

—Continued

2. Take the end of the second section, placing it into the end of the first section. Turn the end of the first section until it clicks into place and locks (Figure 9-41).

FIGURE 9-41

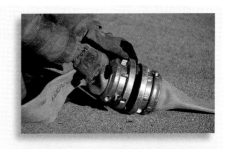

3. Before disconnecting the couplings, assure that the water pressure is released from the supply line and no water is flowing. To disconnect the couplings, place spanner wrenches on each coupling and turn them in a counterclockwise direction. You should operate the coupling lock releases at the same time (Figure 9-42).

FIGURE 9-42

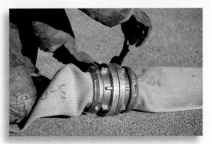

Coupling and uncoupling quick-connect hose couplings with two firefighters:

1. With two people, bring each end together and fit the couplings into the reception slots (Figure 9-43).

FIGURE 9-43

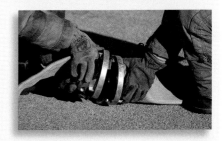

2. Turn the couplings in a clockwise direction to connect them (Figure 9-44). The couplings will fit together snugly, clicking as the locks on each coupling snap into place. If necessary, use spanner wrenches to turn the couplings.

FIGURE 9-44

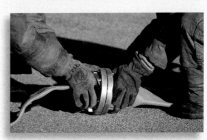

3. To disconnect the couplings, make sure that all water flow has been discontinued to the lines and that the water pressure has been released from them. Each firefighter holds the locking mechanisms down and turns them counterclockwise, releasing each coupling (Figure 9-45).

FIGURE 9-45

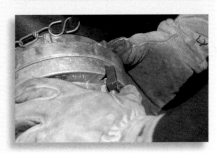

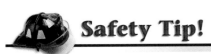 **Safety Tip!**

Never uncouple supply hose unless you are sure it is not pressurized and water is not flowing. Severe injury can occur with a sudden release of water pressure if the hose is uncoupled while under pressure. Always check with the pump operator and release any pressure by opening the nozzle at the end of the attack line.

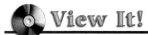 View It!

Go to the DVD, navigate to Chapter 9, and select *Loading Large-Diameter Supply Hose.*

Practice It!

Loading Large-Diameter Supply Hose

Large-diameter hose, like regular supply hose, can be loaded in several configurations. Use the following steps as a guideline for loading large-diameter supply hose:

1. Follow the directions of the Company Officer when loading large-diameter hose. He or she will direct you regarding the proper placement of each section as it is loaded (Figure 9-46).

FIGURE 9-46

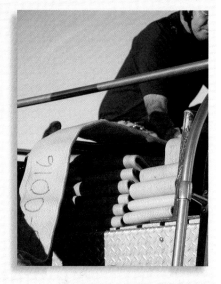

2. Large-diameter hose is usually loaded one section at a time, with each section connected to the next section at the back of the fire apparatus. Position yourself at the back of the apparatus, on the tailboard of the apparatus, or on the hose bed of the apparatus to help feed and place each section of hose (Figure 9-47).

FIGURE 9-47

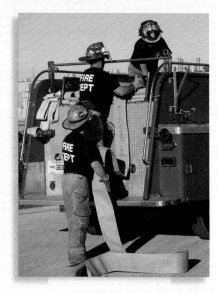

—Continued

3. The sections of hose must be loaded so that they will deploy (flake off) easily during the hose lay. In addition, the hose couplings need to be positioned in the load so that they fit. Both of these items require a short fold known as a *Dutchman* to occasionally be placed in the load (Figure 9-48).

FIGURE 9-48

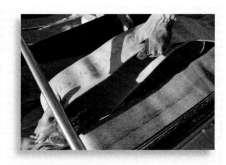

4. The load is finished by placing the last coupling into position. Secure the last coupling in the manner approved by your department (Figure 9-49).

FIGURE 9-49

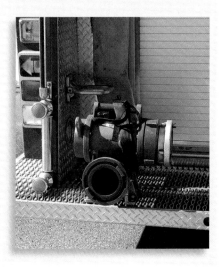

Safety Tip!

When climbing onto the hose bed of a fire apparatus, always use the handholds provided for that purpose. Always check overhead when mounting the top of the hose bed. Look for obstructions and overhead electrical power wires. Never touch these items. If the apparatus needs to move during the reloading process, dismount it, staying clear of it and any traffic lanes that may be present. When the apparatus has repositioned, go back to your previous spot and continue loading the hose.

Supply Hose Layouts

When fire apparatus start arriving on the scene of an active fire, among the first things to be accomplished is the rapid establishment of an initial water supply and a sustained firefighting water supply. The initial supply will more than likely come from the booster tank on your apparatus. The sustained water supply may come from hooking your apparatus into a substantial water supply, laying the water supply line to the fire scene. Alternately, another apparatus can lay a water supply line from a substantial water supply to your unit on the scene, flowing water to the initial fire attack lines. The two general ways to lay supply hose are with a forward lay and a reverse lay.

Forward Lay

A forward lay of supply hose is a very common fire ground operation. It involves the apparatus stopping at the water supply source and leaving a firefighter, who takes a supply line hose end and a hydrant wrench off the hose bed of the apparatus and secures the hose end at the water source.

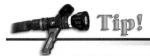

Tip!

Many agencies keep a bag of tools they call the *hydrant bag* on or near the tailboard. This bag makes it easy to grab the hydrant wrench and any other tools, such as a rope, spanners, or adapters, as you remove the line from the rig.

The fire apparatus then proceeds to the desired location at the fire scene as the hose deploys off the back of the hose bed. Simultaneously, the firefighter at the water source connects the end of the supply hose at his location into the water supply source. This water supply can be a fire hydrant on a water main system, a portable pump or tank, or another fire apparatus. On a signal from the apparatus that laid out the supply hose, the firefighter opens the water source. Water flows to the fire scene and apparatus from the water source, and a sustained water supply is established.

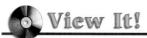

Go to the DVD, navigate to Chapter 9, and select *Forward Lay from a Hydrant*.

Practice It!

Forward Lay from a Hydrant

Probably the most common method of establishing a sustained water supply system on a fire scene is laying hose from a fire hydrant to the scene of the fire. This operation can be accomplished by doing the following:

1. As the firefighter designated to make the hydrant connection, you must wait for the apparatus to come to a full stop. Check for traffic hazards, dismount the fire apparatus, and proceed to the hose bed area.

FIGURE 9-50

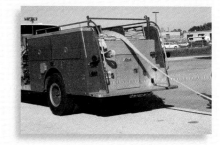

2. Grasp the designated supply line. Loop the hose end around the fire hydrant starting from the street side, and stop on the backside of the hydrant barrel. Position yourself away from the street and place a foot on the end of the looped hose end where it crosses the hose line, a few feet down from the hydrant (Figure 9-50).

FIGURE 9-51

3. When you are ready, signal the apparatus driver to proceed toward the fire scene. The supply hose lines will flake off the rear of the apparatus hose bed (Figure 9 51).

4. You can step off the hose section after a few sections have cleared the rear of the hose bed. Take a cap off one of the small discharge outlets on the hydrant. Open the hydrant with the hydrant wrench until some water flows and shut off the hydrant (Figure 9-52). Note that this step is precautionary. It assures that the hydrant works and that it is free of debris that could clog the line.

FIGURE 9-52

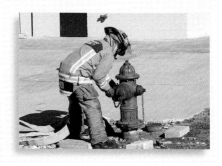

—Continued

5. Connect the supply hose line to the hydrant. Wait for either a predesignated signal or a radio transmission from the apparatus driver requesting that the hydrant and supply hose line be charged with water. On his or her signal, open the hydrant completely and walk with the hose line back to the apparatus, checking for and undoing any kinks in the supply hose line (Figure 9-53).

FIGURE 9-53

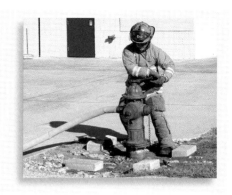

Reverse Lay

A reverse lay involves laying a water supply line from the scene back to the water supply source. This source may be a fire hydrant on a water main system or another apparatus. In this instance, a firefighter may or may not be dropped off at the fire scene to assist the crew in securing the end of the supply line as it is laid out. To secure the line, the hose end can be chocked under a front or rear tire of an apparatus remaining on the scene. When a few hose line sections have come off the apparatus, pull the line from under the truck's tire and connect it to the supply intake outlet on the apparatus at the scene.

 View It!

Go to the DVD, navigate to Chapter 9, and select *Reverse Lay*.

Practice It!

Reverse Lay

Use the following steps when laying a supply hose line from a fire scene to the fire hydrant water source:

1. Your apparatus will come to a stop at the fire scene where another apparatus needing water will be. Alternately, it will stop at a spot where the supply hose line will be used as a fire attack line. Safely dismount the apparatus, checking for traffic hazards. Gather several loops of the supply hose and pull them from the hose bed (Figure 9-54).

2. If you are connecting to another fire apparatus on the scene, pass the hose to the operator of the apparatus and she will slide the hose under a wheel of her apparatus. When you have remounted your apparatus, the operator of the other apparatus will signal for the hose lay to begin.

FIGURE 9-54

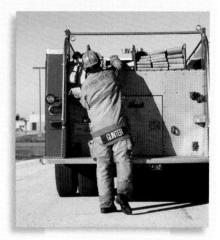

—Continued

3. If you are merely leaving the supply line at the scene to be later used to connect to attack hose lines and nozzles, pull the loops of supply hose to the street behind the apparatus. Then turn them over to a firefighter on the scene to anchor with one knee. On his signal, your apparatus should proceed to the fire hydrant (Figure 9-55).

FIGURE 9-55

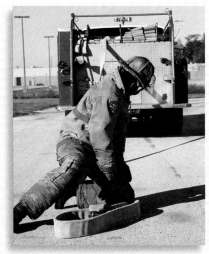

4. Make the connection to the fire hydrant. Alternately, if the line was laid to the attack pumper, hand the supply hose to that pumper's engineer (Figure 9-56).

FIGURE 9-56

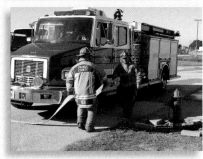

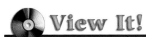

View It!

Go to the DVD, navigate to Chapter 9, and select *Large-Diameter Supply Hose Lay.*

Practice It!

Laying Large-Diameter Supply Hose

The steps for assisting with laying a large-diameter supply hose are similar to the procedures outlined for laying a smaller-diameter hose, with the following exceptions:

Forward lay:

FIGURE 9-57

1. The hydrant wrap can be accomplished by wrapping the hydrant as described. To secure the hose while the apparatus begins the lay, you may use a hose-pulling rope or strap handle to hook the hydrant (Figure 9-57).

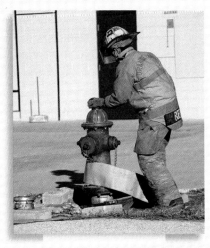

—Continued

2. With a large-diameter hose, there may or may not be a hydrant valve that needs to be hooked into the hydrant (Figures 9-58 and 9-59).

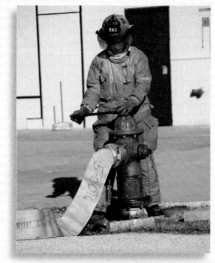

FIGURE 9-58 A hydrant without the hydrant valve attached.

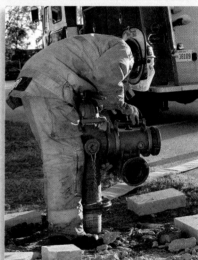

FIGURE 9-59 A hydrant with the hydrant valve attached.

3. The large-diameter hose is hooked into the large discharge opening of the hydrant (Figure 9-60).

FIGURE 9-60

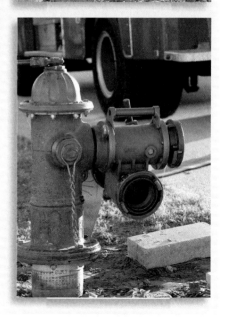

Reverse lay:

1. Use the same procedure that is used for regular-diameter hose lines. However, at the fire scene, the large-diameter hose may be connected into a manifold that will reduce the line to several smaller-diameter hose lines.

2. The large-diameter hose may be connected into a fitting on the apparatus at the water supply. If the apparatus is not able to discharge one large-diameter hose line from its pump panel, the fitting will take in two smaller supply lines, combining them into one large-diameter line.

WARNING: Never place your foot between the hydrant and the hose. If the line becomes snagged in the pumper's hose bed as it travels down the road, your foot or leg could easily be crushed. Keep your feet out of the loop and stand away from the line of travel if the hose snags in the bed.

Hydrant Valves

Hydrant valves are appliances that allow a fire apparatus to hook into the water supply at the fire hydrant without interrupting the flow of water to the fire scene. These valves are commonly used with large-diameter water supply hose but can also be provided on smaller-diameter water supply hose (Figure 9-61). These appliances are attached to the large discharge opening on the fire hydrant, before the first section of supply hose is attached. They can be preconnected to the first section of hose coming off the hose bed. Once they are in place and the water supply from the fire hydrant is turned on, the fire apparatus can return to

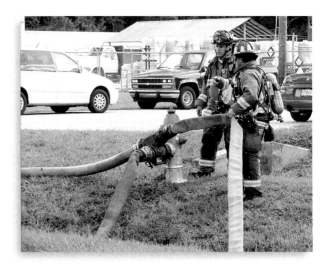

FIGURE 9-61 A Humat valve is a type of hydrant valve used for large-diameter hose.

the hydrant and hook into the hydrant valve. This arrangement allows the apparatus to become an in-line pump, which increases the flow of water through the supply line. This setup is good for fires that require a larger water supply to be controlled. It is also useful if the supply line is a longer layout to the fire scene.

View It!

Go to the DVD, navigate to Chapter 9, and select *Hydrant Valves*.

Practice It!

Applying Hydrant Valves

Use the following procedure to connect a large-diameter hose hydrant valve to a fire hydrant:

1. After the fire apparatus has come to a stop, safely dismount the apparatus and go to the rear hose bed area. Remove the hydrant valve and hose line, looping the hydrant as previously described (see the section "Laying Large-Diameter Supply Hose").

2. Remove the large-diameter discharge outlet cap and flow a small amount of water, checking for any debris inside the opening. Shut down the hydrant and connect the hydrant valve (Figure 9-62).

FIGURE 9-62

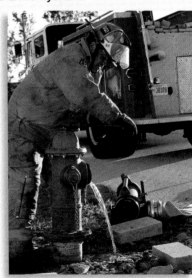

—Continued

3. Make sure that the hydrant valve is connected properly and is in line with the large-diameter hose. Also ensure that the valve is in the proper position to supply the hose line from the hydrant (Figure 9-63). On signal, charge the hose line with the hydrant.

4. Walk along the supply line to the fire, checking for and undoing any kinks in the supply hose line. If needed, you may be required to remain at the fire hydrant so that you can assist the apparatus driver with connecting the supply line to the hydrant valve. Follow your department's operating practices and guidelines for this procedure.

FIGURE 9-63

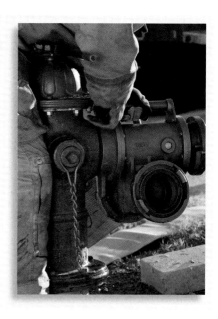

Hose Clamps for Supply Hose

As with fire attack hose lines, there may be times when a section of pressurized supply hose needs to be replaced or extended during a fire and the water cannot be shut off from the pump or water supply. For this reason, hose clamps have been designed to help shut off a hose line in order to stop the flow of water (Figures 9-64 and 9-65). These clamps can be used as a clamping device, operating as a lever with a handle that closes over the hose and locks into place. They can also be used as a screw-down clamp that stops the flow of water. As with all Fire Service tools, hose clamps can be dangerous if not used properly. Be sure to practice and train with them often.

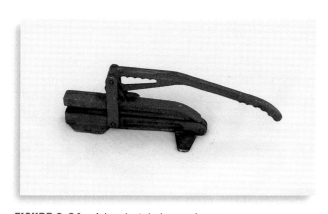

FIGURE 9-64 A level-style hose clamp.

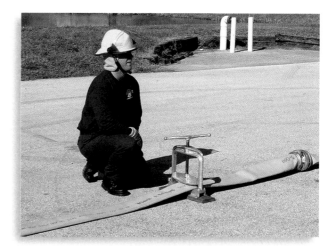

FIGURE 9-65 A screw-style hose clamp.

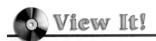
View It!

Go to the DVD, navigate to Chapter 9, and select *Hose Clamps for Supply Hose.*

Practice It!

Applying a Hose Clamp to Supply Hose

Use the following procedure to apply a hose clamp on a supply side hose line:

1. Apply the hose clamp at least 5 feet from the couplings, toward the supply side of the hose line (not toward the fire attack side). Place the appropriate size clamp so that all of the hose will fit inside the hose clamp when it is applied (Figure 9-66).

2. To avoid creating a water hammer in the supply system, slowly apply the hose clamp. When it is fully applied, remove the section of hose, nozzle, or appliance and replace it with the desired replacement.

3. When ready, slowly open the hose clamp to allow the water supply to flow freely again. Make sure your body is not directly over a lever-type clamp when you open it, as the lever can spring up suddenly, causing significant injury.

FIGURE 9-66

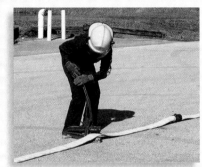

Do It!

Practicing Skills Related to Securing a Water Supply

No single job is more or less important to the safety and efficiency of the mission than others. However, few tasks are more critical during a fire than developing a proper water supply to protect firefighters, contain and extinguish the fire, and protect adjacent property. Practice the steps described in this chapter until you can perform them safely and without hesitation. Practice each step periodically to hone your skills so that, when the need arises, you can safely work as a valuable team member in establishing the water supply needed to extinguish the fire.

Prove It

Knowledge Assessment

Exterior Operations Level Firefighter—Chapter 9

Name: _____

Fill out the ten-question quiz below, the Knowledge Assessment Sheet, by circling the correct answer for each question. When finished, sign it and give to your instructor/Company Officer for his or her signature. Turn in this Knowledge Assessment Sheet to the proper person as part of the documentation that you have completed your training for this chapter.

1. The water supply that is carried on the fire apparatus in what is generally referred to as a _____ .
   a. holding tank
   b. booster tank
   c. hose bed
   d. portable tank

2. The fire truck that pumps the water to the fire attack hose lines at the fire is commonly called the _____ pumper.
   a. first-due
   b. supply
   c. initial
   d. attack

3. On a typical fire hydrant, there will be two or three _____ ports.
   a. intake
   b. inspection
   c. suction
   d. outlet

4. Some fire departments utilize tender water shuttle operations in which several tenders in rotation supply the fire scene, each refilling as the other deploys its load of water, thus establishing a sustained water supply.
   a. True
   b. False

5. _____ hose is a specially designed fire hose that, when deployed into the body of water, can draw water to provide a sustained water supply for the fire scene.
   a. Soft suction
   b. Large-diameter
   c. Hard suction
   d. Fiber jacketed

6. The main difference between a portable pump and a float pump is that the float pump has no _____ hose attached.
   a. soft suction
   b. large-diameter
   c. hard suction
   c. fiber jacketed

7. Firefighters can use a _____ to divide one supply line into two smaller supply lines.
   a. gated manifold appliance
   b. hydrant valve
   c. gated hydrant valve
   d. hard suction hose

8. A supply hose layout operation that begins at the fire and proceeds toward the water supply is called a _____ lay.
   a. supply
   b. reverse
   c. forward
   d. preconnected

9. A 3- to 6-inch-diameter supply hose is considered large-diameter supply hose.
   a. True
   b. False

10. _____ are appliances that allow a fire apparatus to hook into the water supply at the fire hydrant without interrupting the flow of water to the fire scene.
   a. Gated manifolds
   b. Siamese appliances
   c. Hydrant valves
   d. Hose straps

Student Signature and Date _____   Instructor/Company Officer Signature and Date _____

214

Skills Assessment

Signed Documentation Tear-Out Sheet

Exterior Operations Level Firefighter—Chapter 9

Name: _____

Fill out the Skills Assessment Sheet below. Have your instructor/Company Officer check off and initial each skill you demonstrate. When finished, sign it and give to your instructor/Company Officer for his or her signature. Turn in this Skills Assessment Sheet to the proper person as part of the documentation that you have completed your training for this chapter.

Skill	Completed	Initials
1. Explain the elements of an initial and a sustained water supply.	_____	_____
2. Help establish a water supply from different static sources, including portable tanks, lakes, and streams.	_____	_____
3. Describe how to work safely around a static water supply.	_____	_____
4. Work as a member of a team to refill a booster tank.	_____	_____
5. Operate a fire hydrant.	_____	_____
6. Work as a member of a team to establish a drafting operation.	_____	_____
7. Work as a member of a team to establish a sustained water supply from a hydrant using various hose configurations and layouts.	_____	_____
8. Explain the differences among hard suction hose, conventional supply hose, and large-diameter supply hose.	_____	_____
9. Demonstrate setting up a floating portable pump (if applicable).	_____	_____
10. Work as a team member loading 2½- or 3-inch supply hose.	_____	_____
11. Demonstrate safe procedures for coupling and uncoupling quick-connect hose couplings.	_____	_____
12. Work as a team member loading large-diameter supply hose.	_____	_____
13. Demonstrate safe procedure for applying a hydrant valve.	_____	_____
14. Demonstrate how to apply a hose clamp to a hose line.	_____	_____
15. Work as a team member hooking into a water tender for a water supply.	_____	_____

Student Signature and Date _____   Instructor/Company Officer Signature and Date _____

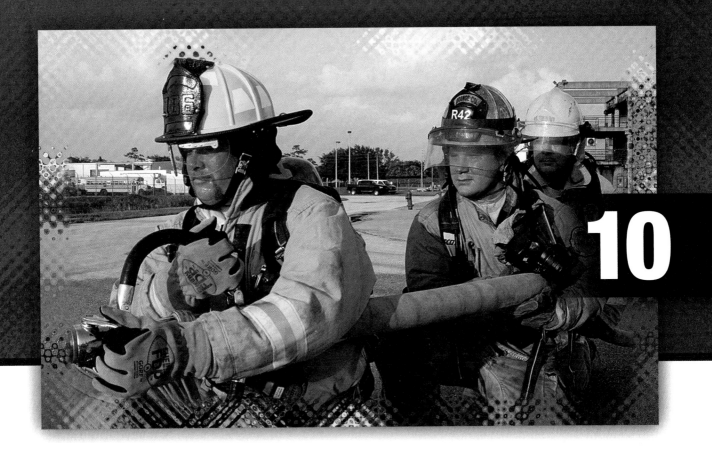

Large Attack Lines

What You Will Learn in This Chapter

In this chapter you will learn about the fire hose lines used to deliver large amounts of water onto large fires. We'll discuss how to pull and stretch large hose lines as well as methods for assembling and extending them. We will also present steps for handling these large and heavy hose lines as well as drills so that you can practice for loading large attack hose lines onto the fire apparatus. Finally, we will introduce you to some basics of master stream appliances.

What You Will Be Able to Do

After reading this chapter and practicing the skills in a classroom setting, you will be able to

1. Demonstrate how to pull and stretch a large pre-connected attack hose line.
2. Demonstrate how to assemble a large attack hose line.

3. Explain and demonstrate the steps for flowing a large attack line, one-person method.
4. Explain and demonstrate the steps for looping a large attack line, one-person method.
5. Discuss and demonstrate the steps for advancing a large attack line as a hose team member.
6. Discuss and demonstrate how multiple firefighters, as hose team members, handle a large attack line in the kneeling position.
7. Demonstrate and explain how to extend a line with a gated wye.
8. Demonstrate how to extend a charged hose line with a hose clamp.
9. Demonstrate how to extend a line through the nozzle.
10. Explain and demonstrate how to set up a monitor-deck gun master stream appliance.

Exterior Fire Attack—Large Attack Lines

There is an old saying in the Fire Service: "Big fire, big water." This phrase is a very commonsense approach to basic fire facts. Simply put, the larger the fire and therefore the greater the release of heat, the more water that is needed to be applied to the fire in order to absorb the heat. Fire attack lines for "big water" are generally 2½- to 3-inch diameter hose lines with associated nozzles. As with small fire attack lines, the nozzles are either fog or smoothbore type and operate similarly. One of the main differences between large and small attack lines is that large attack lines flow much more water volume and require more people to operate them safely. Their reach is farther and they can extinguish much more fire. They also use up the water supply much faster and should therefore be connected to a sustained water supply as soon as possible after they are deployed and operated.

Pulling and Stretching Large Attack Lines

Maneuvering a large attack line is much more cumbersome than using a small attack line. A charged large attack line can be moved, but you will probably need more help to do it (Figure 10-1). These attack lines are often used on exterior fire attacks due to their capacity to flow large amounts of water on **exposures** to the original fire as well as rapidly extinguish fires. When extended to the interior of a structural fire, they can flow much more water. However, they use up manpower and can be difficult to maneuver inside the building.

Large attack lines can be configured in two main ways: (1) they can be preconnected, like small attack lines, or (2) they can be put together as needed off the supply hose bed of the fire apparatus. We will discuss the various methods of establishing a large attack line utilizing both configurations.

KEY WORDS

exposure Anything that has the potential of catching fire as a result of its proximity to something that is already on fire.

Preconnected Large Attack Lines

Often referred to as blitz lines, preconnected large fire attack lines are loaded in a similar manner as small attack lines. Because of the increased size and overall weight of the hose, you should consider getting help to pull the preconnected load (Figure 10-2). Getting assistance is especially important if you need to move a *charged* hose line to a certain placement to apply a fire stream. However, pulling an *uncharged* line across level ground with no obstructions can be accomplished by one firefighter.

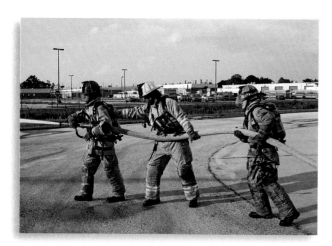

FIGURE 10-1 Large attack lines are more cumbersome and require more people to maneuver than small attack lines.

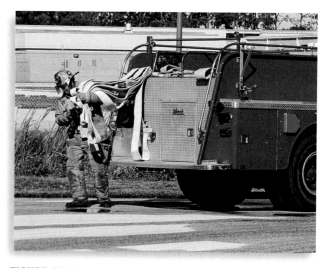

FIGURE 10-2 Preconnected, large attack lines are often referred to as *blitz lines*.

TABLE 10-1	Weights of Uncharged and Charged Fire Hoses		
Hose Size (in inches)	Hose and Coupling Weight (in pounds)	Water Weight (in pounds)	Total Weight (in pounds)
1.5	30	80	110
1.75	35	105	140
2	40	135	175
2.5	55	225	280
3	70	305	375
4	85	545	630
5	100	850	950

Safety Tip!

Obviously, the larger the hose line, the heavier it is, especially when it is filled with water. Strained muscles and sprained joints can occur when we underestimate the weights we are working with and try to do too much without asking for help. Look at Table 10-1 to get an idea of exactly how the diameter of the hose affects its weight when it is charged and ready to flow. The weights given have been rounded off to the nearest 5 pounds and are for each 100 feet of hose.

View It!

Go to the DVD, navigate to Chapter 10, and select *Stretching a Preconnected Large Attack Line.*

Practice It!

Stretching a Preconnected Large Attack Line

Use the following general steps when pulling and deploying any large preconnected attack hose line:

1. Go to the hose bed where the preconnected load is located. Grab the nozzle and one or two loops of hose line, and turn. As you turn, position the hose over one shoulder (Figure 10-3).

2. With the nozzle and hose loops over your shoulder and facing in your direction of travel, walk in that desired direction, feeding off the loops when you feel a substantial tug in the hose. Quickly check to see that the hose is stretched out with no kinks in the line. Also make sure that the hose is not passing under, over, or against any obstructions that may restrict water flow.

FIGURE 10-3

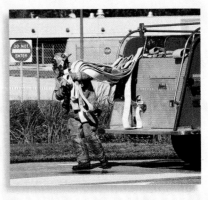

—Continued

3. Get into position to support the nozzle and hose, and signal the pump operator to charge the attack line (Figure 10-4). If possible, plan to have at least one other person assist in holding and maneuvering the charged attack line. Without the help of another firefighter, you will need to slowly shut down the flow at the nozzle, reposition the hose, and then slowly reopen the nozzle flow.

FIGURE 10-4

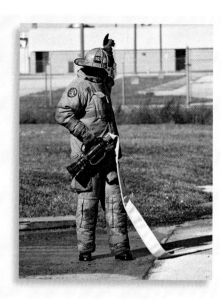

Assembling a Large Attack Line

Oftentimes, the large attack line must be assembled from lengths of hose from the supply hose bed on the apparatus and a large attack nozzle located on the apparatus. This assembly is usually more the norm rather than the exception, so you must know how to quickly assemble these parts to make it work.

⇨ Practice It!

Assembling a Large Attack Line

Follow these steps when assembling a large fire attack line on the fire scene:

1. Grab a large attack nozzle from the apparatus. From the supply hose bed, pull enough of the desired amount of hose to complete the stretch. Place the hose sections over your shoulder as you remove them from the hose bed (Figure 10-5). Disconnect the hose at the last coupling.

FIGURE 10-5

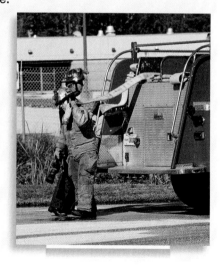

2. Hand the female end to the pump operator, who will connect it to a discharge port on the truck.

3. Continue by carrying the hose, flaking it off as you proceed, to near the area where you want to start flowing water. The male coupling should lead to the fire. Drop the last section of hose and connect the nozzle to the hose line (Figure 10-6).

FIGURE 10-6

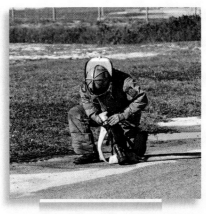

4. Open the nozzle about halfway, pointing it away from any other firefighters, and signal the pump operator to charge the line. Bleed off excess air, adjust the nozzle to the desired pattern, shut it off, and get into position (Figure 10-7). If possible, get a second or third firefighter to assist you in holding the large attack line.

FIGURE 10-7

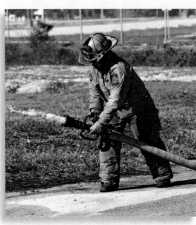

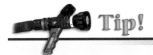
Tip!

When assembling any attack line, make sure you have more than enough hose played out to reach your target and to move around a little. Otherwise, once the hose is stretched full length, you will be held in one spot.

Flowing Large Attack Lines

Large attack lines flow much more water than small attack lines. However, the result is a higher gpm rate of water delivered to the seat of the fire. The greater flow rate means that more people are needed to operate and maneuver the flowing lines. In addition, a more substantial sustained water supply is needed to keep it flowing. Remember that the reaction forces at the nozzle from the larger volumes of flowing water tend to create a greater kickback on the nozzle team.

We'll present steps for positioning and flowing large attack lines with a single firefighter, with multiple firefighters, and in standing and kneeling positions. We will also present looping techniques for line operation.

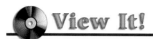

Go to the DVD, navigate to Chapter 10, and select *Flowing a Large Attack Line—Single Firefighter.*

Practice It!

Flowing a Large Attack Line—Single Firefighter

Use the following steps as a guide when flowing and operating a large attack line alone:

1. Position the hose under your arm, using your hip and leg as support for the line. Grasp the nozzle at the handle with one hand and the operating gate valve with the other. Keep your feet at a comfortable width and stay well balanced (Figure 10-8). The nozzle should be a little bit ahead of you so that you will have room to move it up, down, and sideways without having to turn your body.

2. The rest of the attack line should be in a half loop behind you, on the ground. This position provides some slack for a little bit of maneuvering. Slowly open the gate valve on the nozzle until the desired flow is reached and the valve is entirely open. Adjust the gallons-per-minute flow if available and the pattern (if a fog nozzle) as needed. If the reaction force is too great, you can partially close the gate valve and then ask the pump operator to reduce the flow pressure on your attack line. Remember—reducing the flow reduces the amount of water reaching the fire and can produce less extinguishment than desired.

3. Move the nozzle back and forth or up and down as desired while water is flowing. Lean into the line with your hip and leg (Figure 10-9).

FIGURE 10-8

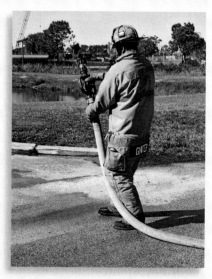

FIGURE 10-9

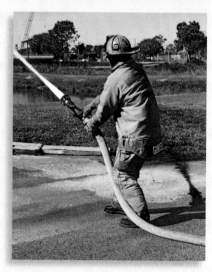

Safety Tip!

Remember: While flowing a large attack line by yourself, you are stuck in the spot where you are standing. Don't try to walk with a large line while it is flowing. Shut down the flow, move, and then start the flow again. Keep the nozzle a little bit ahead of you and the hose close to your body so that you can maneuver the nozzle without twisting your body. This positioning will go a long way toward preventing back strain.

Looping a Large Attack Line

If a large attack line is being used by one or two firefighters, is going to be mostly stationary, and is a safe distance from the fire, the hose line can be looped on the ground. This positioning saves the firefighter's energy and allows for a longer application of water using one firefighter (Figure 10-10).

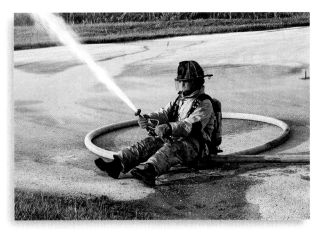

FIGURE 10-10 Looping a large attack line allows for positioning one firefighter on the line.

View It!

Go to the DVD, navigate to Chapter 10, and select *Ground Loop—Single Firefighter.*

Practice It!

Ground Loop—Single Firefighter

Use the following steps to create a loop while operating a large attack hose line:

1. Shut down the flow of water at the nozzle and walk the line in a curve over itself, creating a loop that is about 10 feet in diameter (Figure 10-11).

FIGURE 10-11

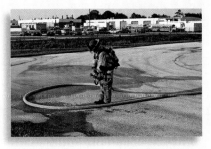

2. Slip the nozzle end under the running end of the hose line where it crosses over it (Figure 10-12). Pull through the nozzle end with about 2 feet of line.

FIGURE 10-12

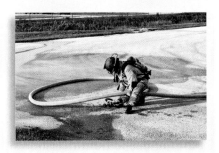

—Continued

3. Sit on the hose on top of the nozzle end. Get into a comfortable position and open the nozzle slowly. To properly apply the water stream, adjust the nozzle flow, the pattern, and the direction as needed (Figure 10-13).

FIGURE 10-13

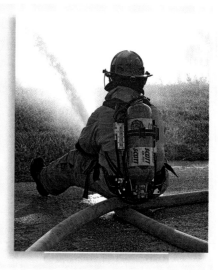

 Safety Tip!

Use the loop method only when you are located in a safe area. Stay away from building collapse zones. Be alert. If you are called upon to retreat rapidly, be ready to shut down the line and leave it.

Advancing Large Attack Lines

When large attack lines need to be advanced to different positions, it is best to have a two- to three-firefighter crew attending the line. As we mentioned earlier, these lines flow tremendous amounts of water and, due to their increased diameter and volume, these lines can become very unwieldy for one firefighter.

 View It!

Go to the DVD, navigate to Chapter 10, and select *Advancing Large Attack Lines—Multiple Firefighters.*

 Practice It!

Advancing a Large Attack Line—Multiple Firefighters

The following steps can be used to maneuver a large attack line with multiple firefighters:

1. The firefighter at the nozzle is positioned as described in "Practice It! Flowing a Large Attack Line—Single Firefighter."

2. A second firefighter positions himself behind the first firefighter on the same side of the hose line. The second firefighter leans into the first firefighter as he bends the hose line over his hip. He should assist the firefighter on the nozzle to maneuver the hose as the first firefighter aims the nozzle (Figure 10-14). The second firefighter should take as much weight of the hose as possible so that the person at the nozzle can concentrate on controlling and directing the stream.

FIGURE 10-14

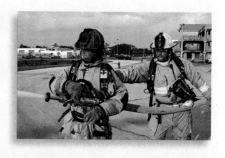

3. A third firefighter can also assist by positioning himself on the same side of the hose line a few feet behind the second firefighter. In this position he can handle the trailing line as well as assist in aiming the hose line with the firefighter at the nozzle (Figure 10-15).

4. On a signal from the firefighter at the nozzle, the large attack line is advanced carefully.

FIGURE 10-15

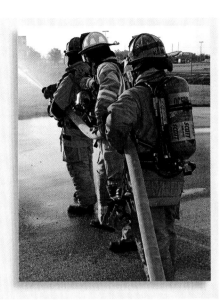

Safety Tip!

It is always better to shut down the nozzle on a large fire attack line before repositioning the line. However, there are occasions when doing so is not possible. If the line must be moved while flowing, the firefighter at the nozzle should be ready to shut down the nozzle if he or she stumbles or loses balance.

View It!

Go to the DVD, navigate to Chapter 10, and select *Kneeling Position on a Large Attack Line—Multiple Firefighters.*

Practice It!

Using a Kneeling Position for a Large Attack Line—Multiple Firefighters

Use the following steps to position yourself in a kneeling position with other firefighters on a large attack line:

1. The first firefighter positions himself at the nozzle as described previously, assuming a kneeling position. The nozzle and line should still be positioned to one side, under the firefighter's arm and on his hip (Figure 10-16).

FIGURE 10-16

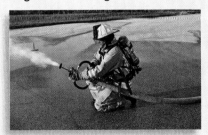

2. A second firefighter positions himself behind the first firefighter, in a kneeling position and on the same side. The second firefighter should be close enough to provide backup assistance in holding the hose line, taking as much of the weight as possible (Figure 10-17).

FIGURE 10-17

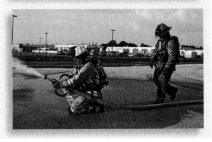

—Continued

3. A third firefighter positions a few feet behind the first two firefighters, in a kneeling position and on the same side of the hose line. From this position he can maneuver the trailing hose line and assist the first two firefighters with maneuvering the nozzle and hose line (Figure 10-18).

FIGURE 10-18

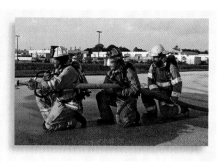

Extending a Line Using a Gated Wye

Large attack lines can also be used to extend the reach of smaller lines when a **gated wye** is used at the end. A gated wye is an appliance that takes in water from a large attack line and then distributes it through two outlets that are controlled by gate valves (Figure 10-19). A typical gated wye has a 2½-inch inlet and two 1½-inch outlets.

Many areas call this operation a garden apartment stretch because the evolution is frequently used to reach courtyard areas and long corridors in garden apartment buildings. However, this evolution is useful almost anytime the fire is beyond the reach of the preconnected attack lines on the pumper.

A gated wye uses quarter-turn valves. When a handle on the appliance is in line with the discharge port, the valve is open and the water is flowing. When the handle is perpendicular to the discharge port, the valve is closed and no water will flow. As with any other valve, open these valves slowly to avoid creating a water hammer.

Some departments have an appliance that closely resembles the gated wye, but in addition to the two 1½-inch discharge ports, it has a single 2½-inch discharge port in the middle. This appliance is called a **water thief.** The water thief allows you to stretch to a certain point, deploy two small attack lines, and then extend further with more large attack lines where either another gated wye or a nozzle is attached. A firefighter should be stationed at each appliance to control the valves (Figure 10-20).

■■■ KEY WORDS ■■■

gated wye　An appliance that takes in water from a large attack line and then distributes it through two outlets that are controlled by gate valves.

water thief　An appliance that closely resembles a gated wye. In addition to the two 1½-inch discharge ports, it has a single 2½-inch discharge port in the middle.

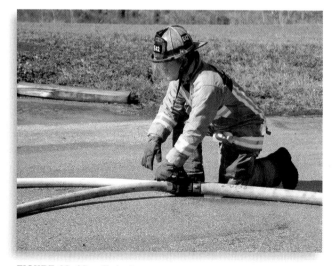

FIGURE 10-19　Gated wye.

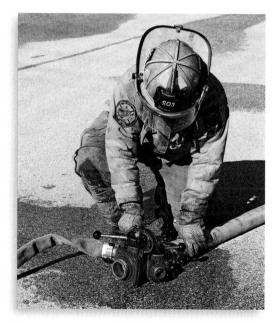

FIGURE 10-20　Water thief.

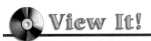 **View It!**

Go to the DVD, navigate to Chapter 10, and select *Extending a Line with a Gated Wye.*

Practice It!

Extending a Line with a Gated Wye

Use the following steps to extend a line with a gated wye:

1. Assemble and extend a large attack line to the connection point—usually within 50 feet of the fire.

2. Attach a gated wye or water thief and attach at least two lengths of small attack line with a nozzle attached (Figure 10-21).

FIGURE 10-21

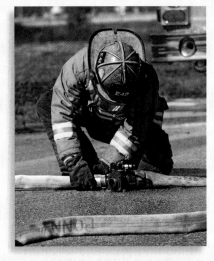

3. Assure that the valves are closed and signal to the pump operator to start the water flow.

4. Once the line is charged, open the appropriate valves slowly (Figure 10-22).

FIGURE 10-22

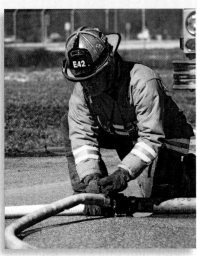

Extending Large Attack Lines— Hose Clamp Method

When you find that the length of line you are flowing falls short, extending its length is a fairly straightforward task. The simplest method to extend the line is to have the pump operator shut down the line, bleed off the pressure at the nozzle, add a section or two of hose, reconnect the nozzle, have the pump operator charge the line, and go back to work. However, this is time-consuming and sometimes impractical. This is where using a hose clamp comes into play.

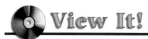

View It!

Go to the DVD, navigate to Chapter 10, and select *Extending a Line—Hose-Clamp Method*.

Practice It!

Extending a Line—Hose-Clamp Method

Use the following steps to extend a line using a hose clamp:

1. Lay out the appropriate amount of hose you want to add to the line so that the female end is 4 or 5 feet behind the nozzle where it is presently located (Figure 10-23). This gives you enough slack in the hose to make the connection.

FIGURE 10-23

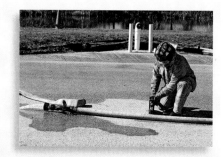

2. Position the hose clamp one section back on the charged line, making sure that the clamp is positioned just to the "engine" side of the coupling (Figure 10-24).

FIGURE 10-24

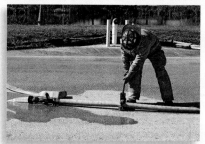

3. When ready, clamp the line, bleed the pressure and remove the nozzle, attach the extended hose, and place the nozzle at the end of the new line (Figure 10-25).

FIGURE 10-25

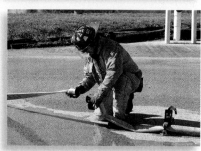

4. Assure that the nozzle is closed and open the hose clamp slowly, reestablishing flow to the nozzle (Figure 10-26).

FIGURE 10-26

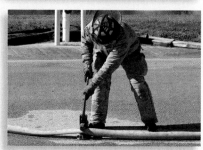

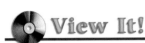

Safety Tip!

Never stand over a lever-type hose clamp. Make sure your body is not in line with the handle, especially when opening the clamp, so that it doesn't fly up and hit you in the chest or face.

Extending Large Attack Lines— Through-the-Nozzle Method

Once a fire is knocked down, it is often time to switch from a large attack line to a smaller one. Since the large line is already in place, it is often better to simply extend the smaller line from the large one instead of pulling a preconnected line all the way from the engine to the fire. This is especially easy if the nozzle you are using is designed to break down at the tip. The gate valve on a typical large stream has a 2½ inch inlet and a 1½ inch outlet. This allows you to simply close the gate valve, remove the nozzle's tip, and replace it with the smaller attack line.

View It!

Go to the DVD, navigate to Chapter 10, and select *Extending a Line—Through-the-Nozzle Method.*

Practice It!

Extending a Line—Through-the-Nozzle Method

Use the following steps to extend a line with a smaller line:

1. Lay out the appropriate amount of hose you want to add to the line so that the female end is 4 or 5 feet behind the nozzle where it is presently located (Figure 10-27). This gives you enough slack in the hose to make the connection. This smaller line should have a nozzle attached that is in the off position.

FIGURE 10-27

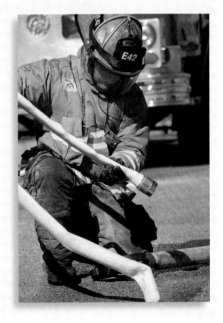

—Continued

2. Stop the flow at the large nozzle and remove the nozzle's tip (Figure 10-28). That nozzle now becomes both a gate valve and a reducer. Attach the smaller line to the male coupling on this gate valve (Figure 10-29).

FIGURE 10-28

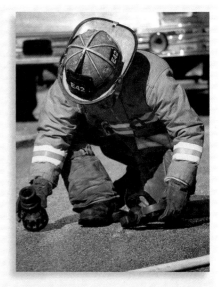

FIGURE 10-29

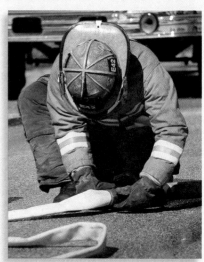

3. Reestablish the flow to the nozzle by opening the gate valve (Figure 10-30).

FIGURE 10-30

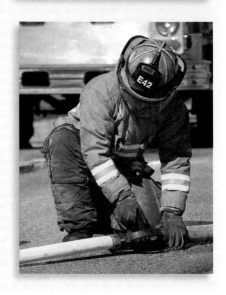

Loading Large Attack Lines

As we mentioned earlier in this chapter, large attack lines are either preconnected or they are assembled as needed from the supply hose on the fire apparatus. After the incident is over, the hose should be reloaded onto the apparatus. As with all fire hose that has been charged with water on the fire incident, large attack lines must be shut down at the pump discharge gate valve, pressure must be relieved at the nozzle, and the hose sections must be disconnected. Each section of hose is then drained and the nozzle is placed at the apparatus in preparation for reloading the hose.

View It!

Go to the DVD, navigate to Chapter 10, and select *Loading Large Attack Lines.*

Practice It!

Loading Large Attack Lines

Use the following steps to load a preconnected large attack line:

1. With the hose drained and disconnected, start at the female end of a section of hose at the apparatus and stretch it away from the opening of the hose bed section into which it is to be loaded (Figure 10-31).

FIGURE 10-31

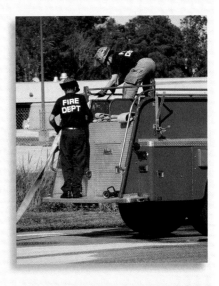

2. Reconnect the female end to the discharge port of the preconnected hose bed. Load the hose, folding it at each end of the hosebed and reconnecting each section as you go, until all the hose is lying in a single stack, flat loaded (Figure 10-32).

FIGURE 10-32

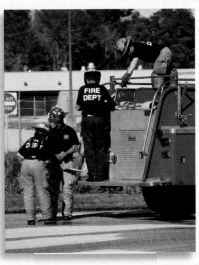

—Continued

3. Reattach the nozzle and take up any slack in the last section of hose (Figure 10-33).

FIGURE 10-33

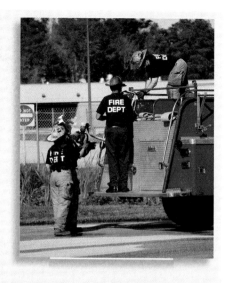

Every department has its own methods of loading preconnected large attack lines. Learn and follow the guidelines that your department utilizes.

If the large attack line was assembled from supply hose on the apparatus, do the following:

1. With the hose drained and disconnected, start at the female end of a section of hose at the apparatus and stretch it away from the opening of the hose bed section into which it is to be loaded. Reconnect each section.

FIGURE 10-34

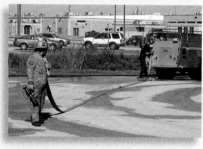

2. Connect the female coupling to the male coupling on the supply hose bed on the apparatus and reload the hose sections (Figure 10-34).

3. When this has been done, return the large attack line nozzle to its storage place on the apparatus (Figure 10-35).

FIGURE 10-35

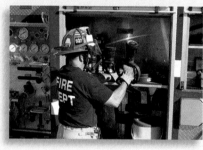

Master Stream Appliances

When a large fire occurs and the greatest possible volume of water must be applied to cover exposures, confine the fire, and extinguish it, master streams are put into action (Figure 10-36). Any appliance that flows over 500 gpm is considered to be a master stream appliance. These large-volume streams of water can be delivered by any one of several appli-ances. Master stream appliances can be positioned and flowed from the ground, from preconnected positions on an engine, or from an elevated position, such as the end of an aerial ladder apparatus. A master stream appliance that is portable and can be located on the ground is often called a *deluge gun*. A master stream appliance located on an engine is often called a *deck gun*. A master stream appliance connected to an aerial ladder or platform is usually called an *aerial stream*. As a member of the outside firefighting team,

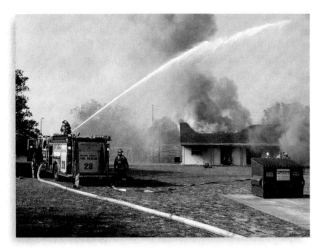

FIGURE 10-36 A master stream appliance flowing water to protect an exposure.

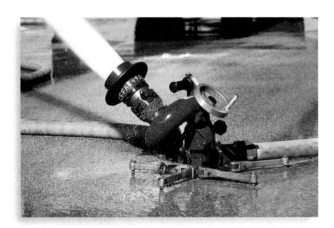

FIGURE 10-37 Deluge gun.

you may be assigned to set up and operate a master stream appliance located on ground level or to assist in flowing a master stream appliance that is on the fire apparatus. Operating master stream devices from aerial ladders is a more advanced skill that is unique to each type of aerial apparatus.

Ground-Level Master Stream Appliances—Deluge Gun

The **deluge gun** (also called a *monitor*) is a master stream appliance set up primarily for use at ground level (Figure 10-37). It has a base with two or three inlets (with female swivels) and a swivel nozzle mount. Attached to the nozzle mount is a nozzle—either an adjustable fog nozzle or an open-tip master stream

nozzle. Supply lines (usually large attack lines) are attached from the pump panel discharge outlets into the base of the unit and charged when ready.

KEY WORDS

deluge gun A type of master stream appliance that is set up primarily for use at ground level; also called a *monitor*.

Master Stream Nozzles

Master stream nozzles are similar to fire attack line nozzles (Figure 10-38). They deliver much higher volumes of water at a far greater distance than other types of nozzles. The firefighter can easily adjust the nozzle pattern (on adjustable-flow fog nozzles), aiming the fire stream by raising and lowering the nozzle and rotating the nozzle from side to side. Master stream nozzles provide a great deal of reach for the master stream and deliver large volumes of water to the desired location.

Master Stream Deployment

Once placed into position and operational, master streams can provide excellent exposure protection at large fire scenes in which exposures to the original fire are at risk. Because they are intended to stay in place while flowing, master streams can be attended by only one firefighter after they are set up. This is their most common application.

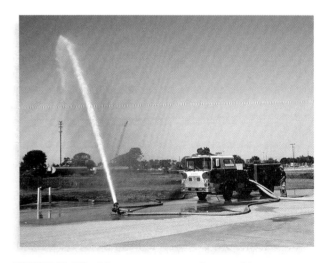

FIGURE 10-38 Master stream nozzles provide a great deal of reach for the master stream and deliver large volumes of water to the desired location.

They can also be set up and then left working in place, which is useful with fires of long duration and especially with hazardous fire situations (Figure 10-39).

Any significant change in location requires the master stream appliance to be shut down and relocated to the next position. It may also require the lines to be extended. In addition, it requires the hose lines supplying the appliance to be shut down, drained of pressure, disconnected, and extended after the appliance is repositioned.

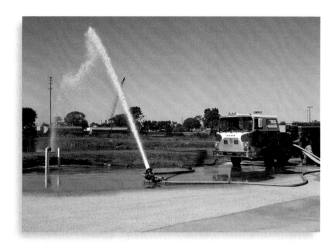

FIGURE 10-39 Unattended master stream.

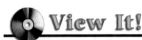

View It!

Go to the DVD, navigate to Chapter 10, and select *Setting Up a Monitor-Deck Gun.*

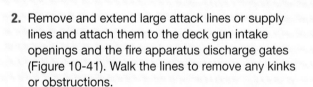

Practice It!

Setting Up a Monitor-Deck Gun

Use the following steps when setting up the deluge gun for operation:

1. Remove the deck gun from its storage place on the fire apparatus and place it where it will provide the best coverage for the effect desired (Figure 10-40).

FIGURE 10-40

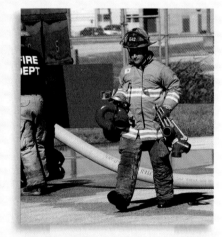

2. Remove and extend large attack lines or supply lines and attach them to the deck gun intake openings and the fire apparatus discharge gates (Figure 10-41). Walk the lines to remove any kinks or obstructions.

FIGURE 10-41

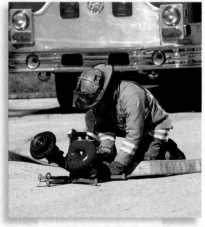

3. Signal the pump operator to charge the lines, aiming the stream away from any firefighters nearby. After the air has been bled from the deck gun and hose, position the height and direction of the master stream and adjust the flow of the nozzle and pattern (with an adjustable fog nozzle) (Figure 10-42).

FIGURE 10-42

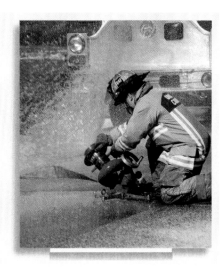

 Safety Tip!

Due to the volume and force of the water coming out of any master stream appliance, you must avoid allowing the stream of water to hit other firefighters. These streams can also knock down weakened building structural parts and push loose debris long distances. In addition, the volume of water can add significant weight to the location it is applied, increasing the chances of structural collapse in fire-weakened buildings. These streams are usually applied to structural fire areas evacuated of any firefighters.

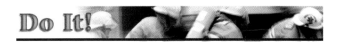 **Do It!**

Deploying and Operating Large Attack Lines

Deploying and operating large attack lines is always a team effort. A charged line holds quite a volume of water and is heavy. In addition, the backpressure of a nozzle flowing a large amount of water can be straining. Practice working as a team and rotate positions often to conserve your energy when working with these lines. One of the main values of using a large attack line is found in the reach they have when flowing water. The extended distance between you and the fire makes the large-diameter line a good choice during a defensive fire attack; this distance keeps firefighters clear of the collapse zone. Take advantage of this safety feature and do not "creep" closer to the fire than necessary. Like any other aspect of fireground operations, working with large attack lines takes practice, so practice often.

Prove It

Knowledge Assessment

Signed Documentation Tear-Out Sheet

Exterior Operations Level Firefighter—Chapter 10

Name: _____

Fill out the ten-question quiz below, the Knowledge Assessment Sheet, by circling the correct answer for each question. When finished, sign it and give to your instructor/Company Officer for his or her signature. Turn in this Knowledge Assessment Sheet to the proper person as part of the documentation that you have completed your training for this chapter.

1. Large fire attack lines are generally _____ diameter hose lines with associated nozzles.
   a. 1- to 3-inch
   b. 2½- to 3-inch
   c. 1½-inch
   d. 5-inch

2. Large, preconnected fire attack lines can also be referred to as _____ lines.
   a. red
   b. quick
   c. blitz
   d. black

3. Large attack lines deliver a greater gallons-per-minute rate of water to the seat of the fire. The greater flow rate means that more people are needed to operate and maneuver the flowing lines. A sustained water supply is also needed to keep it flowing.
   a. True
   b. False

4. If a large attack line is being used by one or two firefighters, is going to be mostly stationary, and is at a safe distance from the fire, the hose line can be _____ on the ground.
   a. twisted
   b. held
   c. flaked
   d. looped

5. When large attack lines need to be advanced to different positions, it is best to have one firefighter attending the line.
   a. True
   b. False

6. If the line must be moved while flowing, the firefighter at the nozzle should be ready to _____ if he or she stumbles or loses balance.
   a. shut down the nozzle
   b. reloop the hose line
   c. advance the hose line
   d. open the nozzle

7. A _____ is an appliance that closely resembles the gated wye, but in addition to the two 1½-inch discharge ports, it has a single 2½-inch discharge port in the middle.

    a. deck gun

    b. water thief

    c. monitor

    d. hydrant valve

8. A typical _____ has a 2½-inch inlet and two 1½-inch outlets.

    a. water thief

    b. deck gun

    c. gated wye

    d. hose clamp

9. Operating _____ from aerial ladders is a more advanced skill that is unique to each type of aerial apparatus.

    a. small attack lines

    b. master stream appliances

    c. a gated wye appliance

    d. a water thief

10. _____ are intended to stay in place while flowing. They can be attended by only one firefighter after they are set up.

    a. Large fire attack hose lines

    b. Gated wye appliances

    c. Water thief appliances

    d. Master streams

Student Signature and Date _____   Instructor/Company Officer Signature and Date _____

238

Skills Assessment

Signed Documentation Tear-Out Sheet

Exterior Operations Level Firefighter—Chapter 10

Name: _____

Fill out the Skills Assessment Sheet below. Have your instructor/Company Officer check off and initial each skill you demonstrate. When finished, sign it and give to your instructor/Company Officer for his or her signature. Turn in this Skills Assessment Sheet to the proper person as part of the documentation that you have completed your training for this chapter.

Skill	Completed	Initials
1. Demonstrate how to pull and stretch a large preconnected hose line.	_____	_____
2. Demonstrate how to assemble a large attack line.	_____	_____
3. Explain and demonstrate the steps for flowing a large attack line, one-person method.	_____	_____
4. Explain and demonstrate the steps looping a large attack line, one-person method.	_____	_____
5. Discuss and demonstrate the steps for advancing a large attack line as a hose team member.	_____	_____
6. Discuss and demonstrate how multiple firefighters handle a large attack line in the kneeling position.	_____	_____
7. Demonstrate and explain how to extend a line with a gated wye.	_____	_____
8. Demonstrate and explain the hose-clamp method for extending a line.	_____	_____
9. Demonstrate and explain how to extend a line using the through-the-nozzle method.	_____	_____
10. Explain and demonstrate how to set up a master stream appliance.	_____	_____

Student Signature and Date _____   Instructor/Company Officer Signature and Date _____

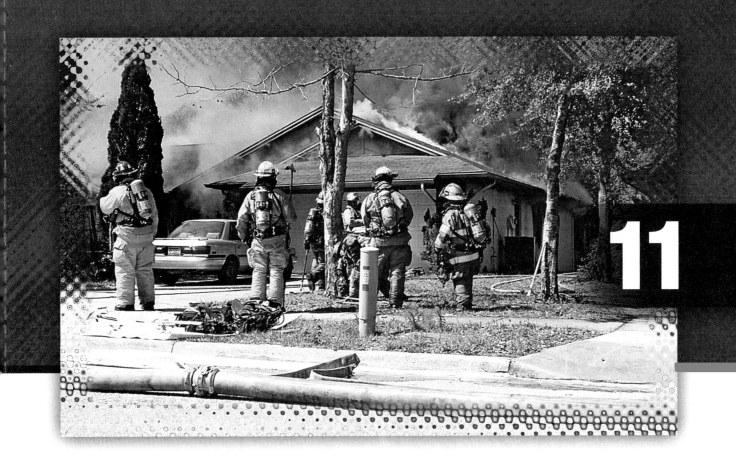

Single-Family-Dwelling Fires

What You Will Learn in This Chapter

In this chapter you will be introduced to one of the most common fire situations faced by today's firefighters, the single-family-dwelling fire. We will introduce you to some construction and burn characteristics of manufactured housing and site-built structures. You will review safe response and arrival practices as well as command personnel accountability needs. Safety practices on the dwelling fire scene will be discussed. We will explain the fire attack team and the various jobs that they may be assigned. You will learn about roof and extension ladders, which are commonly carried and used by engine company units. We'll talk about exposures and making an exterior fire attack on a dwelling fire situation. Finally, you will practice what you have learned with three drills for dwelling fire situations.

What You Will Be Able to Do

After reading this chapter and practicing the skills in a classroom setting, you will be able to

1. Explain the differences between manufactured and site-built dwellings as they relate to construction and fire conditions.

2. Describe safety zones on the dwelling fire emergency scene.

3. Explain how to check in with command using your fire department's personnel accountability system (PAS).

4. Define the different job functions that a typical fire attack team may be called upon to perform on the scene of a dwelling fire.

5. Demonstrate forcible entry techniques on an exterior door that swings inward.

6. Demonstrate forcible entry techniques on an exterior door that swings outward.

7. Explain techniques for using a Halligan bar and flathead axe to force a lock.

8. Explain how to assist interior firefighters with extending hose while stationed at the doorway to a dwelling.

9. Describe how to safely break and clear glass from a window frame on a dwelling.
10. Define what is meant by the term *intervention team.*
11. Describe how and where a tool staging area might be set up and its main purpose on the dwelling fire scene.
12. Demonstrate how to place ventilation fans for negative- and positive-pressure ventilation on a single-family dwelling.
13. Describe a lockout/tagout system and how it is used on the fire ground.
14. Demonstrate how to control utilities in a dwelling.
15. Demonstrate how to deploy, place, and stow a roof ladder.
16. Demonstrate how to prepare a roof ladder for use on a roof.
17. Demonstrate how to deploy, place, and stow an extension ladder.
18. Explain what is meant by the term *exposure* and the best methods of protecting an exposure with an attack line stream.
19. Demonstrate dwelling fire operations for Exterior Operations level firefighters as a member of a fire attack team.
20. Demonstrate dwelling fire support operations for Exterior Operations level firefighters.

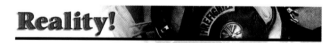

Structural Firefighting and Teamwork

Some of the most complex and inherently dangerous operations a fire department undertakes involve the duties associated with a structural fire. A lot goes on during the first few minutes after the Fire Department arrives on the scene, and for someone uninformed about Fire Department procedure, at first glance our actions can appear chaotic. However, nothing could be farther from the truth. The safety and success of everyone on the scene of a structural fire is dependent on an integrated system of safety, equipment, tools, and the actions of teams of people working as part of a command structure toward the common goal—to save *savable* lives and protect *savable* property. Nothing on a properly staffed and controlled fire scene is accomplished through an individual effort. Safe firefighters work in teams of two or more, depending on the task, and are actively involved in either directly extinguishing the fire or supporting those who are. There is no room for any freelance operations on a fire scene. For everyone's safety, all activities *MUST* be coordinated

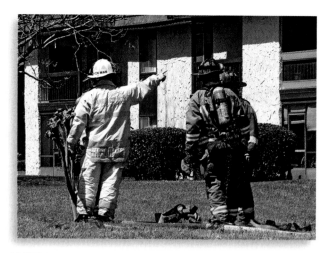

FIGURE 11-1   An Incident Commander is essential on any fire scene.

through the Incident Commander, who orchestrates the actions (Figure 11-1).

Because this is your initial exposure to working at a structural fire, your training at this point will focus on the functions that are conducted *outside* the burning structure—in this case, a single-story, single-family dwelling. A fire in a single-family dwelling is the most common type of structural fire to which we respond. Those who enter the dangerous atmosphere contained in a burning structure should be trained to at least the Level 1 standard. However, there are dozens of essential actions that you can perform outside the building in support of the interior attack team.

Single-Family-Dwelling Fires

The most common kind of structural fire you will respond to as a firefighter is fire in a single-family dwelling. These buildings are where most people live and, consequently, where most structural fires occur. Vast areas of subdivisions surround densely populated cities in the United States. There are also large areas where homes are intermingled with wildland areas, where the risk of a structural fire is no less common.

The normal routine for the Fire Service is to make an aggressive interior fire attack on these structures when the risk is justified by the potential to save a life or to save *savable* property (Figure 11-2). If there are unburned areas in the structure where fire victims may be located, or if the fire is small and the building can be saved for repair, then this option is usually

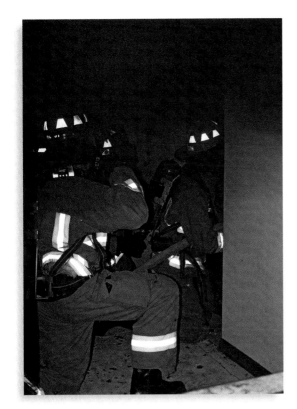

FIGURE 11-2 An aggressive interior fire attack is often referred to as an offensive fire attack.

called for. This practice is referred to as an offensive fire attack.

An Exterior Operations level firefighter does not have the training to enter a burning structural fire. You must first successfully complete the next curriculum, Level 1, to be able to take part in an interior offensive fire attack.

However, as an Exterior Operations level firefighter, you are able to assist an interior fire attack operation from the outside. Essential work is needed on the outside to support interior firefighting crews. After completing this training section, you will be able to assist fire crews in opening locked or blocked doors (forcible entry) as well as removing glass from windows from the outside. During a fire, secondary fire attack hose lines need to be deployed and all hose lines need to be set up and advanced into the structure from the outside. Supply hose lines need to be set into operation and ladders raised (especially on multistory dwellings). All of these jobs can be accomplished by the Exterior Operations level firefighter.

In addition, when the building fire has extended throughout the structure and an exterior fire attack, also referred to a **defensive fire attack,** has been called for, then you will be able to use your skills to extinguish the fire as a member of the exterior firefighting team.

Manufactured Homes

In the years since its inception, the house trailer evolved into the mobile home and has now evolved further into today's **manufactured home.** A manufactured home that was built after the mid-1990s meets a strict building code that makes it much safer than its predecessors. However, there are plenty of the older mobile homes still in use. The greatest difference between the two types is in the time it takes for the fire to travel through the structure. In today's better-built manufactured home, a fire is often contained in one or two rooms inside the structure. Before the code changes, mobile homes were likely to be totally engulfed by rapidly spreading fire.

Manufactured homes usually have an exterior metal cladding and are built with a wood frame and floor. They are mounted on a chassis that allows the home to be transported from the manufacturer to the final home site (Figure 11-3). The chassis arrangement means that the finished floor can be 2 or 3 feet above grade level, with a large void space underneath the home. When properly installed, the manufactured

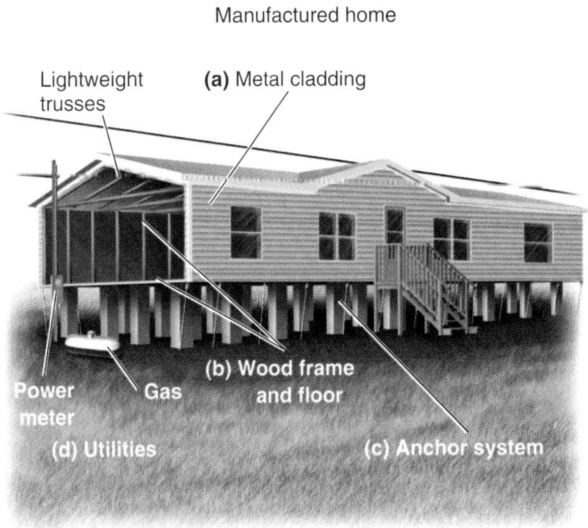

Manufactured home

Lightweight trusses

(a) Metal cladding

(b) Wood frame and floor

(c) Anchor system

Power meter

Gas

(d) Utilities

FIGURE 11-3 A typical modern manufactured home consists of the following elements: (a) metal cladding, (b) wood frame and floor, (c) chassis, (d) anchor system, and (e) utilities.

home is held in place by ground anchors and straps that help prevent wind damage to the structure. Just like a site-built home, most manufactured homes are served by electricity, water, and propane or natural gas utilities.

KEY WORD

manufactured home A building that is assembled in a factory and then transported to its final location for use as a single-family dwelling. This type of building can also be used as nonpermanent housing.

Site-Built Homes

Most single-family dwellings are built on site (Figure 11-4). **Site-built single-family homes** can range from small wood-framed buildings that are less than 1000 square feet in size to vast estates with multiple buildings enclosing many thousands of square feet. They may have large basement areas, multiple levels above ground, and open attic areas under the roof. The fires you encounter involving single-family dwellings will vary greatly between incidents, so our focus at this point is on the skills and abilities that are common to fighting most single-story, single-family-dwelling fires.

KEY WORD

site-built single-family home A building that is built on the site location. This type of building is not designed to be moved and is therefore a permanent structure used for single-family dwelling.

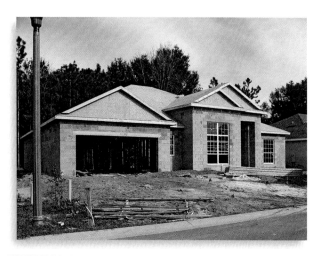

FIGURE 11-4 Single family site built homes are very common throughout North America.

Safe Response and Arrival

When the alarm sounds, dispatching units to a structural fire, it is only natural that your adrenaline flows and you get excited, especially if this type of work is new to you. However, it is extremely important that everyone focuses on the firefighter's first responsibility for any mission: to get to the scene safely. We discussed the steps for a safe response in Chapter 5. However, it cannot be stressed enough that one of the most dangerous aspects of any emergency work is the response phase. Whether you are responding from the fire station to the incident, from home to the fire station, or from home directly to the incident, your safety is your responsibility. ***Wear your seatbelt, and focus on the traffic and safe driving.***

If you respond directly to the scene in your personally owned vehicle (POV), make sure to park your vehicle out of the way when you arrive. Keep in mind that other arriving vehicles may need room to stretch supply hose from the hydrant to the fire and to deploy attack lines, ladders and equipment. Therefore, they need as much room in the street or road as they can get. Remember to remain aware of your surroundings when choosing the proper parking spot for your POV. Keep away from overhead power lines that stretch from the power pole to the burning structure. It is very common for a line to burn free from the house and drop to the ground, creating an extreme electrical hazard to anyone below or near the energized wires.

Incident Command Framework

The elements of a good Incident Command System call for the first trained person who arrives on the scene to establish command of the incident. This person is usually the Company Officer of the first arriving unit. However, it could very well be you if you are the first to arrive in your POV. Your role in this case is to gather information and be prepared to relay that information to the first arriving crew. In most instances, however, you will arrive as part of a crew or after the first responding unit arrives and establishes command. In this case, report to the Incident Commander and wait for instructions before taking any action. There is no room for freelancing on any fire scene, so expect to be teamed up with other firefighters or crews.

One of the most important elements of a command structure is the personnel accountability system (PAS). This system enables the Commander to know where on the fire scene each individual firefighter is working and what they are doing at any given time

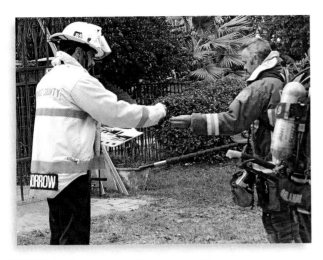

FIGURE 11-5 Personnel accountability systems are important for firefighter safety on the fire scene.

during the operation. It is important that you take whatever action is required by your department's procedures for "tagging in" with the Personnel Accountability Officer and then stay with your assigned crew throughout the incident (Figure 11-5).

Overall Scene Safety

For our purposes at this point, we will divide the job assignments for a dwelling fire into two categories: exterior and interior. Individuals who work inside a burning building are working in an atmosphere that is **Immediately Dangerous to Life and Health (IDLH)** (Figure 11-6). However, this isn't the only hazard they face. Many of the line-of-duty deaths of firefighters working inside a structure occur when the firefighter becomes disoriented and runs out of fresh air supplied by his or her SCBA. Therefore, just knowing how to wear PPE and breathe from an SCBA does not qualify a person to work inside a structural fire. This type of competency will come later, during your Level 1 training. For the rest of this chapter we will focus on exterior operations.

By now you are probably noticing a common theme to most emergency operations we discuss in this book. Everyone's safety at most incidents depends on a few common factors: a safe response, a safe arrival and setup, the observation of safety zones around the hazard, and the proper use and wearing of PPE. Working at a structural fire is no different in this respect. We must observe traffic safety zones in the street around the apparatus. We must also observe the hot, warm, and cold zones around the structure so that everyone is working where they should be and employing the proper level of PPE according to their job task.

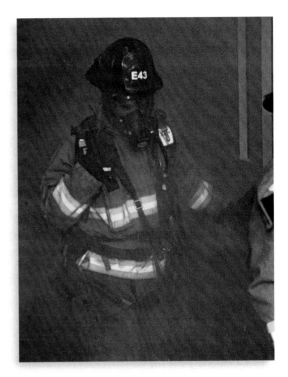

FIGURE 11-6 The interior of a burning building is considered an atmosphere that is Immediately Dangerous to Life and Health (IDLH).

KEY WORD

Immediately Dangerous to Life and Health (IDLH) A term used to define for firefighters the conditions of an atmosphere in a confined area, like a building fire, that can result in serious injury or death.

Traffic Control Zone

The traffic control zone for a structural fire is not much different from a vehicle crash. The main differences are the amount of apparatus staged in the work area and the length of the control zone that is necessary for the supply hose stretched from one or more hydrants (Figure 11-7).

In many areas, laws make it illegal for a civilian to even drive on the same block as a parked fire truck that is working at a fire. However, very few people are aware of such laws. The reality is that most people become excited when they see the activity around a fire and the fire itself. They often drive in an erratic manner, very close to you and the hose or apparatus—so be especially careful.

Onlookers gather at any type of emergency and can become a problem if they are allowed to venture too close to the action. It is best that you speak in a respectful but firm tone when asking bystanders to step back and remain out of the way. The key is to ask for their help and not shout out any orders. And, for the most part, you will get the cooperation you are seeking. Establish a clear, safe area using banner tape when possible, and seek the assistance of law enforcement personnel to control the crowds that gather at the scene.

Safety Zones

The hot, warm, and cold zones associated with a structural fire vary in size and shape depending on the size structure and fire. The zones also differ according to whether the fire attack is offensive or defensive. These zones should be designated by the Incident Commander on each emergency (Figure 11-8).

The Hot Zone

During an offensive, interior attack, the hot zone usually includes any area inside the structure where an IDLH incident in an enclosed area is encountered. Any-

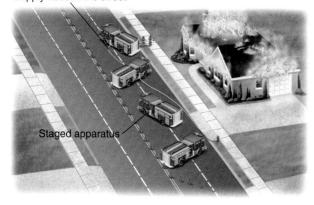

FIGURE 11-7   The traffic control zone for a structural fire includes (a) staged apparatus and (b) a supply hose in the street.

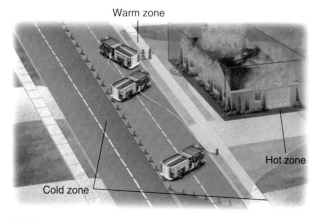

FIGURE 11-8   The safety zones for a typical single-family-dwelling fire consist of (a) the hot zone, (b) the warm zone, and (c) the cold zone.

one working in the hot zone should be fully protected with PPE and a charged hose line. These individuals should also be trained to the Level 1 standard.

If the fire is well-advanced and the fire attack becomes defensive, the hot zone is expanded to anything within the area that could be hazardous if the building was to collapse.

There are conflicting opinions as to how large this area should be, but for safety's sake we consider the collapse area to extend out for a distance of twice the height of the building. Walls seldom fall out any farther than their height, but doubling that potential allows for any errors in judgment.

Another exception to the hot zone area includes areas around any downed or dangerous electrical lines that could possibly fall to the ground as they burn away from the structure. Keep clear of these areas by a distance of at least the length of the wire in all directions. Because the hot zone can be irregular in shape and size, many agencies mark the dangerous areas with traffic cones early in the operation as a warning to firefighters working in the area.

The Warm Zone

In a single-story, single-family-dwelling fire in a residential area, the warm zone typically starts at the doorway and extends outward several feet. The warm zone is usually anything on the property, extending to and including the traffic control areas outside the property line boundaries. Anyone working in the warm zone should also be protected in full PPE during the active fire. However, because a firefighter may work in a support role independent of a charged hose line, once the fire has been controlled the PPE requirements can be relaxed at the Incident Commander's order.

The Cold Zone

The cold zone is obviously anything outside the hot and warm zones. This area is any place beyond the scope and control of the Incident Commander. Therefore, it is generally of no concern to you. Although the PPE requirements for the warm zone are relaxed once the fire has been controlled, the warm zone does not convert to a "cold zone" due to the need to restrict civilian access to the area around the equipment and the hazards that may remain.

Unit Assignments

The type and amount of equipment dispatched to a single-family-dwelling fire varies drastically throughout North America. Fire departments in urban areas tend to send more equipment of various types to a house fire than departments in rural areas because the equipment available in a rural setting is often more limited. Our focus here will not be on the type of truck or trucks that respond to the scene, but on the number of firefighters that should respond and their job functions on the scene.

Any work done on a fire scene should be accomplished in teams of at least two individuals. The work is assigned by the type of job the team is charged to perform. For example, the **fire attack team** is charged with forcing open any locked doors that are in the way of the advancing hose team, while the ventilation team is responsible for opening windows to vent the smoke and hot gases from inside the structure. More than one job can be assigned to a team. In the absence of extra support staff on the scene in the first moments of the fire, the initial hose team may be assigned the tasks of both the fire attack team and the ventilation team so that these important functions are not overlooked. When staffing permits, most of these jobs are performed simultaneously.

KEY WORD

fire attack team A group of firefighters who perform various firefighting functions on the scene of a fire emergency in order to mitigate the situation and return it to a safe condition.

Fire Attack Team

The fire attack team is responsible for deploying the proper size hose line, forcing open any locked doors or windows (forcible entry), and advancing a hose line to the seat of the fire. If the scope of the fire calls for an offensive, interior attack, the team operates inside the burning structure. Although the Exterior Operations level firefighter's job stops at the front door, there are several duties you can perform to assist with the fire attack team's mission. Forcing a locked door, helping to straighten any kinks in the hose line, and feeding hose from the outside to the fire attack crew can help conserve the fire attack team's energy for the hose work inside.

If the fire attack team is working in a defensive, exterior mode, then their duties are performed outside the structure. The Exterior Operations level firefighter may therefore be called upon to help staff the hose line or operate the nozzle (Figure 11-9).

Forcible Entry

The most common tools used to force a door are the flathead axe and the Halligan bar. The flathead axe used for the Fire Service has both a cutting surface and a pound-

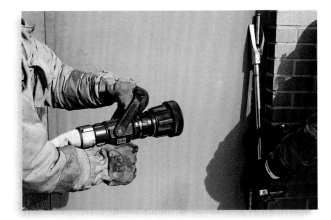

FIGURE 11-9 An Exterior Operations level firefighter may be working on a hose line while other firefighters work on forcing the door.

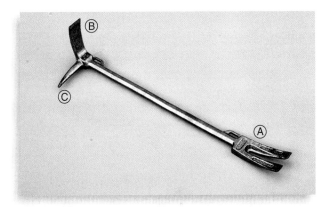

FIGURE 11-10 Halligan bar: (a) forked end, (b) adze, and (c) pick.

ing surface. The Halligan bar is a tool that was specially designed for forcible entry. The Halligan tool is forked on one end and has an adze and pick on the other end. Each of these features can be adapted to almost any use (Figure 11-10). A typical Halligan-style bar provides quite a bit of leverage, so prying a door is well within the range of the tool and a person of average strength. The flathead axe serves as a pounding tool to pound the Halligan bar into place, which then allows the leverage provided by the bar to pry open the door. It is important that you view these two tools as being almost "married" together as a two-piece tool. You should carry them together whenever you are assigned the duty of performing forcible entry. A good way to carry these two tools is to "marry" them together by placing the forked end of the Halligan bar over the axe blade and folding the bar against the axe handle so that you can pick up both tools in one hand (Figure 11-11).

Forcible entry is a skill worthy of an entire textbook of its own. There are two basic maneuvers that help you force open most conventional residential doors; the method used depends on the direction in which the door swings. When sizing up a door that you are about

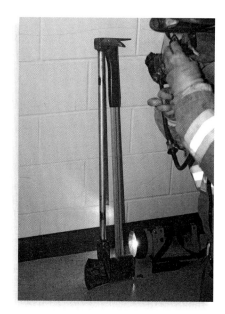

to force open, look closely at whether the door swings inward (away from you) or outward (toward you). Generally, if the hinges are visible on the outside, the door swings outward. Next, try the doorknob. The door may not be locked; if it isn't, report this to your team's Officer and be ready for another order. If the door is locked, then be prepared to force entry when told to do so and not before. Before you take action, it is important that a charged hose line is in place and that the fire attack team is ready for the door to be opened.

FIGURE 11-11 The Halligan bar and axe "married" together.

 View It!

Go to the DVD, navigate to Chapter 11, and select *Forcible Entry—Inward-Swinging Door.*

 Practice It!

Forcible Entry—Inward-Swinging Door

Working as part of a two-person team, use a flathead axe and Halligan bar to perform the following steps:

1. Size up the door, and check to see if it is locked, the direction it swings, and the location of the lock(s) (Figure 11-12).

   FIGURE 11-12

   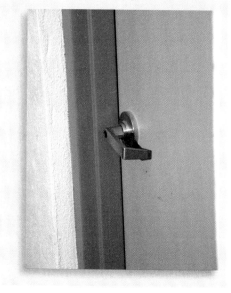

2. Confirm that the hose team is in place with a charged line and is ready for the door to be forced.

3. Position the adze end of the Halligan tool in the gap between the jamb and the door, just above or below the lock(s) (Figure 11-13).

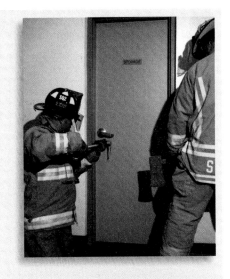

FIGURE 11-13

4. Use the flat of the axe to pound the adze end in place until it is well seated between the door and the jamb (Figure 11-14).

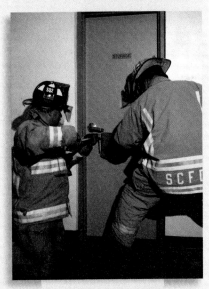

FIGURE 11-14

5. Apply force to the bar, moving the bar toward the door until the door opens (Figure 11-15).

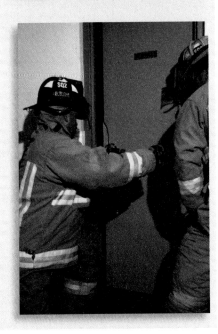

FIGURE 11-15

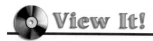

View It!

Go to the DVD, navigate to Chapter 11, and select *Forcible Entry—Outward-Swinging Door.*

Practice It!

Forcible Entry—Outward-Swinging Door

Working as part of a two-person team, use a flathead axe and Halligan bar to perform the following steps:

1. Size up the door, assuring that it is locked, the direction it swings, and the location of the lock(s).

FIGURE 11-16

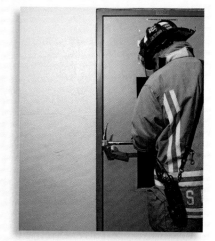

2. Confirm that the hose team is in place with a charged line and is ready for the door to be forced.

3. Position the adze end of the Halligan tool in the gap between the jamb and the door, just above or below the lock(s) (Figure 11-16).

FIGURE 11-17

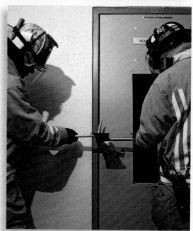

4. Pound the adze in place until it is well seated between the door and the jamb (Figure 11-17).

5. Apply force to the bar, pulling the bar outward until the door opens (Figure 11-18).

FIGURE 11-18

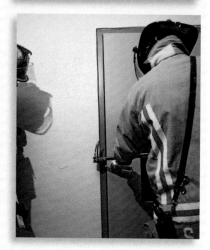

Forcing Locks

Doors to outbuildings, such as storage sheds or barns, may be locked with a padlock and hasp. The pick feature of the Halligan bar is useful when you encounter this situation. While the lock seldom breaks under the force of the Halligan bar, it makes a good purchase point for the Halligan bar to apply force on the hasp. Place the pick into the lock's shackle and pound down sharply on the back of the Halligan tool (Figure 11-19). This action usually strips away any screws that are holding the hasp in place, breaking the assembly free and thus opening the door.

 Safety Tip!

Anytime you use a striking or prying tool, always wear full protective gear, including eye protection. Forcible entry during fire conditions should be performed wearing full PPE with an SCBA in place. Stand to one side of the door and avoid standing directly in the doorway to avoid the hot smoke and flames that may come from the opened door. Stay as low as possible and apply just enough force to open the door, controlling the door so that it doesn't fly open. It is not uncommon to find a victim collapsed just inside a locked door, so be prepared as the door opens.

Advancing Hose

Once the door is opened, the fire attack team advances toward the fire. As an Exterior Operations level firefighter, you won't be part of the crew inside but you are still part of the team. Dragging a charged hose line through a house is difficult, especially if the interior crew is crawling on their hands and knees. This task can be made quite a bit easier if someone stages at the doorway, outside the building and the IDLH environment, to feed the hose into the building. This helps the interior team because they will only have to drag the 20 or so feet of line that is inside the building and not the entire 150 to 200 feet of charged hose line that extends all the way back to the pumper.

It is also important that the hose line be free of kinks and snags. Get in the habit of straightening any kinks in the line so that the maximum water flow is available at the nozzle when needed. Snags occur when the hose is dragged around obstacles such as fence posts, trees, plants, and even the wheels of the pumper. Pull the line free of any obstacles before the line becomes snagged and the interior crew is forced to stop (Figure 11-20).

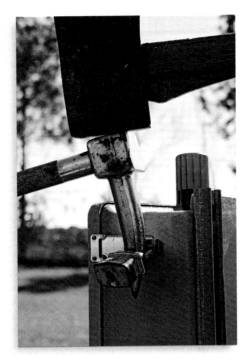

FIGURE 11-19 When you encounter a padlock and hasp, place the pick of the Halligan bar in the shackle and strike the back of the tool with the flat side of an axe.

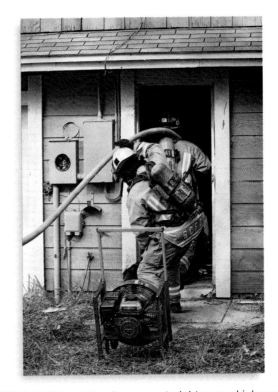

FIGURE 11-20 At the doorway, straighten any kinks and assure that the line is free of obstacles that may snag it while it is being pulled inside.

Ventilation Team

The ventilation team is responsible for opening windows to vent the smoke and hot gases from inside the structure. They may also place specialized fans to ventilate smoke-filled areas.

Although some ventilation methods involve working on a roof, the Exterior Operations level activities are limited to ventilation techniques that can be accomplished from the ground and from outside the building.

Ventilation

The smoke and hot fire gases inside a structure can be more dangerous to the firefighters and occupants inside the structure than the flames. The products of combustion not only are toxic but can be explosive under certain conditions. It is important that the heat and smoke be ventilated from the structure. This ventilation is often accomplished by breaking glass or opening windows in a controlled and systematic manner. The ventilation efforts may occur through the natural process of the hot, pressurized gases that move from the building to the cooler, lower pressure outside. Alternately, ventilation may be augmented by the use of large fans that can either add pressure and fresh air to the structure or, when possible, pull the smoke out.

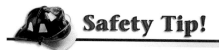

Safety Tip!

Ventilation is conducted under the control and orders of the Incident Commander. Several factors are considered when the order is given to ventilate the structure, including hose line placement, team positions, and the location of the fire inside the structure. *DO NOT* ventilate the structure without an order to do so. The Incident Commander gives the order to ventilate and advises about the location of the openings and the type of ventilation that is to be used.

Breaking Glass   At first glance, it may seem to be excessive damage to break the glass in a window to vent the smoke from a building. If the fire is small enough and the smoke is fairly cool inside, the Incident Commander may give the order for the interior team to just open the windows from the inside as they proceed through the structure. This is usually the case when the fire is confined to a mattress or a pot on the stove in the kitchen. However, when the fire involves one or more rooms inside, the volume of smoke and heat far exceeds the amount that can be ventilated through a small, open window. In this case, the Incident Commander may call for exterior ventilation, which can

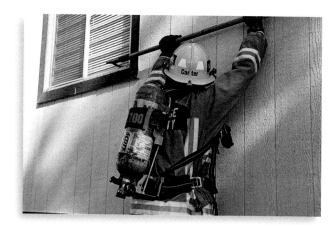

FIGURE 11-21   Positioning with a ceiling hook to break glass.

usually be conducted by crews standing in a safe area on the ground outside the building.

The tools of choice for outside ventilation through windows include an axe, a Halligan bar, and a ceiling hook. As a rule of thumb, the ceiling hook is usually the better choice because it allows you a chance to stand to one side of the window, preferably upwind, and keep your hands away from the glass shards that fall when you strike the window. Regardless of the tool used, keep your hands as far away from the glass as possible. Remember to keep the tool as close to horizontal as you can so that glass shards don't slide down the handle of the tool, striking you or gathering inside your coat sleeve. It takes a little force to break the glass, especially if it is mounted in a thermal-pane window in which the glass is thicker and possibly made of double layers. Strike the glass with minimal force at first and swing the tool quicker with subsequent blows if it doesn't break the first time (Figure 11-21).

Take the time to clear out all of the glass in the window by raking the tool around the window frame. This action removes the sharp, jagged edges that could injure someone later. Many agencies prefer that you simply pull the entire window assembly out of the frame so that the hole left behind can be used as an emergency escape route for the interior crew if something goes wrong. In reality, once you break the glass out of a typical residential window, the damage has been done and the most cost effective way to repair the window later is to replace the entire assembly. Therefore, no further damage is done when you pull the entire assembly out of the frame.

Once the glass and window frame have been cleared, use the tool to reach in and clear away any window treatments that can block smoke, such as curtains or blinds. Even something as porous as a wire screen across a window can hold back a lot of smoke, especially when it becomes clogged with soot, so clear away anything that can slow the ventilation process or get in the way of an exiting firefighter.

Ventilation Fans Ventilation fans come in two basic styles: gasoline powered and electric powered. Like all other aspects of the ventilation process, the placement and use of these fans is conducted only under the direct orders of the Incident Commander.

Negative-Pressure Ventilation Fans Electric-powered ventilation fans are most often used for **negative-pressure ventilation.** The fan is set up in a window or doorway with the inlet side facing toward the fire and the outlet side facing toward the open air. This type of fan is also called a **smoke ejector.** Smoke ejectors have hooks on cables and can be secured in place using an expanding door bar, hanging from a door or ladder, or by being placed on the ground. The key is to place the fan in as small an opening as pos-

sible so that the air pulled into the inlet comes from inside the structure and is not simply recirculated air from outside the building.

▦ KEY WORDS ▦

negative-pressure ventilation A method of ventilation used to remove smoke from a building. An electric-powered fan is set up facing out of a building's opening. The fan is then activated to draw out smoke from inside the building.

smoke ejector A type of electrically powered smoke ventilation fan used on buildings for negative-pressure ventilation.

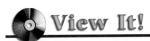 **View It!**

Go to the DVD, navigate to Chapter 11, and select *Negative-Pressure Ventilation.*

▷ Practice It!

Negative-Pressure Ventilation

Use the following steps to position a smoke ejector fan for negative-pressure ventilation:

1. Remove the electric smoke ejector fan from the apparatus and plug it into the power cord from the apparatus generator. Turn it on and off quickly to check for operation. Then carry it to the desired location as directed by your Company Officer.

2. Hook the fan onto an open door, to an expanding door bar, or place it securely in a window (Figure 11-22). Switch it on.

3. Advise your Company Officer that you have accomplished the assignment.

FIGURE 11-22

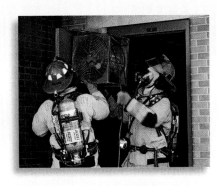

Positive-Pressure Ventilation Fans Gasoline-powered fans are usually much more powerful than the electric versions and are also heavier in weight. Therefore, these fans are almost exclusively restricted to remaining on the ground outside the structure. They blow inward to fill the building with fresh air and positive pressure that forces the smoke and gases out of the building. You will also hear these fans referred to as **PPV (positive-pressure ventilation)** fans. When using a PPV fan on a typical structure, position it about 10 or 12 feet from the doorway so that the "cone" of air exiting the fan fills the entire doorway, forming a positive-pressure seal. This seal, in turn, forces more of the bad air out of the building through the other openings. Setting the PPV fan too close to the doorway causes the

inlet air to fill only part of the doorway, allowing smoke to exit the upper part of the door, which is then sucked into the fan and recirculated back into the structure.

▦ KEY WORD ▦

positive-pressure ventilation (PPV) A method of ventilation used to push smoke out and fresh air into a building. A specially designed fan is positioned outside the building at an opening, facing into the building. The fan is then operated and the building fills with fresh air under pressure, pushing out the smoke and gases.

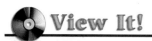
Go to the DVD, navigate to Chapter 11, and select *Positive-Pressure Ventilation*.

Practice It!

Positive-Pressure Ventilation

Use the following steps to position a gasoline-powered fan for positive-pressure ventilation:

1. Remove the fan from the apparatus and carry it to the desired location as directed by your Company Officer. This location is usually 10 to 12 feet from a doorway (Figure 11-23).

FIGURE 11-23

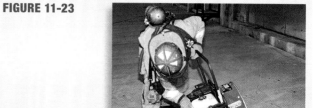

2. Turn the fan to one side, away from the doorway, and start it, checking its operation.

FIGURE 11-24

3. Turn the fan so that it is blowing air toward the doorway and into the structure (Figure 11-24).

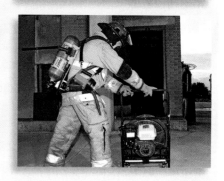

4. Advise the Company Officer that you have accomplished the assignment.

Intervention Team

In an effort to provide backup and protection on the fire scene, the Fire Service has developed the concept of an Intervention Team. This team consists of a small group of firefighters who stand by in the warm zone outside the fire area with full PPE, tools, and attack hose line. They are prepared to quickly enter the fire area to locate, defend, and rescue any downed firefighters inside (Figure 11-25). This team has become a very important aspect of the fire control operation. It provides rescue and safety backup for the firefighting team inside.

Tool Staging

There may be several places on the emergency fire scene where tools and equipment are placed either for use by firefighting teams or returned to after their use. These areas are referred to as tool staging areas. They are provided for the inside firefighting teams, the outside firefighting teams, and the rescue and intervention teams. These staging areas are placed near a fire truck located at the fire scene.

The tool staging areas are where tools and equipment from one or several fire trucks can be placed for later use by firefighters as needed. They are also

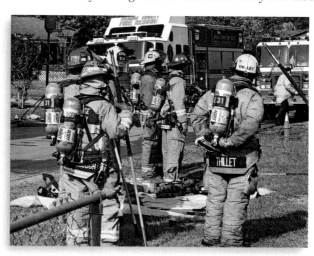

FIGURE 11-25 Intervention teams are prepared to enter the fire area to locate, defend, and rescue any downed firefighters.

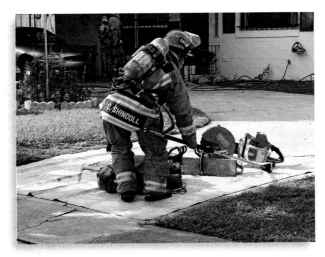

FIGURE 11-26 Outside firefighters assist in setting up the tool staging area.

a place that tools and equipment can be returned for replacement onto the fire trucks after the emergency is over. In this way, staging areas help organize tools and equipment as well as allow an organized movement of these items from the fire apparatus to the staging area to the fire scene and back again.

Part of your job as an outside firefighter is to assist in setting up the staging area, and moving tools from the apparatus to the tool staging area and back to the apparatus (Figure 11-26). Examples of tools that may be placed in these areas include forcible entry tools, ventilation tools, spare SCBA air bottles as well as exhausted SCBA air bottles, salvage tarps, and any other tools deemed necessary by the Company Officer. You must learn the location and types of tools and equipment located on the apparatus to which you are assigned.

When you arrive at the scene of a house fire, your Company Officer and driver will determine the location of the tool staging area as well the types and amount of tools to be placed there. You can be assigned to assist in staging these tools. Generally, a tarp is laid out as an indicator of a tool staging area, and the tools and equipment are placed on the tarp. It is important that you listen closely to your Company Officer and apparatus driver and quickly get the tools out and ready for use.

When the fire emergency is over, you must return the tools and equipment to the tarp and then to the fire apparatus. It is critical that you inspect each tool and piece of equipment for damage as you return it to the apparatus from the tool staging area. It is also very important that the apparatus driver be told that the tool has been placed back into its proper location on the apparatus.

Utilities Control

Almost every building has some sort of utility connection that may need to be controlled during the fire emergency. This control usually means shutting off the utility in some manner. As an outside team member, the utilities that you might encounter and be asked to assist in controlling are the electrical system, gas service, fuel oil supply, and water main.

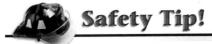

When dealing with flammable or energized utilities it is important to remember to wear full PPE.

Lockout/Tagout Systems Some utility or electrical companies use a utility security system called lockout/tagout. This system ensures that any switch or valve that is meant to remain in its present position is locked into that position with a lock. The person locking the valve is identified on a tag that is attached to the locking device (Figure 11-27). If you encounter these locks and tags when asked to control utilities on a dwelling fire, don't take any action until you check with your Company Officer for advice on whether to break the lock and tag and move the switch or valve to a new position (Figure 11-28).

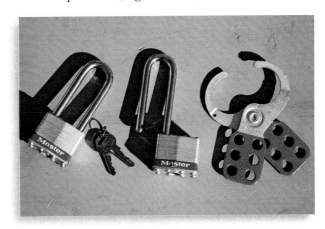

FIGURE 11-27 A typical lockout/tagout kit.

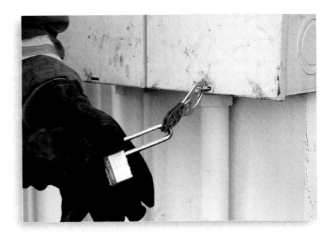

FIGURE 11-28 A lock and tag applied to a switch.

Electricity The electricity provided to most dwellings in the United States is 110 and 240 volts, alternating current. This electricity is delivered to most homes via aboveground or belowground electrical main feeds coming into or near the power meter, which usually is located on the outside of the building. There should be a main disconnect switch that can be switched into the *off* position to cut off power to the building. This disconnect switch is usually near the power meter.

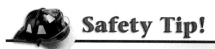

Safety Tip!

Pulling the power meter to disconnect the power is a technique that is best left to the power company. Typically, firefighters do not have the proper safety equipment to pull a meter safely and should avoid this dangerous practice.

The circuit breaker box inside the building is another place switches to cut the power can be found. This box has several individual switches that control power to various room circuits in the home. All of these switches should be placed in the *off* position

to cut off power to the dwelling. Because you are not able to enter a burning building with Exterior Operations level skills, this will be assigned to a firefighter with Level 1 skills.

Because after-construction electrical circuits may have been added or alterations may have been made to the electrical system, you should always remember that disconnecting the electrical power to the building in the ways just described may *NOT* ensure that the power has been completely disconnected. Therefore, any wiring that you encounter should be dealt with as if it is still live.

It is also important to remember that main electrical feeds coming into the house from outside power lines are still energized. Any overhead electrical wires should be avoided and their location relayed to the Incident Commander or your Company Officer. In severe building fires, these electrical feeds can disconnect and fall away from the burning building. For this reason, it is important to mark the location of these feeds during the fire emergency. Use fire-line tape or traffic cones to do this. If the power line does fall on the ground, widen your security around the wire and notify your Company Officer or Incident Commander of the downed wire and its location.

Practice It!

Controlling Electrical Utilities

The electrical power service for most single-family homes is commonly located at the outside meter box. Use the following steps to control the electrical power service to a dwelling:

1. When given direction by your Company Officer, locate the electrical meter and service junction outside the building. If the electrical service is provided by an overhead power line, follow it as it will direct you to the most likely area of the meter on the outside wall (Figure 11-29).

FIGURE 11-29

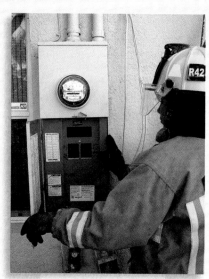

2. Take a good look at the meter and breaker box area. If it is flooded with water or the ground below it is wet, do not touch the main switch. Also, look for a lockout/tagout. If either of these conditions is present, do nothing and report the situation to your Company Officer.

3. If the meter and breaker box area are clear, then shut down the main switch. Report to your Company Officer that you accomplished the task. Remember, full protective clothing should be in place prior to performing this function (Figure 11-30).

FIGURE 11-30

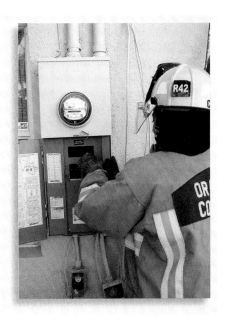

 Safety Tip!

Remember that any energized electrical equipment can kill and should be handled with extreme care. Water conducts electrical current very well, so never handle electrically energized equipment that is wet. Don't stand in water or snow while doing any of these procedures. Always consider all electrical wiring as energized unless you know for sure that it is not.

Gas   Many homes in North America have gas service that is used for heating and cooking as well as for hot water heaters. The type of gas provided is usually natural gas that is piped in or liquid propane gas that is stored in a gas tank on the property. We'll take a look at each of these types of gas and discuss the methods used to shut them down.

Natural gas is a flammable gas that is lighter than air. It is delivered to the dwelling by in-ground pipelines. Because natural gas is lighter than air, it rises when released into the air. The gas feeds to the building are normally located outside along an exterior wall of the house. A meter and/or pressure-regulator diaphragm and cutoff valve is usually placed above or below ground level, where the gas line enters the building. If the valve is belowground, an access cover has to be opened to get to the valve. The valves have a flange that operates the valve. When the flange is turned so that it is perpendicular to the gas piping, the flow is shut off.

Liquid propane gas is also a flammable gas but it is heavier than air. Because of this, liquid propane gas seeks its lowest level when released into the atmosphere. As a liquid, propane is extremely cold. This type of gas is usually contained in pressurized storage tanks, either aboveground or belowground on the dwelling property. These tanks contain liquid propane at the bottom of the tank and gaseous propane above the liquid. The top of the tank features a relief valve as well as a fill valve. The shutoff control valve is located near the fill valve on the top of the storage tank. Turn this valve clockwise to shut off the flow of gas.

KEY WORDS

liquid propane gas   A flammable gas that is heavier than air. Because of its weight, this gas seeks its lowest level when released into the atmosphere. As a liquid, propane is extremely cold. This type of gas is usually contained in pressurized storage tanks, either aboveground or belowground on the dwelling property.

natural gas   A flammable gas that is lighter than air. Because of its weight, this gas rises when released into the air. It is delivered to a dwelling by in-ground pipelines.

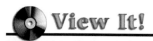 **View It!**

Go to the DVD, navigate to Chapter 11, and select *Controlling Utilities—Gas.*

➡ Practice It!

Controlling Gas Service

Use the following steps to shut off the flow of natural gas:

1. Locate the service meter and flow-regulator piping on the property (Figure 11-31). These items are usually found along an exterior wall. If the meter and piping are belowground, there will be an access lid on the property.

FIGURE 11-31

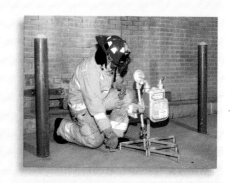

2. Find the valve on the piping. Turn the valve so that the valve flange is perpendicular to the flow pipe. To do this, you may need a hand tool, like a pair of large pliers (Figure 11-32). Most spanner wrenches have a slot designed to fit over a gas valve.

3. Notify your Company Officer when you have accomplished this task.

FIGURE 11-32

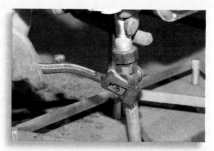

Use the following steps to shut off the flow of liquid propane gas:

1. Locate the gas tank. It will be next to the building or elsewhere on the property. If it is safe to approach, do so from the side. Make sure to wear full protective clothing.

2. Lift the access lid on the tank and locate the shutoff valve. Turn it in a clockwise direction to shut down the flow (Figure 11-33).

3. Notify your Company Officer when you have accomplished this task.

FIGURE 11-33

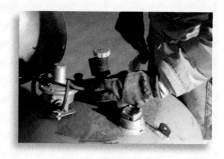

🪖 Safety Tip!

Flammable gas is very dangerous for firefighters, especially if it is located nearby and is an exposure to a burning building. During a building fire, always wear full PPE when working around these tanks. Stay clear of the ends of aboveground tanks and approach from the side. If fire is near the tank or if the tank is being heated by the building fire, do nothing. Retreat and immediately notify your Company Officer of the situation, including that you did not shut down the gas flow.

Fuel Oil   Many dwellings use fuel oil heaters for warmth. This type of heating is most prevalent in the northeastern United States, where 7.7 million homes heat with oil. Fuel oil is lighter than water and floats on any water surface. The fuel oil provided for these heaters is usually stored in an outdoor storage tank. However, the tank can also be located in the basement. This tank can be aboveground or belowground. Aboveground tanks have a shutoff valve located at the bottom, at one end of the tank. Turn this valve clockwise to shut off the fuel flow. Belowground tanks have an access lid and the fuel may be pumped out of the tank at this lid. A shutoff valve may be located in this area. Turn the valve clockwise to stop the flow of fuel. Because the fuel is pumped from a belowground tank, shutting off the electricity to the home usually stops the flow from a belowground tank and no further action is necessary (Figure 11-34).

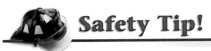 **Safety Tip!**

Fuel oil can be very dangerous for firefighters, especially if it is located nearby and is an exposure to a burning dwelling. During a building fire, always wear full PPE when working around these tanks. Stay clear of the ends of aboveground tanks and approach from the side. If fire is near the tank or if the tank is being heated by the building fire, do nothing. Retreat and notify your Company Officer of the situation, including that you did not shut down the oil flow.

Water   Controlling the water supply to a burning dwelling may seem a bit odd. However, the damage from water to a dwelling can be just as severe and costly as damage from fire. Water pipes in a home are often broken during the fire and water flows freely. The easiest way to control the water service to the home is to locate the water meter. These meters are usually located toward the street or on the side of the home facing the local water main distribution system. They are belowground and can be located under a water department lid. Raise the lid and you will see a small water meter and a shutoff valve. Move the valve so that the operating flange is perpendicular to the water service pipeline (Figure 11-35). Some water service valves require a special tool called a **water key**

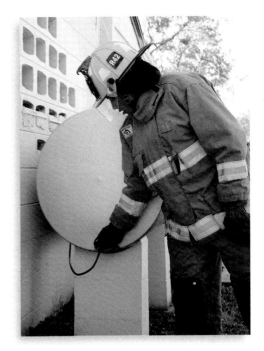

FIGURE 11-34   Fuel oil tank and shutoff valve.

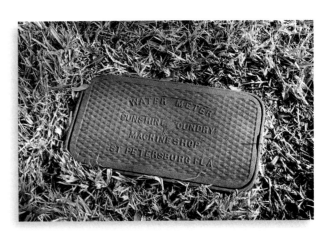

FIGURE 11-35   Move the water valve handle perpendicular to the pipeline.

to operate the valve flange. Your fire apparatus may carry the proper size water key.

KEY WORD

water key   A special tool used to operate shutoff valves on municipal water systems.

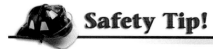 **Practice It!**

Controlling Water Service

Use the following steps to control the water service to a dwelling:

1. Find the water service meter and control valve. They are usually located toward the street or on the side of the home facing the local water main distribution system. They are belowground and can be located under a water department lid. Raise the lid to locate a small water meter and a shutoff valve (Figure 11-36).

FIGURE 11-36

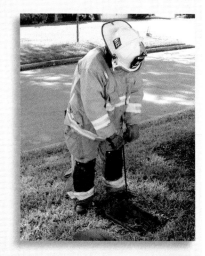

2. Move the valve so that the operating flange is perpendicular to the water service pipeline (Figure 11-37). Some water service valves require a special tool called a water key to operate the valve flange. Your fire apparatus may carry the proper size water key onboard.

3. Notify your Company Officer when you have accomplished this task.

FIGURE 11-37

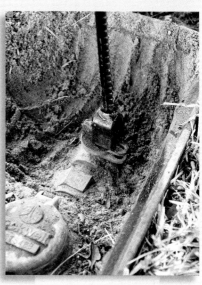

Safety Tip!

Always notify your Company Officer or the Incident Commander when you have shut down any utilities to the dwelling. It is equally important to notify your Company Officer if you are unable to shut down the utility.

Scene Lighting

Most fire units are equipped with portable generators and powerful lights that are used to illuminate the scene and the interior of the structure. It is important to everyone's safety that these lights are deployed early during a nighttime operation. Even during daylight fires, it can become very dark inside a burned building, even after the fire has been knocked down and the smoke has cleared. Everything inside be-

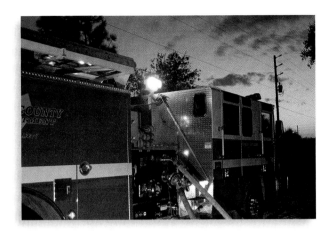

FIGURE 11-38 Most fire units are equipped with portable generators and powerful lights that are used to illuminate the scene and the interior of the structure.

comes charred or covered in a flat, black soot that absorbs light. Therefore, most emergency scene lights we use employ light bulbs that are between 250 and 500 watts (Figure 11-38). These bulbs produce a lot of heat and should not be placed within 12 inches of flammable products. In addition, the lights are not safe to use in flammable or explosive atmospheres.

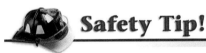 **Safety Tip!**

The generators we use can be very powerful, so don't underestimate the danger of the electrical shock they can provide just because they look like a small device powered by a small engine.

Portable Lighting Exterior lights used to illuminate a scene are usually positioned on all four sides of the structure, if possible. Be careful when dragging long cords from the generator. Keep connections away from accumulating water. Inspect the cords for frays or loose connections before you pick them up. It is often a good idea to plug the cord and light into the generator to be sure that the light operates before you take it to where it is needed. This action not only saves you a trip back to the truck for another light, but it also allows you to illuminate your way as you go (Figure 11-39).

Interior lights should be deployed as soon as possible. If possible, deploy a working light with the initial fire attack crew or as soon as possible after they enter. As an Exterior Operations level firefighter, you can accomplish this by taking a working light to the point of entry and pulling loops of extra cord so that the interior crew can take the light without much effort on their part.

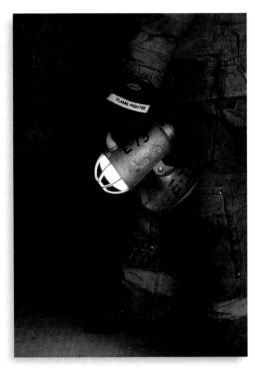

FIGURE 11-39 Plug in the floodlight to see that it works. You can then use it to illuminate your way into position.

Ladders at Dwelling Fires

Firefighters often need to access elevated areas in a dwelling fire. They may need to provide an emergency escape route for interior firefighters in a multilevel building or they may need to rescue occupants from upper levels. Ladders can also be placed to position firefighters for ventilation and fire extinguishing work. For Exterior Operations level firefighters, we are going to limit our discussion of ladders to roof access of single-story dwellings and window access of two-story dwellings. Most engine company apparatus carry a **roof ladder** and an **extension ladder**. At this point in your training, we will limit our discussion to these two types of ladders.

KEY WORDS

extension ladder A specialized Fire Service ladder used for greater height capability by firefighters accessing and working in upper levels of a building fire.

roof ladder A specially designed straight ladder that has two rails connected by rungs and specialized folding hooks at the tip. These hooks are moved to the open position when the ladder is to be placed on a roof surface and hooked over the ridge of the roof. This type of ladder provides access support for firefighters working on a roof.

Ladder Basics

Ladders are made up of rails and rungs (Figure 11-40). The rails run along the sides and are connected by the rungs that are the steps of the ladder. The top end of the ladder is called the tip. The bottom end of the ladder is called the butt.

Ladders are provided in many configurations. Some are single, straight ladders with two rails connected by rungs. Straight ladders can also feature special designs. For example, a roof ladder is a straight ladder with folding hooks at the tip. These ladders are used to hook the ladder in place on a rooftop.

Extension ladders have two or more sets of straight ladders, called **fly sections,** with ropes and pulleys used to extend the fly sections (Figure 11-41). The rope on extension ladders is the **halyard.** Pulling the halyard extends or retracts the fly sections. Ladder-locking devices located on each rail are referred to as dogs or pawls. The fly sections are locked into place by the dogs.

Whether Exterior Operations level firefighters work alone or as part of a team, they need to be able to remove a ladder from its storage location on the fire apparatus, carry the ladder to the desired location under the direction of a Company Officer, and place the ladder for the desired use on a single-family dwelling. Firefighters must also be able to safely replace ladders onto the fire apparatus after use. This needs to be done in a safe manner, using proper body positioning. A good rule of thumb for determining the number of people needed to place a ladder is to check the ladder length tags at the ends of the ladder rail. The first digit indicates the number of people needed to handle the ladder. A

14-foot roof ladder requires one person, a 35-foot extension ladder requires three people, and so on.

Ladders are stored in many different configurations and places on fire apparatus. Be sure to review with your instructor safe methods for removing, deploying, and reloading ladders from the fire appara-

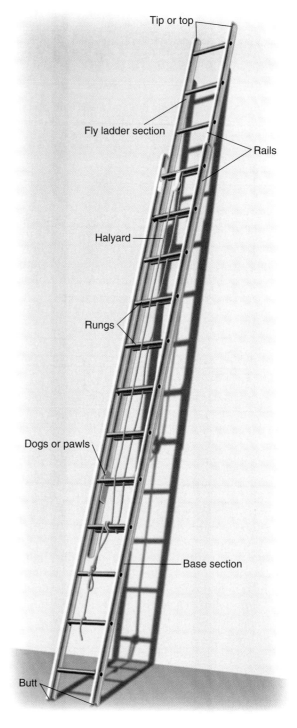

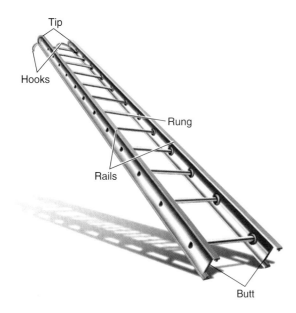

FIGURE 11-40 Parts of a roof ladder: (a) tip, (b) butt, (c) rails, (d) rungs, and (e) folding hooks.

FIGURE 11-41 Parts of an extension ladder: (a) tip, (b) butt, (c) rails, (d) rungs, (e) fly section, (f) base section, (g) halyard, (h) dogs or pawls.

tus you will be using for training. If you need further assistance, the driver should be well informed about ladder removal as well as storage on the apparatus.

KEY WORDS

fly sections Additional ladder sections combined on a single ladder to create an extension ladder. They are the parts of an extension ladder that extend and retract.

halyard A rope located on an extension ladder used for raising and lowering the fly sections of the ladder.

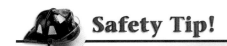
Safety Tip!

Wear the proper safety gear when handling ladders, even during practice. A helmet, eye protection, gloves, and foot protection are the minimum safety equipment to wear during ladder drills.

View It!

Go to the DVD, navigate to Chapter 11, and select *Removing and Stowing Ladders*.

Practice It!

Removing and Stowing Ladders

Use the following steps when removing ladders from fire apparatus:

1. Unlatch any restraining devices that hold the ladder in place on the apparaturs.

FIGURE 11-42

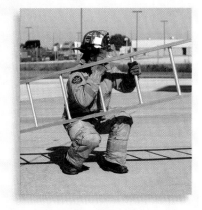

2. If you are alone, find the balance point of the roof ladder by positioning yourself at its center. Lift the ladder from the rack and, bending your knees, place it on the ground next to the apparatus.

3. Pick up the roof ladder at the center. Place your carrying arm and shoulder between the rungs and grasp one rung ahead to control it (Figure 11-42). This technique is commonly referred to as a shoulder carry (Figure 11-43). Carry the roof ladder to the desired location.

FIGURE 11-43

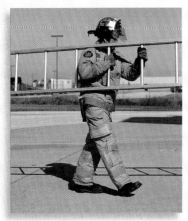

Stow the ladders onto the apparatus using the following steps:

1. Lift the ladder and place it back into its storage rack. Remember proper body positioning. Your feet should be placed shoulder-width apart, with your arms and hands close to the body for support.

—Continued

2. Latch any securing devices (Figure 11-44).

FIGURE 11-44

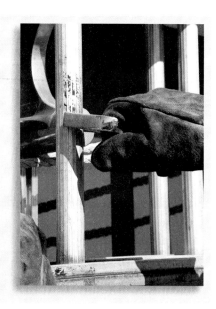

Straight Ladders and Roof Ladders

 View It!

Go to the DVD, navigate to Chapter 11, and select *Straight Ladders.*

Practice It!

Straight Ladders

Use the following steps to place a straight ladder:

1. Check for overhead power lines and obstructions. Then place the ladder flat (against the building), with the butt touching the building.

FIGURE 11-45

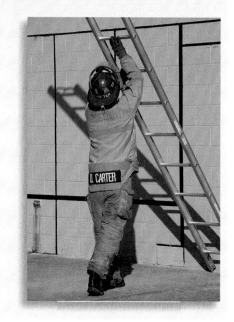

2. Grasp the rung closest to the tip and move toward the building, walking hand over hand on the rungs as you raise the ladder over your head (Figure 11-45).

3. Adjust the ladder for climbing by moving the butt away from the building by about one-fourth of the ladder's height from the building. Place the butt of the ladder at your feet, grasping the rung nearest shoulder height at arm's length (Figure 11-46). This should be the proper climbing angle.

4. If requested, you can support the ladder in place by positioning yourself outside the ladder with your feet at the butt of each rail and your hands straight out on each rail (Figure 11-47). This will help protect your face from falling debris.

Take down a straight ladder using the following steps:

1. Check again for any overhead obstructions and then adjust the ladder by scooting the butt up to the wall.

2. Move to the outside of the ladder and slowly back away from the building using the hand-over-hand method on the rungs as you lower the ladder.

3. At the tip, grasp the last rung and lower the ladder flat on the ground.

4. Pick up the ladder at the center. Place your carrying arm and shoulder between the rungs and rest the rail on your shoulder. Grasp one rung ahead for control. Carry it back to the apparatus.

FIGURE 11-46

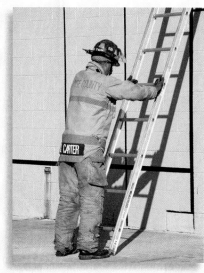

FIGURE 11-47

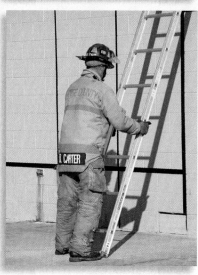

 View It!

Go to the DVD, navigate to Chapter 11, and select *Roof Ladders.*

 Practice It!

Deploying a Roof Ladder

Use the following steps to deploy a roof ladder for use on the roof:

1. At the desired location, place the roof ladder on the ground and open the two roof hooks located at the tip (Figure 11-48).

FIGURE 11-48

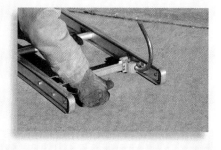

—Continued

2. Lift at the tip and carefully pass this end to a firefighter positioned in place on the ladder (Figure 11-49). The roof ladder will be passed on, hooks away from the building, and positioned by other firefighters at the roof.

FIGURE 11-49

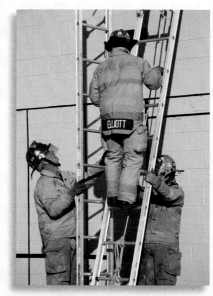

3. The firefighters slide the roof ladder up the slope of the roof with hooks at the top, facing upward. The ladder is adjusted and then turned over, with the hooks beyond the ridge of the roof. The roof ladder is pulled back with the hooks securing the ladder at the ridge (Figure 11-50).

FIGURE 11-50

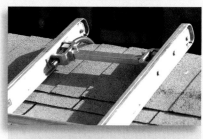

 ## View It!

Go to the DVD, navigate to Chapter 11, and select *Extension Ladder—Single Firefighter*

Practice It!

Extension Ladder—Single Firefighter

The following steps can be used by a single firefighter to place an extension ladder:

1. Pick up the extension ladder at the center. Place your carrying arm and shoulder between the rungs and rest the rail on your shoulder, grasping one rung ahead for control. Proceed to the building (Figure 11-51).

FIGURE 11-51

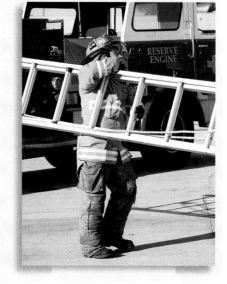

2. Check for overhead power lines and obstructions. Place the extension ladder flat on the ground. Grasp the extension ladder rung at the tip of the ladder and move toward the building. Walk hand over hand on the rungs as you raise the ladder over your head toward the building until it is flat against the wall.

3. At this point, position yourself at the rungs with the extension ladder between you and the building. Pull the butt of the ladder a couple feet from the wall. Untie the halyard, pull the tip away from the wall, and raise the fly section to the desired height (Figure 11-52). Support the ladder with your shoulder and hip while extending it. At the desired height, allow the fly section to lock into the dogs and tie the halyard in place in the middle of a rung in front of you.

FIGURE 11-52

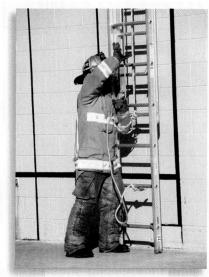

4. Adjust the extension ladder for climbing by positioning about one fourth of the ladder's height from the building (Figure 11-53). Place the butt of the ladder at your feet, grasping the rung nearest shoulder height at arm's length. This should be the proper climbing angle. If needed, you can support the ladder in place by positioning yourself outside the ladder with your feet at the butt of each rail and your hands straight out on each rail. Don't look up.

FIGURE 11-53

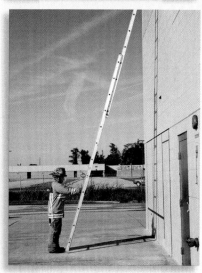

The following steps can be used by a single firefighter to take down an extension ladder:

1. Check again for overhead obstructions and adjust the butt of the ladder inward to within a couple feet of the wall.

FIGURE 11-54

2. Untie the halyard and position the ladder the same way as when you extended the fly section. Pull the halyard to raise the fly section slightly to unlock it from the dogs (Figure 11-54). Then lower the fly section into place for storage and retie the halyard if necessary.

3. Push the butt of the ladder against the building and lower the extension ladder. Slowly back away from the building using the hand-over-hand method on the rungs as you lower the ladder. At the tip, grasp the last rung and lower the ladder flat on the ground.

4. Pick up the extension ladder at its center. Place your carrying arm and shoulder between the rungs, resting the rail on your shoulder. Then grasp one rung ahead for control. Carry it back to the apparatus.

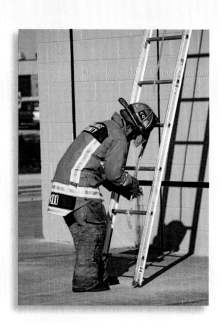

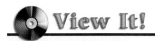

Go to the DVD, navigate to Chapter 11, and select *Extension Ladder—Two Firefighters.*

 Practice It!

Extension Ladder—Two Firefighters

The following steps can be used by two firefighters to place an extension ladder:

1. Position on the same side of the ladder, facing the same direction. The firefighter at the tip gives all of the commands. Pick up the extension ladder, placing your carrying arms and shoulder between the rungs. Rest the rail on your shoulders, grasping one rung ahead for control (Figure 11-55). This action can be better coordinated with a simple command such as *"Ready, lift."* Now proceed to the building.

FIGURE 11-55

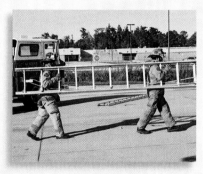

2. Check for overhead power lines and obstructions as you walk toward the building. Lay the ladder flat on the ground with the fly section on top of the ladder. Position at the tip, on the outside of each rail. Grasping the rung closest to the tip, lift the end of the extension ladder and move toward the building, walking hand over hand on the rungs and rails until the ladder is flat against the wall (Figure 11-56). A good signal to coordinate this move is, *"Ready, raise."*

FIGURE 11-56

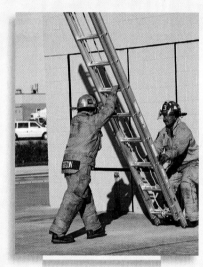

3. Both firefighters position to the side, supporting one rail of the extension ladder. Pull the butt of the ladder a couple feet from the wall. Untie the halyard, pull the tip away from the wall, and raise the fly section to the desired height, allowing the fly section to lock into the dogs. Remember to support the ladder with a shoulder and hip as you pull the halyard (Figure 11-57). Tie the halyard in place in the middle of a rung near waist level.

FIGURE 11-57

4. Adjust the extension ladder for climbing by positioning about one-fourth of the ladder's height from the building and placing the butt of the ladder at your feet. This should be the proper climbing angle. If needed, one of you can support the ladder in place by positioning outside the ladder, your feet at the butt of each rail, and hands straight out on each rail. Don't look up.

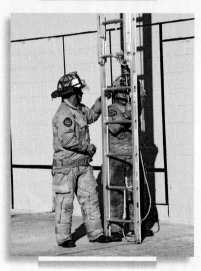

The following steps can be used by two firefighters to take down an extension ladder:

1. Position on each side of the extension ladder at the rails. Check again for overhead obstructions and adjust the butt of the extension ladder inward to within a couple feet of the wall (Figure 11-58).

2. Standing outside the ladder so that the ladder is between you and the wall, pull the halyard to raise the fly section slightly in order to unlock it from the dogs. Lower the fly section into place for storage and retie the halyard if necessary.

3. Push the butt of the extension ladder against the building and lower the extension ladder. Slowly back away from the building, using the hand-over-hand method on the rungs and rails to lower the ladder. Grasp the last rung and lower the ladder flat on the ground.

4. Position at each end and pick up the extension ladder. While resting the rail on your shoulder, grasp one rung ahead for control. A good signal for this is for the firefighter at the tip to say, "*Ready, lift*." Now take the ladder back to the apparatus.

FIGURE 11-58

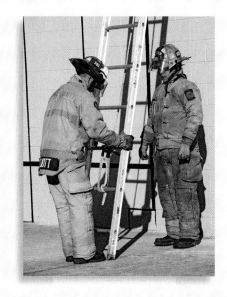

Protecting Exposures

Any material that ignites as a result of fire coming from another source is technically an exposure fire. An **exposure** is anything that has the potential of catching fire due to its proximity to something that is already on fire. In building fires, an exposure is an item in a room that has the potential of catching fire because it is exposed to something already on fire in the room. This definition can be expanded to large fires in a building that have the potential of spreading to adjacent buildings. The adjacent buildings become exposures to the original building fire and must be protected *before* they catch fire.

There are situations in which the fire is so big that the fire department units on the scene do not have the resources to extinguish the fire or the original building is beyond saving. It may be determined that it is best to allow this building to burn while firefighting efforts shift to keep the fire from spreading to exposures around it. Fire attack hose lines are deployed to flow water onto exposures until the fire burns enough of the fuel so that it begins to lessen in intensity. Attack hose lines can then again be applied directly on the fire to extinguish it (Figure 11-59).

Because heat spreads in more than one way (refer to Chapter 6), including by conduction, convection,

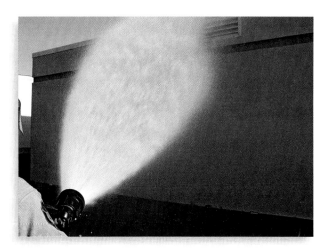

FIGURE 11-59 If the fire is beyond the extinguishing capability of the fire department, water may be flowed onto exposures to keep the fire from spreading.

and radiation, applying a water stream is important in protecting exposures. As an outside team member, you may be assigned to deploy a fire attack hose line to protect an exterior exposure. Protecting an exposure by applying water cools it, keeping the temperature of the exposure below the temperature necessary for fire ignition.

It is also important to position in a **safe area** while protecting exposures. A safe area is any place that is free of hazards to you and your team. Many hazards can result from your position yourself too close to the fire. The building can collapse as it weakens and is consumed by fire. Other hose streams can unintentionally be directed toward you, causing you serious injury. Heat from the fire can be so intense that you can become an exposure yourself and receive thermal burns, even if you have full PPE in place. If you do not have your SCBA on and in use, intense, low-lying smoke can become a health hazard. When possible, Exterior Operations level firefighters should remain in safe areas on the fire scene.

▆▆ KEY WORDS ▆▆

exposure   Anything that has the potential of catching fire as a result of its proximity to something that is already on fire. In building fires, an exposure is an item in a room that has the potential of catching fire because it is exposed to something already on fire in the room. This definition can be expanded to large fires in a building that have the potential of spreading to adjacent buildings. The adjacent buildings become exposures to the original building fire and must be protected *before* they catch fire.

safe area   Any place on an emergency scene that is free of hazards to you and your team.

Exterior Fire Attack

As a member of the firefighting team outside the building, at times you may be directed to apply water from the exterior of a dwelling fire. Always follow your Company Officer's directions regarding the pattern, shape, and direction of the water stream (Figure 11-60). If you need to protect yourself from the heat of the fire, either switch the pattern to a wide-angle fog on the line or back away from the fire, still flowing water toward the fire. Again, Exterior Operations level firefighters should remain in safe areas during firefighting operations on dwelling fires.

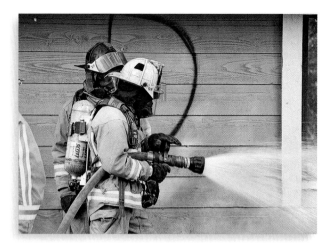

FIGURE 11-60   Follow the Company Officer's orders regarding the pattern, shape, and direction of the fire stream.

Do It!

Performing Safely at Single-Family-Dwelling Fires

Everyone working at the scene of a structural fire has a responsibility for the safety of the operation. By this point in your training, you should be able to perform well as an effective member of a team, performing several of the functions that are inherent to a safe, efficient operation. The key word to remember is *team*. Nothing on a safety-conscious operation is an individual effort, nor is it performed freelance, without the knowledge and direction of the Incident Commander. Your role starts with a safe response, arrival, and proper tagging in to the personnel accountability system. It continues with the efficient and proper use of tools and equipment to support the fire attack crews working inside the structure. Performing all of these tasks takes practice and repetition. Listen to your instructors and to more experienced firefighters, absorbing their knowledge.

There is plenty to be done between now and your first actual fire. Spend time learning all about the tools on the rigs in your station. Participate in all the drills and read everything you can about the Fire Service—twice. The learning process is never-ending, especially when public safety is concerned.

Evolution 11-1

Maneuvering a Small Attack Line During an Exterior Attack

This drill has been developed to practice the skills necessary to establish a water supply and to apply water from the exterior to a simulated single-family-dwelling fire using a small attack line. The firefighters will be working either to establish the water supply or to deploy, set up, and apply a fire stream to the simulated building fire (Figure 11-61). The drill should be repeated, switching firefighter positions so that each person can practice the training drill in both positions.

Training Area: Open area; level ground free of trip hazards

Equipment: Equipped pumper

Training burn building or other acquired building

Sustained water supply source, or static or water main system with hydrant

PPE: Full protective clothing and scba, on and ready for use

1. A fully equipped pumper with a crew consisting of a driver, a Company Officer, and two firefighters is positioned away from the water supply and simulated dwelling fire. All individuals are appropriately protected in PPE with their seatbelts on and ready to respond. A signal is given and the pumper responds to the simulated fire.

2. The pumper positions at the water supply source. A firefighter dismounts safely and removes any equipment necessary to establish a connection to the water supply, including supply hose lines. The firefighter signals for the pumper to proceed with a layout of supply hose while approaching and positioning at the simulated fire.

3. When the pumper positions at the fire, the second firefighter safely dismounts and receives orders from the Company Officer to deploy a small attack line and prepare to flow water onto the building from a safe area.

4. After establishing a connection to the water source, the first firefighter walks next to the supply hose line, straightening it out as he or she approaches the fire scene. This firefighter then arrives at the fire scene, locates the Company Officer, and receives orders to assist the second firefighter on the small attack line.

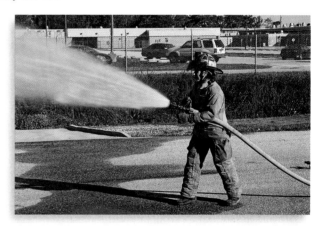

FIGURE 11-61 Using a small attack line, firefighters will establish a water supply or apply water to a simulated building fire from the outside.

5. While the two firefighters are flowing water from the small attack line, they are directed to reposition it several times. They will also be directed to change the flow pattern of the stream.

6. When the drill has been completed, the crew will properly relieve pressure, disconnect, drain, and reload all the supply and attack hose. They should trade positions and repeat the drill.

Evolution 11-2

Maneuvering a Large Attack Line During an Exterior Attack

This drill has been developed to practice the skills necessary to establish a water supply and apply water from the exterior to a simulated single-family-dwelling fire using a large attack line. The firefighters will be working either to establish the water supply or to deploy, set up, and apply a fire stream to the simulated building fire (Figure 11-62). The drill should be repeated, switching firefighter positions so that each person can practice the training drill in both positions.

Training Area: Open area; level ground free of trip hazards

Equipment: Equipped pumper

Training burn building or other acquired building

Sustained water supply source, or static or water main system with hydrant

PPE: Full protective clothing and SCBA, on and ready for use

1. A fully equipped pumper with a crew consisting of a driver, a Company Officer, and two firefighters is positioned away from the water supply and simulated dwelling fire. All individuals are appropriately protected in PPE with their seatbelts on and ready to respond. A signal is given and the pumper responds to the simulated fire.

2. The pumper positions at the water supply source. A firefighter dismounts safely and removes any equipment necessary to establish a connection to the water supply, including supply hose lines. The firefighter signals for the pumper to proceed with a layout of supply hose while approaching and positioning at the simulated fire.

3. When the pumper positions at the fire, the second firefighter safely dismounts and receives orders from the Company Officer to deploy a large attack line, place it in a looped configuration, and prepare to flow water onto the building from a safe area.

4. After establishing a connection to the water source, the first firefighter walks next to the supply hose line, straightening it out as he or she approaches the fire scene. This firefighter then arrives at the fire scene, locates the Company Officer, and receives orders to assist the second firefighter on the large attack line.

5. As the two firefighters are flowing water from the large attack line, they are directed to reposition it several times. They will also be directed to change the flow pattern of the stream.

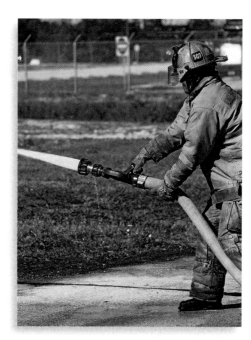

FIGURE 11-62 Using a large attack line, firefighters will establish a water supply or apply water to a simulated building fire from the outside.

6. When the drill has been completed, the crew will properly relieve pressure, disconnect, drain, and reload all the supply and large attack hose. They trade positions and the drill is repeated.

Evolution 11-3

Other Functions During an Exterior Attack

This drill has been developed to practice the skills necessary to demonstrate many of the other functions an Exterior Operations level firefighter will perform at a simulated, typical dwelling fire. The firefighters will be working to assist in forcible entry, stretching a line into a doorway, setting up ventilation, placing ladders, and staging tools for a simulated building fire (Figure 11-63).

Training Area: Open area; level ground free of trip hazards

Equipment: Equipped pumper

Training burn building or other acquired building

Sustained water supply source, or static or water main system with hydrant

PPE: Full protective clothing and SCBA, on and ready for use

1. A fully equipped pumper with a crew consisting of a driver, a Company Officer, and two firefighters is positioned away from the simulated dwelling fire. All individuals are appropriately protected in PPE with their seatbelts on and ready to respond. A signal is given and the pumper responds to the simulated fire.

2. The pumper arrives and is designated to assist in exterior preparations and activities. The crew reports to command and turns over passes for the accountability system.

3. The Company Officer first directs the firefighters to deploy a small attack line from the pumper and stretch it to the simulated front door. He then directs the firefighters to force open the door.

4. A interior fire attack crew pulls the attack line into the building and the firefighters assist until given another assignment by their Company officer.

5. The Company Officer then assigns the firefighters to place ventilation fans for negative or positive ventilation in the doorway area.

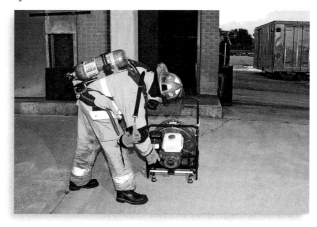

FIGURE 11-63   Assisting with other functions at a simulated building fire from the outside.

6. The firefighters are next assigned to place an extension ladder against the building and prepare a roof ladder for use on the roof, at the extension ladder.

7. Finally, the Company Officer directs the firefighters to set up a tool staging area near the pumper for use by crews operating at the scene. They will stage tools as directed by the Company Officer.

Prove It

Knowledge Assessment
Signed Documentation Tear-Out Sheet
Exterior Operations Level Firefighter—Chapter 11

Name: _____

Fill out the ten-question quiz below, the Knowledge Assessment Sheet, by circling the correct answer for each question. When finished, sign it and give to your instructor/Company Officer for his or her signature. Turn in this Knowledge Assessment Sheet to the proper person as part of the documentation that you have completed your training for this chapter.

1. Many of the line-of-duty deaths of firefighters working inside a structure happen when the firefighter becomes disoriented and runs out of fresh air supplied by his or her SCBA.
   a. True
   b. False

2. Any firefighter working in the hot zone at a structural fire should be fully protected with PPE and a charged hose line. The firefighter should be trained to the _____ standard.
   a. Level 2
   b. Level 3
   c. Level 1
   d. Exterior Operations level

3. If the door of a burning dwelling is locked, firefighters should be prepared to _____ when told to do so and not before.
   a. ventilate
   b. force entry
   c. control utilities
   d. attack the fire

4. Dragging a charged hose line through a house is an easy job, especially if the interior crew is crawling on their hands and knees.
   a. True
   b. False

5. _____ are placed outside a building, blowing inward to fill the structure with fresh air and forcing the smoke and gases outward.
   a. Smoke ejector fans
   b. Negative-pressure fans
   c. Negative-pressure, gasoline-powered fans
   d. Positive-pressure fans

6. A system used to ensure that a switch or valve is secured in its present position is known as a _____ system.
   a. lockout/tagout
   b. lockout/tag-in
   c. lock-in/tagout
   c. personnel accountability

7. If a power line falls on the ground, widen your security around the wire and notify your Company Officer or command of the downed wire and its location.
   a. True
   b. False

8. Most engine company apparatus carry a roof ladder and a(n) _____ ladder.
   a. folding
   b. A-frame
   c. extension
   c. attic

9. By positioning a ladder at about one-fourth of the ladder's height from the building and placing the butt of the ladder at your feet, if you grasp the rung nearest shoulder height at arm's length, you will place the ladder _____.
   a. too vertical for safe climbing
   b. at the proper climbing angle
   c. at an improper climbing angle
   d. at too low a climbing angle

10. Anything that has the potential of catching fire due to its proximity to something that is already on fire is known as _____.
    a. the seat of the fire
    b. an ignition factor
    c. an exposure
    c. a safe position

Student Signature and Date _____   Instructor/Company Officer Signature and Date _____

276

Prove It

Skills Assessment
Signed Documentation Tear-Out Sheet
Exterior Operations Level Firefighter—Chapter 11

Name: _____

Fill out the Skills Assessment Sheet below. Have your instructor/Company Officer check off and initial each skill you demonstrate. When finished, sign it and give to your instructor/Company Officer for his or her signature. Turn in this Skills Assessment Sheet to the proper person as part of the documentation that you have completed your training for this chapter.

Skill	Completed	Initials
1. Explain the difference between manufactured and site-built dwellings as they relate to construction and fire conditions.	_____	_____
3. Describe safety zones on the dwelling fire emergency scene.	_____	_____
3. Explain how to check in to command using your fire department's personnel accountability system (PAS).	_____	_____
4. Define the different job functions that a typical fire attack team may be called upon to perform on the scene of a dwelling fire.	_____	_____
5. Demonstrate forcible entry techniques on an exterior door that swings inward.	_____	_____
6. Demonstrate forcible entry techniques on an exterior door that swings outward.	_____	_____
7. Explain techniques for using a Halligan bar and flathead axe to force a lock.	_____	_____
8. Explain how to assist interior firefighters with extending hose while stationed at the doorway to a dwelling.	_____	_____
9. Describe how to safely break and clear out glass in a window frame on a dwelling.	_____	_____
10. Define what is meant by the term *Intervention Team*.	_____	_____
11. Describe how and where a tool staging area might be set up and its main purpose on the dwelling fire scene.	_____	_____
12. Demonstrate how to place ventilation fans for negative- and positive-pressure ventilation in a single-family dwelling.	_____	_____
13. Describe a lockout/tagout system and how it is used on the fireground.	_____	_____
14. Demonstrate how to control utilities in a dwelling.	_____	_____
15. Demonstrate how to deploy, place, and stow a roof ladder.	_____	_____
16. Demonstrate how to prepare a roof ladder for use on a roof.	_____	_____
17. Demonstrate how to deploy, place, and stow an extension ladder.	_____	_____
18. Explain what is meant by the term *exposure* and the best methods of protecting an exposure with an attack-line stream.	_____	_____

19. Demonstrate dwelling fire operations for Exterior Operations level firefighters as a member of a fire attack team. _____ _____

20. Demonstrate dwelling fire support operations for Exterior Operations level firefighters. _____ _____

Student Signature and Date _____ Instructor/Company Officer Signature and Date _____

278

Answer Key, Knowledge Assessment

Chapter 1

1. A

One of NIOSH's most important functions is the investigation of line-of-duty firefighter injuries and deaths.

2. C

Company Officer is the term more commonly used to describe the person in charge of the engine, truck, or rescue company.

3. B

As its name implies, the Fire Prevention Division conducts fire inspections and enforces fire codes as part of its overall job of preventing fires before they occur.

4. A

In the vast majority of the United States, providing fire protection is the responsibility of local government.

5. C

On larger or complex fire emergency scenes in which several companies are working, the use of an Incident Command System provides a predetermined organization that supervises the units as they arrive and work on the scene.

6. B

The personnel accountability system (PAS) helps the Incident Commander keep track of companies as well as individuals on the fire scene.

7. C

Sector is the term most commonly used to designate different parts of the fireground operation.

8. B

It is never acceptable to allow visitors to roam freely throughout a fire station, especially in the vehicle bay area. This area is probably the most dangerous area to the public, especially when an emergency call is received and units are dispatched.

9. B

As noted in the NIOSH follow-up report included in the chapter, properly placed and secured ladders or lifts are much preferable to and safer than the tops of emergency units for working on the ceiling areas of fire station vehicle bays.

10. A

Right-to-know information is required to be posted in any workplace, including a fire station.

Chapter 2

1. B

To be effective in your first aid efforts, you must first be aware of what caused the problem so that you can maintain a safe attitude in everything you do. If not, you can fall victim to the same fate.

2. C

In most cases you should take the time to seek the patient's permission before you touch him or her. If the person is a minor and his or her parent or guardian is not present to give consent, then it is implied that you have permission to treat the child.

3. A

We take universal precautions when potentially exposed to body substances. These precautions include wearing eye protection (splash-resistant eyewear), hand protection (approved, nonlatex, disposable medical gloves), and other body protection (such as a splash-resistant gown) as needed.

4. C

Life-threatening injuries or conditions almost always involve a person's airway, breathing, and/or blood circulation. The ABCs of emergency care are **A**irway, **B**reathing, and **C**irculation. Assessing the patient's ABCs will alert you to any immediate danger to life.

5. B

When performing abdominal thrusts, stand behind the patient, wrapping your arms around the patient's waist while making a fist with one hand. Grasp your fist with your other hand and place it into the patient's abdomen above the navel while *avoiding* the bottom of the patient's breastbone.

6. D

The head tilt–chin lift maneuver is very simple to accomplish; however, it involves manipulating the patient's head and neck a bit. Therefore, this maneuver is not recommended if the patient has been injured and/or has fallen in such a way as to potentially cause a neck injury. In these cases, a jaw-thrust maneuver should be used.

7. B

To control the bleeding, cover the wound with one or several sterile dressings and apply direct pressure with your hand. This action should slow or stop the bleeding. Once the bleeding has been controlled, leave the pressure dressing in place and wrap it with a gauze bandage.

8. A

Shock occurs when a patient's circulation is compromised. This condition can be due to a heart condition, blood loss, internal bleeding, a head injury, or other medical causes.

9. A

If a patient is vomiting or is about to vomit, the best position is on her side so that no vomit falls back into her airway, causing her to choke. Place the patient on her left side if possible to help prevent vomiting. This is called the recovery position.

10. C

Partial-thickness burns are accompanied by blistering of the burn area. These are deeper injuries of the skin and may take a few weeks to heal.

Chapter 3

1. A

Your protective clothing is a combination of several items, each of which must be in place with all the others before maximum protection is established. For example, if you do not have your gloves on at a fire, you are not fully protected and you are exposing yourself to injury.

2. C

The firefighter coat and pants are made up of three layers of protection. The first layer, the outer shell, is somewhat flame-retardant. The second and third layers of protection are in the inner liner, which is a combination of a thermal barrier and a moisture barrier.

3. B

Your helmet has a pull-down eye shield. This shield provides a low level of eye protection for instances in which you are in a hurry, or you are not wearing goggles or the face piece of your self-contained breathing apparatus (SCBA). Your eyes can still be exposed to objects flying up from underneath the pull-down eye shield. The addition of safety-approved goggles or your SCBA face piece greatly enhances the eye protection you receive from the pull-down eye shield on your helmet.

4. A

Fire Service protective clothing should be cleaned a minimum of every 6 months. It is recommended that this cleaning be done professionally or at least in professional-grade washers operated by the fire department. Dirt and products of combustion will start to degrade the fire-resistance capabilities of the materials.

5. B

Your personal protective clothing is designed to protect your skin. However, to complete your ensemble of personal protective equipment (PPE), you must also protect your respiratory system. A self-contained breathing apparatus (SCBA) completes your protective gear. While every component of your PPE is essential, the SCBA is probably the most critical component of the ensemble when you are exposed to toxic smoke, hazardous gases, and steam.

6. D

The rate at which you use the air in a cylinder depends on several factors, including your physical condition and size, the amount of physical activity you are performing, and the temperature in which you are working.

7. B

Most regulators have an emergency bypass valve, which is red. This valve allows high-pressure air to bypass the regulator in case of a failure. By slightly cracking open the emergency bypass valve, you will receive the remaining air in the cylinder at a fairly fast rate.

8. C

Donning the facemask is the final step you take before breathing from the system. It makes no difference whether you don the mask by placing your chin in first and dragging the straps over your head or whether you use the ball-cap method. In the ball-cap method, you hold the straps on the back of your head and drag the mask down over your face.

9. C

A personal alert safety system, or PASS, is a small electronic device that is designed to detect your movement and your lack of movement. It sounds a very loud alarm if it determines that you have remained stationary for a predetermined length of time. The purpose of this device is to signal to other firefighters that you need help and to give them an audible signal that aids them in locating you rapidly.

10. A

An item that is essential to every firefighter's safety is a personnel accountability system (PAS). In this system, the Incident Commander or a designee accounts for every person as they enter and exit a hazardous area or environment. To keep track of everyone, the Accountability Officer will use some form of a tracking system in which each firefighter reports to his or her Company Officer, who then reports to the Accountability Officer.

Chapter 4

1. B

The fire attack hose line system begins at the pump panel on the fire apparatus and ends when the stream of water coming from the end of the nozzle effectively reaches the base of the fire.

2. C

The size of the fittings, couplings, and hose accessory devices (appliances) that water passes through can reduce the volume of water and pressure of the stream as it flows out the nozzle.

3. A

Small attack lines are those fire attack hose systems in which the diameter of the hose is 3/4 inch to 2 inches in diameter (as measured on the inside opening of the hose).

4. A

Booster hose couplings usually will have small grip points that are recessed. They require a special type of spanner wrench called a Barway spanner for disconnecting and connecting the couplings.

5. A

Most couplings are designed to screw together in a clockwise direction. They should be tightened hand-tight.

6. D

Unlike booster lines, the 1-inch jacketed line needs to be drained of water after use and before loading it. This is done by disconnecting the line from the apparatus, removing the nozzle, and disconnecting each section of hose.

7. C

Spanner wrenches are used to tighten and loosen hose couplings.

8. C

The gated wye usually takes in water from a larger supply, like a 2½- or 3-inch supply, then divides it into two 1½- or 1¾-inch lines.

9. A

Nozzles should be held waist-high at one's side, with the hose under the arm and one hand either on the body of the nozzle (for nozzles without a pistol grip) or on the pistol grip; the other hand should be on the gate valve control (the bale) or the twist valve, depending on the style nozzle you are using.

10. C

The first step in caring for fire hose is to bleed the excess water pressure from the hose after the discharge has been shut off at the fire apparatus. Next, disconnect the nozzle. Then disconnect the hose sections. Finally, walk along the hose, placing it over your shoulder or raising it to your waist, allowing the water to drain as you walk along the line.

Chapter 5

1. A

A defensive driving course, which also instructs course attendees about departmental, local, and state-level laws and regulations related to POV response, should be given to new firefighters as soon as possible.

2. B

The Emergency Vehicle Operator's Course provided by the U.S. Department of Transportation defines a true emergency as *a situation in which there is a high probability of death or serious injury to an individual or significant property loss, and action by an emergency vehicle operator may reduce the seriousness of the situation.*

3. D

In simple terms, negligence is either the act of doing something that a reasonable or prudent person would not do, or not doing something that such a person would do, in a given situation.

4. B

Not using a seatbelt has contributed to many fatalities. Firefighters should set an example for the community by following the law and wearing their seatbelts at all times. It is a proven fact that seatbelt use reduces injury and death in traffic crashes, and greatly reduces the chance of ejection from a vehicle.

5. C

The extent and type of protective clothing you need depends on the type of emergency and the policy of your Company Officer and your department.

6. B

When dismounting from the apparatus, always check in all directions. Look for traffic and obstructions or hazards on the ground below.

7. D

Place a tapering pattern of 5 cones in a stretch of roadway at a distance of about 75 feet from the rear of the apparatus. This placement provides a transition for traffic from the present pattern to the new lane pattern established by your apparatus placement and the placement of cones.

8. C

Keep your eye on the traffic and never turn your back on it. Face traffic when placing cones and be ready to sound an alarm if a vehicle breaks through your blocking cones and heads for the fire apparatus.

9. A

The total stopping distance of an apparatus is the reaction time plus the braking distance.

10. B

There are two methods for estimating a safe following distance. The first method is the 3-second rule. This rule requires that you pick a marker—perhaps a tree or a post on the side of the roadway—and begin a count of three ("1001, 1002, 1003") when the vehicle in front of you passes the marker; you should not pass the marker before having reached the third count. If you are responding to an emergency, this distance (the traveling time) should be increased to allow you more reaction time. The second method is to estimate apparatus lengths. Estimate one apparatus length between your vehicle and the vehicle in front of you for every 10 miles per hour that you are traveling.

Chapter 6

1. C

Four things need to come together for combustion to occur: fuel, heat, oxygen, and the chemical reaction that keeps the flame burning. These four ingredients of combustion are often depicted as the fire tetrahedron.

2. C

Fires grow based on the amount of fuel available to burn. Flames can easily spread to other combustible materials near the original fire through heat transfer; therefore, knowing how flames spread can help you contain a fire.

3. A

Open flames emit heat from the light of the flames by the process of radiation. Radiant heat transfer doesn't depend on air currents or direct contact with the flame to spread a fire. For example, a large fire burning outside a building can ignite the curtains inside the building when some of the energy of the original fire radiates through a glass window.

4. A

Portable fire extinguishers have labels indicating the types of fires they are designed to extinguish. An extinguisher containing only water is usually effective only for a Class A fire.

5. C

Common examples of small, burning liquid fires include cooking oil fires and fires involving spilled gasoline around lawn mowers. Anything larger than these types of fires is beyond the capabilities of most portable fire extinguishers. Class B fire extinguishers include a carbon dioxide (CO_2) extinguisher and a dry chemical extinguisher. Most dry chemical extinguishers are useful for both Class A and Class B fires.

6. D

Regardless of the classification of fire, the extinguishing agent should be applied at the base of the flames and on the material that is burning.

7. B

An energized electrical fire receives its main heat source from electricity and not from what is burning. For example, if a small electrical appliance is on fire, switching off the electrical source at the circuit breaker will usually stop the fire or at least decrease the fire from a Class C fire to a lower-grade fire. By stopping the electrical current, the fire can be switched from a Class C to a Class A or Class B fire, depending on the material that is left burning.

8. B

Class B fire extinguishers include a carbon dioxide (CO_2) extinguisher and a dry chemical extinguisher. Most dry chemical extinguishers are useful for both Class A and Class B fires.

9. A

There are many types of trash containers that you will encounter in responding to trash fires. The most common trash containers at commercial businesses and construction sites are dumpsters. Dumpsters are commonly metal containers of various sizes that have a metal or plastic lid.

10. B

When extinguishing a dumpster fire, always wear full PPE, including an SCBA.

Chapter 7

1. B

Even though we see and hear about massive fires that occur in our wildland areas, the great majority of ground cover fires will be less than an acre in size and are controlled by a small crew of firefighters.

2. A

In hilly or mountainous areas, the fire tends to burn up a slope toward the unburned area until it is affected by winds at the top of the hill.

3. D

There is usually a concentrated, heavy involvement at the leading edge of a fire. This part of the fire is known as the head of the fire.

4. B

The area around the edge of the entire fire area, including both the burned and the still-burning areas, is known as the fire perimeter.

5. C

Examples of manmade firebreaks include roadways, parking lots, and farmlands. Manmade firebreaks also include trenches made by teams of fire crews using hand tools or specially designed forestry tractors in areas well ahead of the fire.

6. A

Keeping fires from jumping a roadway usually involves brand control, in which the original fire is allowed to burn to the "black line" while any spot-over fires are handled quickly with available water.

7. B

Regardless of the type of apparatus you ride in, the safety rules are the same: You should wear your seatbelt, sit in a designated seat, and put on your gear either before leaving the station or after arriving on the scene.

8. B

Be aware of the limited extinguishing capabilities of a small fire attack line and nozzle. Stay out of brush and ground cover that is higher than your knees.

9. C

A council rake is a good tool for clearing vegetation and debris at a ground cover fire.

10. A

If a brush truck goes into the fire perimeter, it enters from the burned side, away from the direction the head of the fire is traveling.

Chapter 8

1. D

Vehicle fires are common, numbering approximately 200,000 or 17% of the fires throughout the United States each year. You will probably respond to more vehicle fires than structural fires.

2. B

Anyone working within 50 feet of a car or light truck that is well-involved in fire must be properly protected with full personal protective equipment, including breathing apparatus. It is never a good idea to breathe smoke, especially when you consider the products of combustion that are liberated from the burning plastics and other manmade materials in a motor vehicle.

3. D

Most accidental fires in light vehicles start in the engine compartment area. The engine compartment is where all the electronics and fuels come together in a single location; therefore, this area can be the most dangerous when on fire.

4. A

The fluids and manmade materials that burn in the engine area liberate thick, black, choking smoke, a single breath of which can incapacitate you. Large amounts of deadly gas, including hydrogen cyanide, are present in the immediate area anytime plastics burn. These gases mix with the other dangerous gases that are by-products of fires involving flammable liquids and caustics.

5. C

When the vehicle's passenger compartment is well-involved in fire, the airbags often deploy from the heat, with a sound like a shotgun blast. The elements that deploy most airbags found in the dash and seat-backs are flammable products that burn rapidly at a relatively low temperature. Side-curtain airbags are usually inflated with an inert gas that is contained in a pressurized cylinder, which can be contained in the A post, the C post, or even the roof rail on some models of cars.

6. A

Fire in the cargo compartment can be unpredictable because the fuel tank of most cars is near the cargo area. In addition, aftermarket alternative fuels such as propane or compressed natural gas might be located in the cargo compartment.

7. A

The entire battery cell in a typical hybrid vehicle can deliver more than 400 volts of power. The high-voltage circuits of hybrid vehicles derive their power from banks of dry-cell batteries, very similar to flashlight batteries. However, unlike a flashlight that uses two or three of the 1.2-volt batteries for power, the rechargeable batteries in a hybrid vehicle are assembled in a series, which means that their voltage is multiplied.

8. B

Begin flowing water from at least 30 feet away when approaching a well-involved fire, using a tight pattern to reach the seat of the fire and overwhelming it with force. First direct the stream toward any fire that is near the fuel tank and then concentrate on each of the three compartments as you go. The passenger compartment will emit a large volume of fire that can be knocked down quickly with a tight stream from a relatively safe position.

9. A

Fires in the engine compartment can be knocked down to some extent by flowing water through the wheel wells. The main obstacle to controlling a fire in the engine compartment is the lack of access to the area. Most passenger vehicles have plastic inner liners placed on their fenders in the engine compartment that usually burn out of the way, making this area a quick path for applying water.

10. D

Overhaul is the process of systematically looking for any hidden fire or hot areas and taking measures to completely extinguish any of these remaining problems. Overhaul begins once the main body of the fire has been extinguished and continues until there is no chance of an accidental re-ignition. Overhaul is an important process in any fire operation; it is the best defense to prevent a rekindling of the original blaze.

Chapter 9

1. B

An initial water supply is usually developed from water carried on a fire apparatus in its booster tank.

2. D

A fire engine that supplies water to the nozzles is called the attack pumper. The engine that delivers its booster tank water to the attack pumper is called the supply pumper.

3. D

A typical fire hydrant has two or three outlet ports.

4. A

Fire departments will utilize several tenders in rotation to supply the fire scene. Each tender is refilled as the other deploys its load of water, thus establishing a sustained water supply. This operation is commonly referred to as a tender water shuttle operation.

5. C

Many fire trucks will have specially designed fire hose referred to as hard suction hose. When deployed into a body of water, this hose can draw water to provide a sustained water supply for the fire scene.

6. C

The main difference between a portable pump and a float pump is that the float pump has no hard suction hose attached. It simply draws water from below as it floats on the surface of the water.

7. A

When one supply line is made into two or more smaller supply lines, firefighters use a gated manifold appliance.

8. B

Fire apparatus will usually lay supply hose in two primary directions: (1) to the fire (a forward lay) or (2) away from the fire toward the water supply (a reverse lay).

9. B

A 4- to 6-inch-diameter supply hose is considered large-diameter supply hose. This type of hose may have quick-connect couplings.

10. C

A hydrant valve is an appliance that allows a fire apparatus to hook into the water supply at a fire hydrant without interrupting the flow of water to the fire scene.

Chapter 10

1. B

Simply put, the larger the fire and therefore the greater the release of heat, the more water that is needed to be applied to the fire in order to absorb the heat. Fire attack lines for "big water" are generally 2½- to 3-inch diameter hose lines with associated nozzles. As with small fire attack lines, the nozzles are either fog or smoothbore type and operate similarly.

2. C

Often referred to as blitz lines, preconnected large fire attack lines are loaded in a similar manner as small attack lines. Because of the increased size and overall weight of the hose, you should consider getting help to pull the preconnected load.

3. A

Large attack lines flow much more water than small attack lines. However, the result is a greater gallons-per-minute rate of water delivered to the seat of the fire. The greater flow rate means that more people will be needed to operate and maneuver the flowing lines. In addition, a more substantial sustained water supply is needed to keep it flowing.

4. D

If a large attack line is being used by one or two firefighters, is going to be mostly stationary, and is a safe distance from the fire, the hose line can be looped on the ground. This positioning saves the firefighter's energy and allows for a longer application of water using one firefighter.

5. B

When large attack lines need to be advanced to different positions, it is best to have a two- or three-firefighter crew attending the line. These lines flow tremendous amounts of water and, due to their increased diameter and volume, they can be very unwieldy for one firefighter.

6. A

If the line must be moved while flowing, the firefighter at the nozzle should be ready to shut down the nozzle if he or she stumbles or loses balance.

7. B

The water thief is an appliance that closely resembles the gated wye, but in addition to the two 1½-inch discharge ports, it has a single 2½-inch discharge port in the middle. The water thief allows you to stretch to a certain point, deploy two small attack lines, and then extend further with more large attack lines where either another gated wye or a nozzle is attached.

8. C

A gated wye is an appliance that takes in water from a large attack line and then distributes it through two outlets that are controlled by gate valves. A typical gated wye has a 2½-inch inlet and two 1½-inch outlets.

9. B

Operating master stream appliances from aerial ladders is a more advanced skill that is unique to each type aerial apparatus.

10. D

Because master streams are intended to stay in place while flowing, they can be attended by only one firefighter after they are set up. This is their most common application.

Chapter 11

1. A

Individuals who work inside a burning building are working in an atmosphere that is Immediately Dangerous to Life and Health (IDLH). However, this isn't the only hazard they face. Many of the line-of-duty deaths of firefighters working inside the structure occur when the firefighter becomes disoriented and runs out of fresh air supplied by his or her SCBA. Therefore, just knowing how to wear PPE and breathe from an SCBA does not qualify a person to work inside a structural fire.

2. C

During an offensive, interior attack, the hot zone usually encompasses any area inside the structure where an IDLH incident in an enclosed area is encountered. Any firefighter working in the hot zone should be fully protected with PPE and a charged hose line, and should be trained to the Level 1 standard.

3. B

When sizing up a door that you are about to force open, first try turning the doorknob. The door may not be locked. If it isn't, report this to your team's Officer and be ready for another order. If the door is locked, then be prepared to force entry when told to do so and not before. Before you take action, it is important that a charged hose line be in place and that the fire attack team is ready for the door to be opened.

4. B

Dragging a charged hose line through a house is difficult, especially if the interior crew is crawling on their hands and knees. This task can be made quite a bit easier if someone stages at the doorway, outside the building and the IDLH environment, to feed the hose into the building.

5. D

Gasoline-powered fans are usually much more powerful than the electric versions and are also heavier in weight. Therefore, these fans are almost exclusively restricted to remaining on the ground outside the structure. They blow inward to fill the building with fresh air and positive pressure that forces the smoke and gases out of the building. You will also hear these fans referred to as PPV (positive-pressure ventilation) fans.

6. A

The lockout/tagout system ensures that any switch or valve that is meant to remain in its present position is locked into that position with a lock. The person locking the valve is identified on a tag that is attached to the locking device.

7. A

In severe building fires, electrical feeds can disconnect and fall away from the burning building. For this reason, it is important to mark the location of these feeds during the fire emergency. Use fire-line tape or traffic cones to do this. If the power line does fall on the ground, widen your security around the wire and notify your Company Officer or command of the downed wire and its location.

8. C

Most engine company apparatus carry a roof ladder and an extension ladder.

9. B

Adjust the extension ladder for climbing by positioning it about one-fourth of the ladder's height from the building. Place the butt of the ladder at your feet, grasping the rung nearest shoulder height at arm's length. This should be the proper climbing angle.

10. C

Any material that ignites as a result of fire coming from another source is technically an exposure fire. An *exposure* is anything that has the potential of catching fire due to its proximity to something that is already on fire. In building fires, an exposure is an item in a room that has the potential of catching fire because it is exposed to something already on fire in the room. This definition can be expanded to large fires in a building that have the potential to spread to adjacent buildings. The adjacent buildings become exposures to the original building fire and must be protected *before* they catch fire.

Glossary

A

abandonment Failing to stay with a patient and/or to continue delivering care until relieved by another medical provider with the appropriate level of training.

abdominal thrusts An emergency maneuver used to clear an obstructed airway.

acquired immune deficiency syndrome (AIDS) A viral disease that attacks the body's immune system. HIV, the virus that causes AIDS, is commonly spread by direct contact with the body fluids of the infected person.

action circle The area encompassed by the warm zone and including the hot zone where the actual rescue activities take place.

American Heart Association An organization that provides certification and training for heart-related prehospital care.

American Red Cross An organization that develops and provides certification of various levels of first aid training.

apparatus Rolling equipment (such as an engine, a truck, or a rescue unit) that is used in the Fire Service.

appliance Any Fire Service–related device through which water flows. These devices include manifolds, master stream appliances, adapters, and others.

attack line The hose that is used to carry the water from the pump to the fire.

attack pumper A fire truck located at the fire scene to which water is supplied from a sustained source during the firefighting operation. This fire truck distributes the supplied water to the fire attack hose lines at the fire.

automatic external defibrillators (AEDs) Devices that are located in many types of public access areas and provide defibrillation (cardiac shock) in case of sudden heart attack with a loss of breathing and pulse.

B

black-line approach A method of controlling ground cover fires that allows the fire to burn to a natural or manmade firebreak, where it runs out of fuel.

body substance isolation (BSI) Procedures and practices used by rescue and fire personnel to protect themselves from exposure to diseases spread by direct contact with body substances.

booster tank The onboard water supply tank on a fire apparatus usually used as an initial water supply at a fire scene.

brush truck A specialized piece of fire apparatus designed to deliver tools, manpower, and some water to the scene of a ground cover fire. It may or may not have off-road capability and can be used to extinguish smaller fires as well as to protect equipment, personnel, and fire lines on larger wildland fire operations.

C

cardiopulmonary resuscitation (CPR) The discipline of resuscitation recognized by the American Heart Association and the American Red Cross for administering aid to someone who has lost breathing and a pulse.

ceiling hook A common hand tool used by firefighters to access inside wall and ceiling areas in light vehicles. It has a handle with a specialized head on one end of the handle that is used to puncture and then cut and pull interior ceiling and wall coverings.

centrifugal force The force that acts upon an object traveling in an arc or circle that pushes the object away from the center of the arc or circle.

chain of command The organization of supervisory levels within a fire department, generally utilized for both emergency and nonemergency operations.

Class A foam A fire-extinguishing additive agent applied to fires involving Class A materials. It provides additional absorption capability to the water to which it is added.

Collision Avoidance Training (CAT) Driver training that specializes in gaining control of vehicles under different adverse situations and roadway conditions.

compressed natural gas A type of fuel found as a gas in nature that is liquefied and stored in compressed gas cylinders for use. As a gas, it is lighter than air and will rise when released. It can be used as an alternative fuel for a gasoline-powered internal combustion engine.

conduction A type of heat transfer in which the hot flame or fire-heated object is in direct contact with another, cooler object and heats it up.

consent Permission granted to a rescuer by an injured or ill patient that allows the rescuer to provide first aid to that patient.

convection A type of heat transfer that occurs when the fire heats the air near it, causing the heated air to rise.

cool zone The area beyond the warm zone on a crash scene (beyond 10–15 feet). Tools, equipment, and extra personnel are staged in this zone until they are needed in the hot and warm zones.

council rake A specialized tool used by firefighters to clear undergrowth and debris in order to create a firebreak at a ground cover fire.

D

defensive driving A method of driving that emphasizes paying closer attention to other drivers on the roadway and anticipating and avoiding driving dangers.

defensive fire attack A term used during fireground operations for a building fire that has extended throughout the structure, necessitating an exterior fire attack.

deluge gun A type of master stream appliance that is set up primarily for use at ground level; also called a *monitor.*

drafting hydrant A specialized fire hydrant adapted for use in order to access a static water supply such as a lake, river, or buried water tank. Because there is no pressurized water flow from the hydrant, an apparatus must access the hydrant with hard suction supply hose and draft the water supply from the hydrant.

E

Emergency Medical Responder (EMR) A designation for an emergency professional trained in very basic first aid and rescue skills.

Emergency Medical Services (EMS) A group of organizations that provide emergency medical prehospital care to the community.

Emergency Medical Technician (EMT) A person trained in emergency prehospital care at a level above basic and advanced first aid.

Emergency Vehicle Operator's Course (EVOC) A driving course given to operators of emergency vehicles that teaches students how to safely operate and control fire and rescue emergency vehicles. This course is provided by the U.S. Department of Transportation.

exposure Anything that has the potential of catching fire as a result of its proximity to something that is already on fire. In building fires, an exposure is an item in a room that has the potential of catching fire because it is exposed to something already on fire in the room. This definition can be expanded to large fires in a building that have the potential of spreading to adjacent buildings. The adjacent buildings become exposures to the original building fire and must be protected *before* they catch fire.

extension ladder A specialized Fire Service ladder used for greater height capability by firefighters accessing and working in upper levels of a building fire.

Exterior Operations level A level of training that, once successfully completed, covers the knowledge, skills and abilities for working safely *outside* a structural fire.

F

fend-off position The positioning of emergency apparatus on a roadway in order to protect the temporary work area in the street by blocking it with apparatus.

fingers Small extensions of fire growth that protrude from the main body of a ground cover fire.

fire attack team A group of firefighters who perform various firefighting functions on the scene of a fire emergency in order to mitigate the situation and return it to a safe condition.

fire hydrant A valve opened and closed by a firefighter that provides the water supply from a water main system for fire department operations. A typical fire hydrant has two or three outlet ports that have male thread ends with female caps. An operating nut on top of the hydrant opens and closes the water flow from the appliance.

fire line The work area around the body of a ground cover fire.

fire perimeter The outside edge of the entire ground cover fire. The inside of the fire perimeter contains the burned area while the area outside the perimeter is unburned.

fire stream A flow of water from the open end of a fire nozzle that reaches the desired location (that is, the fire).

fire tetrahedron A depiction of the four elements required for combustion to occur: fuel, heat, oxygen, and the chemical chain reaction that keeps the flame burning.

firebreak An area, either manmade or natural, that provides no fuel for a spreading ground cover fire. Firebreaks are used to halt the spread of and assist in controlling ground cover fires.

flanks The smaller fire-involved areas on either side of the head of a ground cover fire.

fly sections Additional ladder sections combined on a single ladder to create an extension ladder. They are the parts of an extension ladder that extend and retract.

forcible entry Methods of gaining access into a locked or obstructed building or vehicle by applying tools to physically dislodge and open a gate, doorway, or window.

freelancing Working independently of the Incident Command System, without the knowledge of the Incident Commander. *Freelancing* is seen as a negative term and is usually associated with an unsafe activity.

G

gated manifold appliance An appliance designed for use with large-diameter supply hose. It allows one large supply hose to be branched into two or more smaller supply hose lines. For example, a 5-inch manifold appliance may branch into four 2½-inch supply lines, each with its own gated valve for operation.

gated wye An appliance that takes in water from a large attack line and then distributes it through two outlets that are controlled by gate valves.

ground cover fire A category of brush fire that is smaller than a wildfire—usually less than an acre in size and handled by one firefighting crew. The majority of brush fires in the United States fit this description.

H

Halligan bar A specialized firefighter's hand tool made up of a handle with a pry fork at one end and a combination adze and pick at the opposite end. This tool was developed to aid in forcing entry into buildings through door and window openings. It has since been adapted for many other uses in the Fire Service.

halyard   A rope located on an extension ladder used for raising and lowering the fly sections of the ladder.

hard suction hose   A specially designed fire hose that is deployed into a body of water to draw water into the fire apparatus pump and provide a sustained water supply for the fire scene.

hazardous materials (hazmat)   Materials and processes that present a hazard to human health through poisoning, chemical and thermal burns, radioactivity, explosiveness, chemical reactivity, or carcinogenic exposure.

head   The main burning area of a brush fire that occurs on the perimeter of the fire. It is located on the side in the direction in which the fire is moving and will have the most intense fire characteristics.

hot zone   The area immediately adjacent to the patient or hazard on a crash scene.

hotspot   An area of burning located either within the burned perimeter of a brush fire or outside the fire perimeter where fire has jumped over from the main body of fire. A hotspot continues to burn inside a burned-out area of a ground cover fire. Hotspots can also develop from hot ashes and burning embers that drop from the fire, landing outside the fire area and starting a small fire or hotspot.

human immunodeficiency virus (HIV)   An immune deficiency disease that often is followed by AIDS.

hydrogen cyanide   A highly poisonous gas created when plastic materials burn. This gas is present in the immediate area anytime plastics burn. It mixes with other dangerous gases that are by-products of fires involving flammable liquids and caustics.

I

Immediately Dangerous to Life and Health (IDLH)   A term used to define for firefighters the conditions of an atmosphere in a confined area, like a building fire, that can result in serious injury or death.

Incident Command System (ICS)   An organization of supervision at an emergency that designates supervisory levels and responsibility.

Incident Commander (IC)   The person in charge of an emergency operation command structure and consequently in charge of the emergency incident at hand.

Industrial Fire Brigade   An organization similar to a fire department that protects a single business or business complex. This organization is generally privately funded and operated.

inertia   The law of nature that states that objects set into motion tend to remain in motion and objects that are stationary tend to remain stationary unless acted upon by another object.

initial water supply   The first supply of water that is accessed for extinguishing a fire. This water supply is usually established prior to a sustained water supply. It is usually carried to the scene by the fire apparatus or specially designed tenders.

L

liquid propane gas   A flammable gas that is heavier than air. Because of its weight, this gas seeks its lowest level when released into the atmosphere. As a liquid, propane is extremely cold. This type of gas is usually contained in pressurized storage tanks, either aboveground or belowground on the dwelling property.

M

manufactured home   A building that is assembled in a factory and then transported to its final location for use as a single-family dwelling. This type of building can also be used as nonpermanent housing.

momentum   The law of nature that describes the force that builds in an object in motion that keeps it moving. The more velocity an object has, the more momentum it has and thus the more force it will take to slow down that object and stop it.

N

National Fire Protection Association (NFPA)   An organization that sets fire codes and standards recognized by most fire department organizations in the United States.

National Institute for Occupational Safety and Health (NIOSH)   A national organization concerned with improving employee safety in the workplace.

national standard threads (NST)   A nationally recognized Fire Service specification that established the number and size of threads used in fire hose couplings. This specification is recognized throughout most of the United States.

natural gas   A flammable gas that is lighter than air. Because of its weight, this gas rises when released into the air. It is delivered to a dwelling by in-ground pipelines.

negative-pressure ventilation   A method of ventilation used to remove smoke from a building. An electric-powered fan is set up facing out of a building's opening. The fan is then activated to draw out smoke from inside the building.

nozzle reaction   When water is flowed under pressure from a fire nozzle, there is an opposite reaction of force that pushes in the opposite direction of the water. Nozzle reaction is also sometimes called back-pressure.

O

Occupational Safety and Health Administration (OSHA)   A federal governmental agency that establishes regulations that apply to many aspects of employee safety at the workplace.

open-circuit system   A type of SCBA system that provides clean, dry air from a compressed air cylinder, through a regulator, at a pressure slightly above that of the outside atmosphere. Exhaled air is exhausted through a valve on the face piece.

overhaul   The techniques and methods applied on an emergency fire scene that lessen the progress of the fire damage. The fire scene is checked for fire extension and hidden fires that are then extinguished. These techniques and methods include measures that help make buildings safe after a fire.

P

Paramedic   A prehospital emergency care provider who is trained at a level above Emergency Medical Technician.

personal alert safety system (PASS)   A small electronic device that is designed to detect movement or a lack of movement. This device is designed to help locate separated or downed firefighters. It sounds a loud alarm if it detects that the firefighter has remained stationary for a predetermined amount of time.

personal protective clothing (PPC)   Protective clothing worn by firefighters during emergency fire control operations. This ensemble includes protection for the eyes, head, hands, feet, and body.

personal protective equipment (PPE), *firefighting*   The protective equipment firefighters wear when fighting fires, especially in a hazardous atmosphere. This gear includes a complete set of personal protective clothing with the addition of a self-contained breathing apparatus (SCBA) for respiratory protection.

personal protective equipment (PPE), *medical*   Specially designed clothing and protective equipment that provides overall body protection. It includes head, eye, hand, foot, and respiratory protection. PPE is safety approved for the hazard that a firefighter or rescuer can expect to encounter in a particular working environment.

personnel accountability system (PAS)   An identification system used to track fire department units as well as personnel on the emergency scene.

positive-pressure ventilation (PPV)   A method of ventilation used to push smoke out and fresh air into a building. A specially designed fan is positioned outside the building at an opening, facing into the building. The fan is then operated and the building fills with fresh air under pressure, pushing out the smoke and gases.

posts   The parts of a vehicle's construction that connect the roof of the vehicle to the body. They are constructed of rolled sheet metal and are given alphabetical labels, starting with *A* at the front and continuing with *B* and *C* for each of the next posts on the same side of the vehicle.

propane   A type of fuel found as a gas in nature that is liquefied and stored in compressed gas cylinders for use. As a gas, it is heavier than air and will seek its lowest level when released. This material can be used as an alternative fuel for a gasoline-powered internal combustion engine.

Pulaski axe   A brush-clearing tool used by firefighters in preparing firebreaks.

R

radiation   A transfer of heat through light waves. We receive our heat from the sun through radiation.

radiator   A part of any water-cooled internal combustion engine that provides a coil and air vents to cool fluids that in turn cool the engine as it operates. In most vehicles, the radiator is located at the front of the engine compartment.

rear   The edge of the burned fire area opposite the head.

recovery position   Positioning a patient on his left side so that secretions can drain naturally from his mouth, thus helping to avoid further choking.

roof ladder   A specially designed straight ladder that has two rails connected by rungs and specialized folding hooks at the tip. These hooks are moved to the open position when the ladder is to be placed on a roof surface and hooked over the ridge of the roof. This type of ladder provides access support for firefighters working on a roof.

running   Rapid movement of a ground cover fire.

S

safe area   Any place on an emergency scene that is free of hazards to you and your team.

safe working zone   The designated safety area around a burning vehicle that includes the entire roadway or at least the lanes of travel on a divided highway that are within 50 feet of the fire. This area should be totally blocked while the fire is actively burning.

safety zones   Areas established on any emergency scene that designate the areas of operation and the level of hazard or control required. Examples of safety control zones include traffic control zones as well as *hot, warm,* and *cool* zones.

salvage   Measures taken by firefighting personnel that help reduce property damage to rooms and content during and after a fire.

seatbelt pretensioner   A device designed to automatically retract a seatbelt to better secure the user during a collision.

self-contained breathing apparatus (SCBA)   Personal protective equipment worn by firefighters to provide respiratory protection in an atmosphere that is hazardous to life.

Siamese appliance   A hose appliance that attaches two or more supply lines into one supply line. Normally, this appliance has a clapper valve inside each intake opening that shuts off if only one line coming into the appliance is flowing water. This appliance allows two or more supply lines to combine to provide more water flow and pressure to one supply line, a fire attack line, or a master stream appliance.

site-built single-family home   A building that is built on the site location. This type of building is not designed to be moved and is therefore a permanent structure used for single family dwelling.

smoke ejector   A type of electrically powered smoke ventilation fan used on buildings for negative-pressure ventilation.

stopping distance   The total distance needed to stop a vehicle. This distance is calculated by adding the reaction time plus the braking distance.

supply line   The hose that is used to move water from its source—for example, a fire hydrant, tanker truck (also known as a tender), or pond—to the pump.

supply pumper The fire truck that provides water to the attack pumper, either from its own booster tank or by pumping water in water supply hose lines to the attack pumper.

sustained water supply The water supply established with a substantial water supply system or source, like a municipal water system or a large static water resource, such as a stream or a lake.

T

tanker An airplane equipped to deliver large amounts of water or other extinguishing agents to a ground cover fire via an air drop.

task force A grouping of individual, company-level units within a fire department that is generally used for response designation purposes.

technical rescue Any rescue discipline requiring specialized knowledge, skills, and tools. Technical rescue includes water, vehicle, rope, building collapse, trench, and confined space rescue.

tempered glass A type of glass commonly used in the construction of side and rear vehicle windows. This type of glass is heat-treated and tempered, which add strength to the glass. It is broken by applying a small point of contact with a large amount of force, which breaks it into many small pieces.

tender A piece of specialized firefighting apparatus designed to deliver large amounts of water to a fire scene where a water supply is not readily available. Under the National Incident Management System, wheeled apparatus that had previously been called a tanker is now called a tender. The term *tanker* is now used to refer to an airplane that delivers water or other extinguishing agents via an air drop.

tender water shuttle operation An operation that uses several tenders in rotation to supply water to a fire scene. Each tender is refilled as another deploys its load of water, which creates a sustained water supply.

traffic control area The area around a vehicle crash or vehicle fire incident in which any traffic passing through is safely directed by personnel or traffic cones away from the safety zone.

U

universal precautions Infection control practices, such as using eye and face protection, disposable gloves, and disposable outer garments, that can protect individuals from diseases that may be transmitted through blood and other body fluids.

V

ventilation Techniques applied to building fires that allow smoke and hot gases to escape from a building involved in a fire. These techniques may also be utilized for atmospheres hazardous to health and life (such as a hazardous gas release inside a building).

W

warm zone The work area that extends 10 to 15 feet away from the crashed vehicle(s).

water hammer A reaction to the sudden starting or stopping of water flow through hoses and pipes that momentarily increases the pressure to sometimes dangerous levels in all directions on the line and pump.

water key A special tool used to operate shutoff valves on municipal water systems.

water supply The water used for extinguishing fires that is carried to the fire by apparatus; pumped from static sources like ponds, rivers, and lakes; or obtained from pressurized water delivery systems through water mains and fire hydrant access points.

water tanker Under the National Incident Management System, this apparatus is now called a *tender*.

water thief An appliance that closely resembles a gated wye. In addition to the two 1½-inch discharge ports, it has a single 2½-inch discharge port in the middle.

wildfire A large ground cover fire that involves many acres of open wildland.

wildland firefighter A firefighter trained for fighting fires in open wildland areas.

wildland/urban interface The situation in which urban and suburban growth has intruded into open wildland areas, increasing the exposure to wildfires to homes and businesses in the area.

Index

A

Abandonment, 24
Abdominal thrusts, 27–29
Acquired immune deficiency syndrome (AIDS), 24, 25
Action circle, 122, 123
Administration Division, 6
Advanced Emergency Medical Technician (AEMT), 22
Aerial stream, 232
Airbag systems, 169–170
Airway, in CPR, 33–34
Airway management techniques
  abdominal thrusts, 27–29
  anatomy of airway, 29
  head-tilt-chin-lift maneuver, 29–31
  jaw-thrust maneuver, 31–32
  recovery position, 32
  upper airway management, 29–32
Alarm response
  ground cover fires, 156
  single-family dwelling fires, 244
Alarms, in SCBA, 60
Alcohol use
  fatal vehicle crashes and, 109–110
American Heart Association, 34
American Red Cross, 34
Apparatus
  blind spots, 115–116
  defined, 2, 80
  fend-off position, 119
  physical forces and driving safety, 112–113
  riding safety, 114–116
Appliances
  defined, 198
  gated manifold appliance, 198–199
  master stream appliances, 232–235
  Siamese, 199
Assistant Chief, 6
Attack lines
  booster, 86–88
  carry techniques, 100–101
  connecting hose sections, 89–90
  defined, 79, 80
  general care for, 102
  general hose-handling techniques, 89–90
  hose appliances, 93–94
  hose rolls, 95–99
  hose tools, 90–91
  importance of, 80
  large, 217–235

nozzle operations, 94–95
one-inch jacketed, 89
small, 81–85
tools for, 90–91
trash line, 89
weights of uncharged/charged fire hoses, 219
Attack pumper, 187
Automatic external defibrillators (AEDs), 37–39

B

Backpack-style water extinguisher, 156
Barway spanner, 86
Battalion Chief, 6
Batteries
  disconnecting lead-acid, 169
  hybrid vehicles, 170–171
Biological waste emblem, 27
Black-line approach, 154
Bleeding, controlling, 39–41
Blitz lines, 218
Body substance isolation (BSI), 24
  defined, 25
  overview of, 26
Booster attack lines, 86–88
  characteristics of, 86
  loading, 88
  stretching, 87–88
  uses of, 86
Booster tanks
  overview of, 186–187
  refilling, 191–192
Boots, 54
Braking distance, 112
Branches, 9
Breathing, in CPR, 34
Bruises, 42
Brush axe, 155, 156
Brush truck, 152, 153
  operation of, 157–158
  refilling, 158, 159
Burning liquids, 139–143
  carbon dioxide fire extinguisher, 140–141
  dry chemical extinguisher, 142–143
  overview of, 139–140
Burns
  extent and severity of, 44
  first aid for, 44–45
  types of, 44
Butt, of ladder, 262

C

Captains, 6
Carbon dioxide fire extinguisher, 140–141
Cardiopulmonary resuscitation (CPR), 33–37
  airway, 33–34
  breathing, 34
  circulation, 34
  defined, 22
  steps in, 35–37
Cargo compartment
  extinguishing fires in, 175
  fire hazards, 170
Ceiling hook, 171, 172
  breaking glass for ventilation, 252
Centrifugal force, 113
Chain of command, 5–7
  defined, 5
  department divisions, 6
  fire chief, 6–7
  governing bodies, 7
  mid-management, 6
  upper management, 6
Charged hose line
  advancing charged hose line (1 person drill), 178
  advancing charged hose line (2 person drill), 177
Chief Officer, 6
Circulation, in CPR, 34
Class A fire, 134, 135
  dry chemical extinguisher, 142–143
  using small attack line, 138–139
  using water-type fire extinguisher, 136–137
Class A foam
  ground cover fires and, 152
  vehicle fires, 179
Class B fire, 134, 135
  carbon dioxide fire extinguisher, 140–141
  dry chemical extinguisher, 142–143
  overview of, 139–140
Class C fire, 134, 135, 143
  dry chemical extinguisher, 142–143
Class D fire, 134
Class K fire, 134, 135
Clothing. See Personal protective clothing
Coat, 54
Cold zone
  single-family dwelling fires, 246
  vehicle crashes, 122, 123
Collision Avoidance Training (CAT), 114

Intervention team, 254–261
  protecting exposures, 269–270
  role of, 254
  scene lighting, 260–261
  tool staging area, 254–255
  utilities control, 255–260

J

Jacketed attack line, 89
Jaw-thrust maneuver, 31–32

L

Ladders, 261–269, 264–265
  deploying roof ladder, 265–266
  extension, 261, 266–269
  overview of, 262
  parts of, 262
  placing straight ladders, 264–265
  removing and stowing, 263–264
  roof, 261, 265–266
  straight, 264–265
Land-based fire pump, 197
Large attack lines, 217–235
  advancing with multiple firefighters, 224–225
  assembling, 220–221
  compared to small attack lines, 218
  defined, 80
  exterior fire attack, 272
  flowing with single firefighter, 221
  gated wye to extend, 226–227
  hose-clamp method to extend, 227–229
  kneeling position with multiple firefighters, 225–226
  loading, 231–232
  looping with single firefighter, 223–224
  overview of, 218
  preconnected, 218–220
  safety feature of, 235
  stretching, 219–220
  through-the-nozzle method to extend, 229–230
  uses of, 218
  weights of uncharged/charged fire hoses, 219
Large-diameter hoses, 200–201
  forward lay, 207–208
  loading, 203–204
  reverse lay, 208
Lighting, scene, 260–261
Liquid propane gas, 257–258
Lockout/tagout systems, 255
Locks, forcing, 251

M

Manufactured homes, 243–244
Master stream appliances, 232–235
  deck gun, 232, 234–235
  deluge gun, 232, 233
  master stream nozzles, 233
  uses of, 233–234
Master stream nozzles, 233

Mid-management, 6
Momentum, 113
Monitor, 232, 234–235

N

National Fire Protection Association (NFPA), 10
National Institute for Occupational Safety and Health (NIOSH), 10
National Institute for Occupational Safety and Health (NIOSH) Investigative Report
  F2000-07 (in-station incident), 12–13
  F2002-24 (on the scene collapse), 22
  F99-34 (personal protective clothing), 52
  F2002-04 (seatbelt safety), 108
  F2002-37 (wear your gear, even on small fires), 150
National standard threads (NST), 82
Natural gas, 257–258
Negative-pressure ventilation, 253
NFPA. *See* National Fire Protection Association (NFPA)
NIOSH. *See* National Institute for Occupational Safety and Health (NIOSH)
Nozzle control
  advancing charged hose line and nozzle control (1 person drill), 178
  advancing charged hose line and nozzle control (2 person drill), 177
  stretching dry hose line and nozzle control, 176
Nozzles
  adjusting, 95
  holding, 95
  master stream nozzles, 233
  opening, 94
  through-the-nozzle method, 229–230
  types of, 94–95

O

Occupational Safety and Health Administration (OSHA)
  overview of, 10
  right-to-know requirements, 13
Offensive fire attack, 243
Open-circuit system, 59
Organization of fire departments, 2–6
OSHA. *See* Occupational Safety and Health Administration (OSHA)
Overhaul
  defined, 4
  vehicle fires, 178–179

P

Paid department, 2
Paid-on-call department, 2
Pants, 54
Paramedics, 4, 22
Partial-thickness burns, 44, 45

Passenger compartment
  extinguishing fire in, 171–173
  fire hazards of, 169–170
Passenger vehicle fires. *See* Vehicle fires
Pawls, on ladder, 262
Personal alert safety system (PASS), 70–71
  defined, 70
  inspecting, 71
Personal protective clothing, 52–59
  boots, 54
  cleaning, 58
  coat and pants, 54
  components of, 53–55
  donning, 56–58
  gloves, 54–55
  for ground cover fires, 154–155
  hearing protection, 115
  hood and helmet, 55
  importance of, 52
  inspecting, 58–59
  riding safety and, 114–115
  storing, 58
  types of, 52–53
  wildland gear, 154–155
Personal protective equipment (PPE), 26
  safety zones and, 246
Personnel accountability system
  defined, 9
  ground cover fires, 156–157
  single-family dwelling fires, 244–245
  steps of, 72
Pocket mask, 34
Portable fire pumps, 197
Portable lighting, 261
Portable water tanks, 196
Positive-pressure ventilation, 253–254
Posts, 170
PPV (positive-pressure ventilation), 253
Preconnected attack lines
  large, 218–220
  small, 81–82
Pressure dressing, 40–41
Professional-grade washer, 58
Propane, 170, 257–258
Protective equipment, 52–73
  personal alert safety system (PASS), 70–71
  personal protective clothing, 52–59
  self-contained breathing apparatus (SCBA), 59–70
Pulse check, 33
Pump panel, 80, 81

Q

Quick-connect couplings, 82, 201–202

R

Radiation, 133, 134
Radiators, 168
Rails, ladder, 262
Reaction time, 112
Rear, of ground cover fire, 152

Utilities control, 255–260
  electricity, 256–257
  fuel oil, 259
  gas, 257–258
  lockout/tagout systems, 255
  water, 259–260

V

Valves
  gate, 93
  hydrant, 209–210
  quarter-turn, 226
Vehicle crashes
  alcohol use, 110
  causes of fatal, 109–110
  crashes at intersections, 109–110
  crash scene benchmarks, 123–124
  deaths from, 108
  defensive driving, 108
  defining true emergency, 109
  head-on crashes, 110
  rollover crashes, 109
  safety zone, 122–125
  seatbelt use, 109
  speed and, 109
  traffic control, 118–122
Vehicle fires, 165–179
  advancing charged hose line (1 person
    drill), 178
  advancing charged hose line (2 person
    drill), 177
  cargo compartment hazards, 170
  chocking wheels and removing
    keys, 167
  Class A foam, 179
  disconnecting batteries, 169
  engine compartment hazards, 168–169

extinguishing cargo compartment
    fires, 175
extinguishing engine compartment
    fires, 173–174
extinguishing passenger compartment
    fire, 171–173
hybrid vehicles, 170–171
opening hood, 173
overhaul, 178–179
passenger compartment hazards,
    169–170
putting into perspective, 166
safety zones at, 166–167
safe working zone, 167
smoke from, 166, 167, 168
stretching dry hose line and nozzle
    control, 176
traffic control area, 166, 167
Velocity
  stopping distance and, 112
Ventilation
  defined, 4
  importance of good, 252
Ventilation fans, 253–254
Ventilation team, 252–254
  breaking class, 252
  importance of good ventilation, 252
  negative-pressure ventilation, 253
  positive-pressure ventilation,
    253–254
  smoke ejector, 253
Volunteer department, 2

W

Warm zone
  single-family dwelling fires, 246
  vehicle crashes, 122, 123

Water fire extinguisher
  use of, 134, 136–137
Water hammer, 94
Water key, 259
Water main systems, 198
Water supply
  booster tanks, 186–187
  defined, 4
  engine-to-engine water supply, 187–188
  fire hydrants, 188–191
  importance of, 185–186
  initial, 186–192
  overview of, 186
  portable fire pumps, 197
  portable water tanks, 196
  static, 186, 193–195
  sustained, 186, 192–193
  tenders, 192–193
  water main systems, 198
Water tankers, 152, 153
  defined, 192
  hooking into, 193
Water thief, 93
  using, 226
Water utilities, controlling, 259–260
Wet-barrel hydrant, 188, 189
Wildfires, 151
Wildland firefighter, 151
  protective clothing for, 154–155
Wildland/urban interface, 150, 151
Wild line, 95
Windows
  breaking glass, 252
Work groups
  engine companies, 2–3
  in Incident Command System, 9
  rescue companies, 4
  truck companies, 3